BOTANICAL RESEARCH AND PRACTICES

CITRUS

MOLECULAR PHYLOGENY, ANTIOXIDANT PROPERTIES AND MEDICINAL USES

BOTANICAL RESEARCH AND PRACTICES

Additional books in this series can be found on Nova's website under the Series tab.

Additional e-books in this series can be found on Nova's website under the e-book tab.

BOTANICAL RESEARCH AND PRACTICES

CITRUS

MOLECULAR PHYLOGENY, ANTIOXIDANT PROPERTIES AND MEDICINAL USES

KHIZAR HAYAT
EDITOR

nova publishers
New York

For permission to use material from this book please contact us:
Telephone 631-231-7269; Fax 631-231-8175
Web Site: http://www.novapublishers.com

Library of Congress Cataloging-in-Publication Data

Citrus : molecular phylogeny, antioxidant properties and medicinal uses / editor: Khizar Hayat (Department of Chemistry, COMSATS Institute of Information Technology, Abbottabad, Pakistan).
pages cm. -- (Botanical research and practices)
Includes bibliographical references and index.
ISBN: 978-1-63117-985-3 (hardcover)
1. Citrus fruits--Analysis. 2. Antioxidants--Health aspects. 3. Citrus fruits--Therapeutic use. 4. Citrus--Phylogeny--Molecular aspects. I. Hayat, Khizar. II. Series: Botanical research and practices.
TX558.C5C56 2014
641.3'4304--dc23

2014016918

Published by Nova Science Publishers, Inc. † New York

CONTENTS

Preface

In recent years, the concept of 'Preventive Medicine' has fostered the nutrition research towards the consumption of plant based diet containing non-nutritive bioactive components. Analysis of the recent epidemiological studies indicates that phytochemicals e.g., polyphenols can reduce the risk of a number of diseases. *Citrus* is an important genus of family *Rutaceae* in the plant kingdom and it contains a wide range of metabolites which are beneficial to human health. The genus *Citrus* is characterized by a substantial accumulation of flavanone glycosides, which are not found in many other fruits.

There are a number of research articles published and research projects undertaken on citrus by the academic and research communities as well as the food and pharmaceutical industry. The thirst to improve the yield and quality of fruits and to explore their medicinal value has propelled and will continue propelling the interest on citrus. In addition the varietal and geographical factors also affect the antioxidant potential and medicinal value of citrus cultivars. With this background, this book on '*Citrus: Molecular Phylogeny, Antioxidant Properties and Medicinal Uses*' is compiled and created. This book is intended to equip those who are novice in the field of citrus and its medicinal uses and those who are already immersed in the field with the hope that the topics discussed in the book will trigger future novel ideas and processes to contribute towards healthy nutrition.

This book covers the biological aspects of citrus production and its ecological journey emphasizing on functional traits related to its nutritional and photosynthetic apparatus. The already published data has been reviewed and re-interpreted with an added ecological point of view that, perhaps, is not discussed by most of the textbooks or journals. The enzymes involved in the biosynthetic pathways of citrus bioactive compounds to modulate a variety of plant characteristics are debated. The information about the genetic architecture of citrus genome and the genes specifically involved in fruit development, in particular, related to antioxidant accumulation, are extensively discussed. The phytophenolic composition of citrus fruits with emphasis on their flavonoid and carotenoid content and their related antioxidative potency as well as the prophylactic potential of citrus has been highlighted in this book. The effect of different commonly applied treatments during the postharvest handling of citrus fruits has been examined in one of the chapters in this volume. The medicinal properties of different citrus compounds and extracts have been discussed and reviewed comprehensively in this book. All the chapters have been developed in such a manner that each chapter can stand on its own. Due to the nature and scope of each chapter, overlapping topics cannot be completely avoided. On the other hand, these overlaps are indispensable for each chapter to be able to stand on its own.

A sincere and great appreciation goes to the book chapter authors for their contributions. I am indebted to the excellent staff at Nova Science Publishers for their unfailing encouragement, patience and their whole-hearted support of this book project. I express a heartfelt gratitude to my parents who are the source of my motivation, the flame of my ambitions and foundation of my achievements. Last, but not least, I owe love and special appreciation to my wife and best friend, Dr. Yasmin, for her immeasurable contribution by creating the atmosphere to the successful completion of this book.

Finally, I earnestly hope that the reader will find something interesting.

Khizar Hayat, Ph.D.
Assistant Professor,
Department of Chemistry,
COMSATS Institute of Information
Technology Abbottabad, Pakistan
E-mail: khizaraura@hotmail.com

In: Citrus
Editor: Khizar Hayat

ISBN: 978-1-63117-985-3

Chapter 1

History, Ecology and Challenges of Citrus Production in Tropical and Subtropical Areas

Gustavo Habermann[1,*] and Marcelo Claro de Souza[2]
[1]Departamento de Botânica, IB, Univ Estadual Paulista (UNESP), Rio Claro-SP, Brazil
[2]Programa de Pós-Graduação em Ciências Biológicas (Biologia Vegetal), Departamento de Botânica, Univ Estadual Paulista (UNESP), Rio Claro-SP, Brazil

Abstract

The center of genetic origin of *Citrus* is believed to be southeastern Asia. This includes the areas from eastern Arabia to the Philippines, and also from Himalayas south to Indonesia and northern Australia. The vegetation in that region subsumes rain forests and tropical shaded tall-tree habitats, and *Citrus* species might have thrived for many years in the understory of these forests. Before the fifth century B.C., *Citrus* fruits were recognized by its medicinal uses. First sailors used fresh *Citrus* fruits to prevent scurvy. But when brought to Europe and the Americas after 1500 A.D., *Citrus* fruits were used as a general source of food. After the great voyages, plants of this genus became crop plants outside its natural environment. In South America, it was first introduced in northeast Brazil, and in the Andes. By the middle of the past century, São Paulo and Minas Gerais states in southeastern Brazil became one of the hot spots of *Citrus* production. Differently from lands that had long been used for agriculture, *Citrus* plantations in Brazil required the removal of native vegetation for producing sweet oranges for juice processing. This strategy, although successful, disregarded many morphological and functional traits of native plants on the southern border of the Brazilian savanna (Cerrado), which was displaced by orange tree plantations. These "*invader plants*" had to face the sunshiny plains in the center, north, and northwest São Paulo state, where savanna-type vegetation used to grow on soils that are acidic (pH < 4.0), rich in aluminum (Al), poor in macronutrients, and that are also subjected to five-month seasonal droughts. Cerrado

* Corresponding author address: Departamento de Botânica, IB, Univ Estadual Paulista (UNESP), Rio Claro-SP, 13506-900, Brazil; Email: ghaber@rc.unesp.br.

woody plants possess long and deep roots, with low specific leaf area, traits which possibly help these species survive droughts and fire events. These species also evolved mechanisms to deal with Al in the metabolism. On the other hand, orange trees, which exhibit traits that are typical of forest species, had to be grafted on rootstocks that attenuate such harsh edaphic conditions. In addition, fertilizers and lime are still being used today as a means of overcoming the low fertility of Cerrado soils. In this chapter we rescue biological history and ecology, and revisit differences between *Citrus* and Cerrado woody species, which have developed as forest and savanna species, respectively. We focused on functional traits related to nutritional and photosynthetic apparatus of these plants. We believe that these discussions can provide reflections for *Citrus* breeding programs.

Keywords: Cerrado, Citrus breeding, Environment, Historical Citrus production, Metal toxicity

A Brief History of Citrus

It is known that the primitive habitat of *Citrus* plants is the understory of rain forests and tropical shaded tall-tree environments in southeastern Asia [1,2]. Even before recorded history, movements of distinct *Citrus* species might have occurred, and these plants were probably cultivated in the Middle East, such as Oman, Persia and Palestine, before Christ [3]. Subsequently, many citruses might have been introduced to the Mediterranean region (Italy and surroundings) by the Roman Empire (27 B.C. – 284 A.D.), but greenhouses that were used for cold protection of sweet orange plants (*Citrus sinensis* L. Osbeck) in backyards of rich Roman families must have been destroyed along with *Citrus* introductions, by the end of this era [2,3]. Oranges have been reintroduced between 1400 A.D. and 1500 A.D. through the Genoese trade routes [4]. But it was the Portuguese that brought superior selections of sour orange (*Citrus aurantium* L.) and sweet oranges from China and southeastern Asia to the Mediterranean area, probably around 1500 A.D., during the great voyages. From Mediterranean areas, many citruses were taken to new landscapes belonging to Portuguese and Spanish colonies, such as Brazil and the Hispanic America [2].

Plant genotype introductions aimed for plantations and agriculture in Brazil might have taken place later, after the exploitation of 'Pau Brasil' trees (*Caesalpinia echinata* Lam.) ceased. The 'Pau Brasil' wood maintained an important timber trade market in Europe, and this returned initial economical resources to the Portuguese, which subsidized the continuation of the colonization. Then, after the sugar cane, gold and rubber (in the Amazonian region) economic cycles, coffee plantations were performed in southeastern Brazil, especially in São Paulo and Minas Gerais states [5,6]. In Brazil, *Citrus* plants have arrived through the northern and northeastern harbors, after 1800 A.D. [2]. Not until 1950 A.D. had been *Citrus* plantations mentioned as an important crop for the Brazilian agriculture.

Since the beginning of the *Citrus* industry around the world, massive fruit production is only achieved through the use of the perfect scion/rootstock combinations [7]. Therefore, species, cultivars, hybrids, and varieties of *Citrus* rootstocks must match the perfect scion to be productive under specific conditions or regions, with specific soils, climates, and disease and pest pressures [8].

The *Citrus* industry was established in Brazil specifically in the central, north, northwest and northeast São Paulo state, by 1950. Plantations were established primarily for sweet orange production destined for juice processing. Therefore, combinations of sweet oranges grafted mainly on sour orange and 'Rangpur' lime (*Citrus limonia* L.) rootstocks had been tentatively used for this huge *Citrus* industry that was being formed in São Paulo, Brazil [9].

By the middle of the 20th century, a disease attacked the Brazilian citriculture: the Citrus Tristeza Virus (CTV). Sweet orange scions that had been grafted on 'Rangpur' limes, however, were able to escape that disease. After that episode, 'Rangpur' lime became the most deployed rootstock in the Brazilian *Citrus* industry. Citrus Variegated Chlorosis (CVC) was another disease that spread over *Citrus* groves by 1990, and it was independent of rootstock types, as the bacterium *Xylella fastidiosa*, its causal agent, colonizes the xylem vessels of the canopy [10]. In the years 2000, the Citrus Sudden Death, another disease of still unrevealed causes started affecting sweet orange plants grafted, specifically, on 'Rangpur' limes [11].

More recently, since 2008, *Citrus* groves have been gradually replaced with sugar cane plantations, especially in São Paulo. This time no disease pressures caused such substitution, but prices paid to *Citrus* growers, who realized that profits from sugar cane are more advantageous over *Citrus*, especially when considering costs involved in both economic activities [12].

CITRUS CROPS CONSTRAINTS

One might presume that disease and pest pressures, as well as climate and nutritional status are the most important factors controlling yields. Notwithstanding, Tisdale and colleagues [13] identified 52 factors that affect and influence plant growth and production. Man is able to influence or control 45 out of these 52 factors. However, one should also consider that interactions among these 52 (or 45) factors also play a role in the production capacity of any crop.

For *Citrus* production, these concerns are not exceptions. Many factors interact among them to drive yields. Temperature is a factor that is related to climate, which may be determinant for growing *Citrus*. Although a certain region may be suitable for plant survival, it cannot be chosen for commercial production. For this reason, the heat unit (*hu*) concept has been developed and it more or less explains plant growth rates and fruit quality, with some reflections on yield capacities, if other constraints are not limiting [14]. Heat units are calculated as the amount of time (h) multiplied by the average temperature difference from the minimum temperature for *Citrus* vegetative growth (12.5°C) [15]. Annual *hu* accumulation of tropical regions varies between 5000 and 1000, depending on altitude, whereas in subtropical regions, where most *Citrus* hot spots production are located, *hu* ranges from 1500 to 3000 [15]. High *hu* accumulation in tropical regions is believed to raise plant respiration, which would reduce photosynthetic products available for fruits, but this fact has not been consistently proved yet.

Although *Citrus* plants, in general, come from understories of rain forests in southeastern Asia [1,2], it has been successfully grown between 40° north-south latitudes, in tropical and subtropical regions. However, the most productive regions for *Citrus* are located in the humid subtropics, such as São Paulo state in Brazil and Florida state in the US. In these subtropical regions, average annual temperatures stay between 15 and 18°C, with greater fluctuation in diurnal temperatures as compared to tropical regions. Therefore, subtropical and tropical regions may show similar annual *hu* accumulation, such as Orlando (Florida, USA) – 3700, and Palmira (Colombia) – 3500, but general conditions in the subtropics provide enhanced climatic conditions for large yields. This points out that temperature daily fluctuations and annul *hu* accumulation alone cannot determine agronomic performance for *Citrus*.

Aside from elevated nocturnal temperatures presumably increasing plant respiration and lowering yields, tropical areas are also subjected to excessive relative humidity. This condition pushes disease and pest pressures. Also, it is believed that fogs in tropical regions may reduce sunlight penetration, consequently avoiding large photosynthetic rates. In addition, constant and less fluctuant diurnal temperatures may cause continuous vegetative growth, without contrasting seasons, typical of subtropical areas. Although tropical climate may have rainy seasons, when bloom occurs, some flowering is also observed throughout the year. In subtropical (and temperate) areas, contrasting seasons influence plant physiology tremendously, not only in *Citrus* plants, but also in all plant species, and it really affects flowering [16] and, consequently, yields.

Within subtropical *Citrus* productive areas, especially in humid subtropics, such as in Florida (US) and São Paulo (Brazil) states, it seems that soil water availability is an important yield constraint. In Florida, where most orchards are irrigated, per hectare (ha) sweet orange yields are at least two-fold higher than those in São Paulo state, Brazil [2].

In São Paulo, the northern region possesses greater number of sweet orange plants when compared to the south of this region, and apparently, there are climatic and disease pressure consequences between choosing one of these regions for *Citrus* production. In the "north" (north, northwest and northeast São Paulo state) orange fruits are larger than those produced in the south, but fruit yields per plant seem to be lower than those in the south [17]. Notwithstanding, differences in *Citrus* production between northern and southern São Paulo state are complex, and one must also take the climate and the disease pressure into account. Definitely, the northern São Paulo region faces greater soil water deficit and increased vapor pressure deficits when compared to the southern region (Figure 1). In addition, CVC-affected plants suffer greater physiological damage in the north in relation to southern São Paulo state [17].

These climatic differences have obvious consequences for leaf gas exchanges and net photosynthesis, which are physiologically linked to yields. Although seasons may contribute to important shifts induced in the metabolism of *Citrus* plants, leading to transitions between vegetative and reproductive phenophases, contrasting seasons also play a role in the photosynthetic capacity of *Citrus* plants. Dry and cold winters in the subtropics diminish stomatal conductance (*gs*) and net photosynthesis [17-19]. Cold is also responsible for metabolic responses biophysically perceived by *Citrus* roots during the winter in subtropical conditions [20]; and the summer induces sink demand for vegetative growth, which, in turn, seems to regulate photosynthesis in *Citrus* leaves [21]. Until recently, the absolute concentration of carbohydrate in leaves, rather than sink demand, was believed to control photosynthesis rates in *Citrus* plants [22].

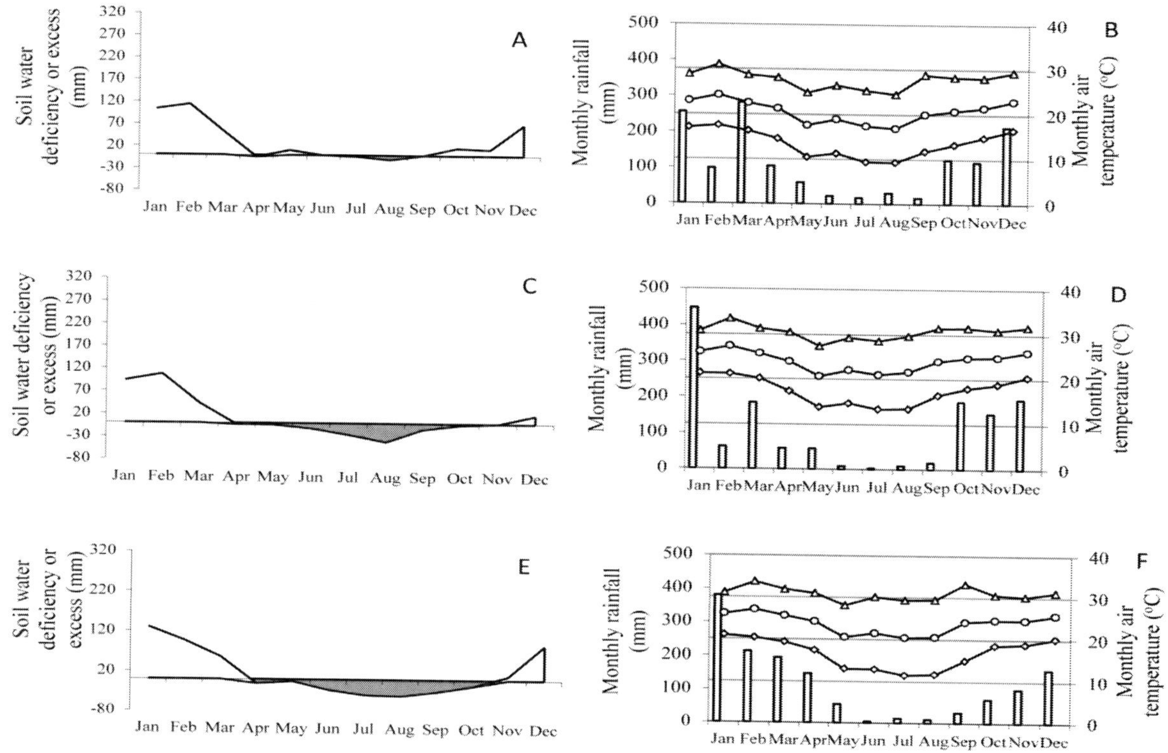

Figure 1. Soil water balance (A, C, E) based on a 12-year (1990-2002) data set, and monthly rainfall, minimum, mean and maximum air temperatures (B, D, F) during 2003. Data were collected in southern (Pratânia), Central (Matão, Cambuhy farm) and northern (Bebedouro, Bebedouro Citrus Experimental Station) São Paulo state, Brazil.

Therefore, *Citrus* plants are highly influenced by seasons in the subtropics, with consequences that may be taken as negative (droughts, cold and growth inhibition) or positive (induction of flowering and variations in disease and pest pressures). However, irrigation appears to be an effective way to overcome 'negative' impacts of drought on yields of orange plants grown in subtropical conditions. Florida state produces around 35 tons oranges per ha, whereas São Paulo state, in Brazil, gets half of those values, but irrigated orchards in São Paulo provide similar yields as compared to those in Florida, US [2].

In contrast, arid or semi-arid subtropical areas, such as Israel, Australia, Portugal, Italy, Spain and South Africa fail to have great yields due to water scarcity and soil salinity. But fresh *Citrus* fruits are of amazingly high quality when produced in Mediterranean areas, mainly in Spain, where *Citrus* growers use irrigation, fertilizers and control diseases and pests in an efficient way.

In conclusion, although many factors may be responsible for yields in *Citrus* plants, some may be more significant than others when considering distinct areas on the globe. While in the tropics yields may be low due to constant climatic conditions throughout the year, under subtropical conditions, contrasting seasons may induce important phenological events on the plant, but droughts and cold may cause growth inhibition. On the other hand, in arid or semi-arid regions, the quality of fruits is greatly enhanced, as long as ferti-irrigation is appropriately applied. Therefore, there are no general conclusions about the control of *Citrus* yields that could be drawn, and further investigations should also address climate change events that have been gradually becoming a threat for *Citrus* production in the tropics and subtropics, both in humid and arid/semi-arid conditions.

BIOLOGICAL HISTORY OF SAVANNAS

Tropical savannas occupy around 20% of emerged lands [23] and comprise xerophytic vegetation composed of trees, shrubs and grasses. Amongst the great savannas (Australian, Brazilian and South African), the Brazilian savanna (locally known as "*Cerrado*", meaning "*closed*" vegetation) is considered the richest savanna in number of plant species. Due to the great number of endemic species, the Cerrado is ranked 25th in a biodiversity hot spot list [24]. The establishment of savannas on the globe started in the late Miocene (~8 million years ago), with the replacement of C_3 grasses with flammable C_4 ones [25,26]. In the same period, increases in the incidence of fires resulted in the replacement of forest species with savanna species [26,27]. The reasons for such transition are not totally clear yet. However, considering that the high incidence of fire is associated with low frequency of rainfall, and that high occurrence of grasses is negatively associated with the presence of wood species [28], it sounds reasonable to suggest that the climate may have changed during the Miocene, possibly resulting in a gradient of savannas, as observed between the South African (dry savanna), Australian (intermediate savanna) and the Brazilian (wet) savanna (Figure 2).

Among species occurring in savannas, an intriguing group of woody plants have evolved: aluminum (Al) accumulating species. These plants, belonging to two botanical families (*Melastomataceae* and *Vochysiaceae*) [8], are able to accumulate more than 10 g of Al per kg of leaf dry mass [32]. However, these two botanical families are much more common in the Cerrado in relation to other savannas on the globe. Aluminum accumulation is observed not only in *Melastomataceae* and *Vochysiaceae* species from the Cerrado, but also in few other families, such as *Myrtaceae* and *Rubiaceae* in Australia and Brazil and *Combretaceae* in South Africa. Considering that Al accumulation is frequently observed in woody species [33], rather than grasses, and that the Cerrado possesses many times more woody species than the other savannas, it is expected that the Cerrado will hold many times more Al-accumulating species than the Australian and African savannas.

According to the Angiosperrn Phylogeny Group (APG) classification system, Al accumulation can be found in 45 botanical families, including savanna and forest species [32]. Phylogenetically, this trait is particularly common in basal branches of fairly advanced groups, such as rosids and asterids, but this trait has been probably lost in the most derived taxa [32]. Considering that the savanna vegetation derives from forest species, then, savannas are millions of years younger than forests, and Al accumulation has been considered an ancient trait [32].

In conclusion, Al accumulation is more commonly observed in plants growing on acidic soils of tropical regions, such as the soils of Cerrado areas (pH 4.0). Acidity can be also found in soils where the South African and Australian savannas grow, but soil pH in these regions ranges between 5.0 and 6.0. We believe that Al accumulation, exhibited by tree species from these three savanna areas in the world, may be considered a non-plastic character, since it is essentially observed in woody species in a restricted number of sites.

In this way, knowing how resistance and tolerance to Al has emerged through millions of years, and understanding the metabolism of Al in these Al-accumulating plants could increase the knowledge useful to overcome Al toxicity in crop plants, as observed in *Citrus* plants [33-36]. *Citrus* is a plant genus that has evolved in the understory of forest environments in southeastern Asia [1,2,19]. Therefore, being sensitive to Al reinforces its low adaptation and unfitness for the sunshiny plains and acidic soils of the subtropics in South America, where Cerrado vegetation used to grow [8].

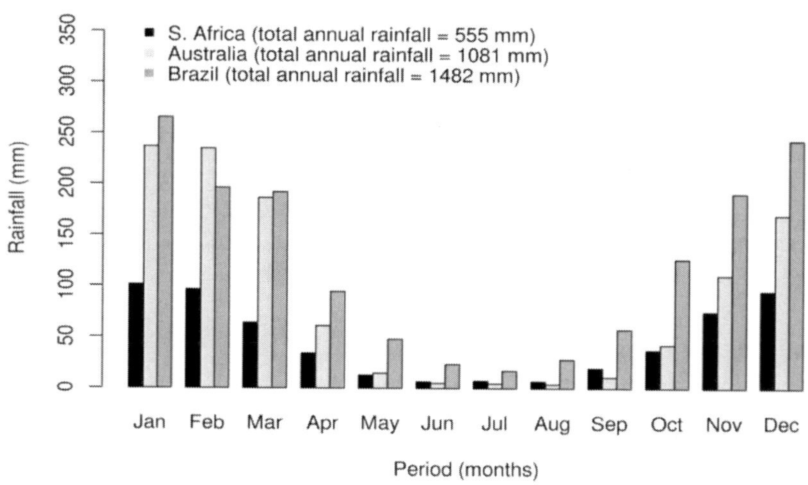

Figure 2. Yearly rainfall distribution in the South African, Australian and Brazilian savannas, based on a 30-year (1980-2010) data set. The climate of each savanna was characterized considering climate peculiarities on the periphery and in the core of each savanna. Monthly rainfall was obtained from already published sources: S. Africa [29], Australia [30] and Brazil [31].

FUNCTIONAL TRAITS FOR BIOLOGICAL PRODUCTIVITY

Citrus trees are evergreen species, densely foliated within three to five years in the field. *Citrus* trees seem to be genetically programed to flush throughout the year, although leaf flushing is intensified between the spring and summer [21]. But visiting vigorous and old (more than 25 years old) groves, especially those in which scions are grafted on the vigorous 'Rangpur' lime, gives everybody the real understanding of this forest species: tall trees, with a shaded micro-environment in the interior of the canopy (between 20 and 80 μmol photons /m^2 /s, or photosynthetic photon flux density – PPFD). In *Citrus* trees the leaf number and total leaf area can increase by approximately 1000% and 600%, respectively, within a 29-year period [37]. Therefore, the problem of shading in the interior of *Citrus* tree canopies points out an intriguing trait. Why does this species actively branch and consistently develop leaves inside the canopy? These shaded leaves have extremely low possibility of capturing sunlight. In natural environments, such as semidecidual and rain forests, sunlight capture is paramount for forest species, and rapidly reaching the canopy forest is critical for survival [38]. Indeed, a robust model applicable to many forest species demonstrates that as plant height increases, the fraction of production allocated to foliage diminishes [38]. In Cerrado areas, congeneric species exhibit this same ecological behavior. Savanna species have low specific leaf area (SLA) and invest in the root system, elongating it for root water access at deep soil layers during droughts, while species from the same genus, but occurring in forest environments have high SLA (for sunlight capture) and invest in shoot growth to reach the forest canopy [39,40].

Therefore, it is clear that *Citrus* plants, when growing on sunshiny plains and planted under organized spacing, emit too many leaves and surpass the critical leaf area index (LAI), and start auto-shading the whole plant [37]. This behavior turns this plant species highly inefficient in terms of carbon balance. Should this behavior be considered a plastic response of *Citrus* plants to excessive radiation? Note that this behavior is exactly the opposite strategy performed by forests (and savanna) species in their natural environments [39, 40]. Studying SLA, LAI and other growth attributes in response to a PPFD gradient makes no sense for *Citrus* research, and consequently would not be supported by most horticultural journals. But for instance, a forest species from the Cerrado area, *Styrax pohlii*, showed higher SLA when cultivated in shaded environments, as compared to when it was cultivated in savanna-type vegetation with high irradiation load [39]. Similar results and interpretations can be drawn from many forest species from Cerrado areas [40]. So, although *Citrus* plants astonishingly increase leaf area and leaf number when planted in a grove [37], how would SLA vary within the same period and across the canopy profile?

Following our reasoning, one may also suppose that *Citrus* trees face excessive radiation in groves, and that it would cause excessive damage (photoinhibition) to its chloroplasts, since it is a forest species not adapted to high irradiance habitats. However, excessive radiation exists for every plant species on earth [41]. For *Citrus* plants, excessive PPFD induces photoinhibition and decreases the quantum efficiency of photosystems in chloroplasts [19]. In addition, these increased photoinhibition and low photochemical efficiency in the field is mainly accentuated between 12:00h and 16:00h [19]. Forest species [42] and even savanna species [43,44] may suffer from photoinhibition, but in general, these are dynamic photoinhibition responses (it recovers at the end of the day), which is similar to photoinhibition responses observed for *Citrus* plants [19]. Nevertheless, for *Citrus* plants, photoinhibition can get worse during droughts in the winter [19].

CONCLUSION

In this chapter, we tried to discuss biological aspects of *Citrus* production around the world. We reviewed and re-interpreted data already published on the subject, and we added an ecological point of view that, perhaps, is not discussed by most horticultural texts in books or journals. The *Citrus* genus has begun its "voyage" from its center of genetic origin, in southeastern Asia before Christ. It is a forest species that was brought to different tropical and subtropical areas to be cultivated under arid/semi-arid and humid conditions as a crop plant. Although the use of rootstocks is essential for attenuating many edaphic conditions that limit yields, from an ecological standpoint, it is evident that fertilization and edaphic limitations to *Citrus* production still applies.

As a forest species, there are questions that are still unresolved, such as resources allocation to different organs of *Citrus* plants, which are perhaps useless from ecological and agronomic standpoints. This turns these plants highly inefficient in terms of carbon balance. Under grove systems, *Citrus* trees are pushed to survive and produce fruits outside a forest or shaded environments, where it supposedly fits better.

Native plants growing in different savannas around the world, but especially in the Cerrado, provide science with important tools and unknown metabolisms still to be investigated. Until now, these species have been replaced with plantations, but their biology and metabolism have been totally neglected, even if these plantations are conducted where this native vegetation used to grow.

Finally, considering the topics discussed above, it would be reasonable to start reflecting on the interaction between horticultural and ecological traits, considering the center of genetic origin of Citrus. Only if working together, and examining different points of views, from ecological to agronomic, will we be able to overcome or at least understand factors controlling plant yields.

REFERENCES

[1] Gmitter, F.G., Jr., Hu, X., (1990). The possible role of Yunnan, China, in the origin of contemporary *Citrus* species (Rutaceae). *Econ. Bot.* 44, 267-277.

[2] Davies, F.S., Albrigo, L.G., (1994). History, distribution and uses of *Citrus* fruit. In: *Citrus*. Wallingford: CAB International. pp. 1-11.

[3] Tolkowsky, S., (1938). *Hesperides: a history of the culture and use of citrus fruits.* John Bales, Sons & Curnow, pp. 371.

[4] Webber, J.H., Reuther, W., Lawton, H.W., (1967). History and development of the citrus industry. In: Reuther, W., Webber, H.J., Batchelor, L.D. (eds.). *The Citrus Industry*. University of California Press, Riverside. pp. 1-39.

[5] del Priore, M., Venâncio, R.P., (1998). O livro de ouro da história do Brasil. Ediouro, São Paulo. pp. 397.

[6] Freire, G., (2005). *Casa Grande & Senzala*. Global Editora, São Paulo. pp. 719.

[7] Calavan, E.C., Mather, S.M., McEachern, E.H., (1978). Registration, Certification, and Indexing of Citrus trees. In: Reuther, W., Calavan, E.C., Carman, G.E. (eds). *The Citrus Industry*. University of California Press, Riverside. pp. 185-222.

[8] Souza, M.C., Habermann, G., (2012). Towards a new ecophysiological approach to understand *Citrus* crop yield under abiotic stresses mirroring in the Brazilian savanna genetic resources. In: Rahman, I.Md.M., Hasegawa, H. (eds). *Water stress*. Intech, Rijeka. pp 151-164.

[9] Castle, W.S., (1987). *Citrus* rootstocks. In: Rom, R.C., Carlson, R.F. (eds). *Rootstocks for fruit crops*. John Wiley and Sons, New York. pp. 361-399.

[10] Rossetti, V., Garnier, M., Bové, J.M., Beretta, M.J.G., Teixeira, A.R., Quaggio, J.A., Negri, J.D., (1990). Présence de bactéries dans le xylème d'orangers atteints de chlorose variégée, une nouvelle maladie des agrumes au Brésil. *Comptes Rendus de l'Academie des Sciences*, 310, 345–349.

[11] Jesus Junior, W.C., Bassanezi, R., (2004). Análise da dinâmica e estrutura de focos da morte súbita dos citros. *Fitopatol. Bras.* 29, 399-405.

[12] Rodrigues, D., Ortiz, L., (2006). *Em direção à sustentabilidade da produção de etanol de cana de açúcar no Brasil*. Porto Alegre, Brazil: Amigos da Terra Brasil; São Paulo, Brazil: Vitae Civilis.

[13] Tisdale, S.L., Nelson, W.L., Beaton, J.D., (1985). Growth and the factors affecting it. In: *Soil fertility and fertilizers*. Macmillan, New York. pp.19-58.

[14] Holmes, R.M., Robertson, G.W., (1959). Heat units and crop growth. *Canadian Defense Agriculture Publication*. pp. 1042-1050.

[15] Mendel, K., (1969) The influence of temperature and light on the vegetative development of citrus trees. *Proc. First Int. Citrus Symp.* 1, 259-265.

[16] Zeevaart, J.A.D., (1976). Physiology of flower formation. *Annu. Rev. Plant Physiol.* 27, 321-348.

[17] Habermann, G., Rodrigues, J.D., (2009). Leaf gas exchange and fruit yield in sweet orange trees as affected by citrus variegated chlorosis and environmental conditions. *Sci. Hortic.* 122, 69-76.

[18] Machado, E.C., Medina, C.L., Gomes, M.M.A., Habermann, G., (2002). Seasonal variation of photosynthetic rates, stomatal conductance and leaf water potential in 'Valência' orange trees. *Sci. Agric.* 59, 53-58.

[19] Ribeiro, R.V., Machado, E.C., (2007). Some aspects of *Citrus* ecophysiology in subtropical climates: re-visiting photosynthesis under natural conditions. *Braz. J. Plant Physiol.* 19, 393-411.

[20] Santos, C.M.A., Ribeiro, R.V., Magalhães Filho, J.R., Machado, D.F.S.P., Machado, E.C., (2011). Low substrate temperature imposes higher limitation to photosynthesis of orange plants as compared to atmospheric chilling. *Photos.* 49, 546-554

[21] Ribeiro, R.V., Machado, E.C., Habermann, G., Santos, M.G., Oliveira, R.F., (2012). Seasonal effects on the relationship between photosynthesis and leaf carbohydrates in orange trees. *Funct. Plant Biol.* 39, 471-480.

[22] Iglesias, D.J., Lliso, I., Tadeo, F.R., Talon, M., (2002). Regulation of photosynthesis through source-sink imbalance in citrus is mediated by carbohydrate content in leaves. *Physiol. Plant.* 116, 563–572.

[23] Scholes, R.J., Hall, D.O., (1996). The carbon budget of tropical savannas, woodlands and grasslands. In: Breymeyer, A.I., Hall, D.O., Melillo, J.M., Agren, G.I., (eds). Global change: effects on coniferous forests and grasslands. Chichester,

[24] Myers, N., Mittermeier, R.A., Mittermeier, C.G., Fonseca, G.A.B., Kents, J., (2000). Biodiversity hotspots for conservation priorities. *Nature* 403, 853-858.

[25] Beerling, D., Osborne, C., (2006). The origin of the savanna biome. *Global Change Biology* 12, 2023-2031.

[26] Simon, M.F., Grether, R., Queiroz, L.P., Skema, C., Pennington, R.T., Hughes, C.E., (2009). Recent assembly of the Cerrado, a neotropical plant diversity hotspot, by in sity evolution of adaptations to fire. *Proc. Nat. Acad. Scien.* 106, 20359-20364.

[27] Pinheiro, M.H.O, Monteiro, R., (2010). Contribution to the discussions on the origin of the cerrado biome: Brazilian savanna. *Braz. J. Biol.* 70, 95-102.

[28] Sankaran, M., Hanan, N.H., Scholes, R.J., et al., (2005). Determinants of woody cover in African savannas. *Nature* 408, 846-849.

[29] Zambatis, N., (2006). Scientific Services, Kruger National Park. Available on <http://www.tydonsafaris.com/climate.htm>. Accessed on 22 august, 2013.

[30] Australian Government Bureau Meteorology, (2013). Available at <http://www.bom.gov.au>. Accessed on 22 august, 2013.

[31] INMET (2003). Available at <http://www.inmet.gov.br/portal/>. Accessed on 22 august, 2013.

[32] Jansen, S., Broadley, M.R., Robbrecht, E., Smets, E., (2002). Aluminum hyperaccumulation in angiosperms: a review of its phylogenetic significance. *Bot. Rev.* 68, 235-269.

[33] Jiang, H.X., Chen, L.S., Zheng, J.G., Han, S., Tang, N., Smith, B.R., (2008). Aluminum-induced effects on Photosystem II photochemistry in Citrus leaves assessed by the chlorophyll a fluorescence transient. *Tree Physiol.* 28, 1863–1871.

[34] Pereira, W.E., Siqueira, D.L., Puiatti, M., Martinez, C.A., Salomão, L.C.C., Cecon, P.R., (2003). Growth of citrus rootstocks under aluminum stress in hydroponics. *Sci. Agric.* 60, 31-41.

[35] Lin, Z., Myhre, D.L., (1991). Differential response of citrus rootstocks to aluminum levels in nutrient solutions: I. Plant growth. *J. Plant Nutr.* 14, 1223-1238.

[36] Lin, Z., Myhre, D.L., (1991). Differential response of citrus rootstocks to aluminum levels in nutrient solutions: II. Plant mineral concentrations. *J. Plant Nutr.* 14, 1239-1254.

[37] Turrell, F.M., (1961). Growth of the photosynthetic area of Citrus. *Bot. Gaz.* 122, 285-298.

[38] Givnish, T.J., (1988). Adaptation to sun and shade: A whole-plant perspective. *Aust. J. Plant Physiol.* 15, 63-92.

[39] Habermann, G., Bressan, A.C.G., (2011). Root, shoot and leaf traits of the congeneric Styrax species may explain their distribution patterns in the Cerrado *sensu lato* areas in Brazil. *Funct. Plant Biol.* 38, 209-218.

[40] Hoffmann, W.A., Franco, A.C., (2003). Comparative growth analysis of tropical forest and savanna woody plants using phylogenetically independent contrasts. *J. Ecol.* 91, 475-484.

[41] Melis, A., (2009). Solar energy conversion efficiencies in photosynthesis: Minimizing the chlorophyll antennae to maximize efficiency. *Plant Sci.* 177, 272-280.

[42] Scarano, F.R., Duarte, H.M., Franco, A.C., Geβler, A., de Mattos, E. A., Rennenberg, H., Lüttge, U., (2004). Physiological synecology of tree species in relation to geographic distribution and ecophysiological parameters at the Atlantic forest periphery in Brazil: An overview. *Trees* 19, 493-496.

[43] Feistler, A.M., Habermann, G., (2012). Assessing the role of vertical leaves within the photosynthetic function of *Styrax camporum* under drought conditions. *Photos.* 50, 613-622.

[44] da Veiga, E.B., Habermann, G. Instantaneously measured traits may detect non-plastic ecophysiological performances in response to drought, explaining distributions of *Styrax* species in the Cerrado. *Trees* 27, 1737-1745.

In: Citrus
Editor: Khizar Hayat

ISBN: 978-1-63117-985-3

Chapter 2

MOLECULAR CHARACTERIZATION OF CITRUS CULTIVARS: INSIGHT FROM RECENT STUDIES

***Jamila Bernardi*[1,*], *Adriano Marocco*[1,2], *Paola Caruso*[3] *and Concetta Licciardello*[3]**
[1]Istituto di Agronomia, Genetica e Coltivazioni Erbacee,
[2]Centro di Ricerca sulla Biodiversità e il DNA Antico,
Università Cattolica del Sacro Cuore, Piacenza, Italy
[3]Consiglio per la Ricerca e la Sperimentazione in
Agricoltura (CRA-ACM), Acireale, Italy

ABSTRACT

Citrus fruits are an important nutritional source for human health and have immense economic value. Fruit development and ripening are key processes in the production of the phytonutrients, which are essential for a balanced diet and for disease prevention. The anthocyanins are responsible for red pigmentation in the flesh of sweet orange and one of the most important antioxidant compounds together with carotenoids (in particular lycopene) and ascorbic acid. These compounds contribute to protect against certain cancers, cardiovascular diseases, and other degenerative processes.

The anthocyanin pathway is well described, and gene coding enzymes of the biosynthesis sequenced and analyzed at the molecular level. The generally identical structure and composition of genes taking part to anthocyanins pathway and their higher expression in blood oranges compared to common ones, suggested the investigation on regulatory network, in particular MYB transcription factors that play an important role in activation of the biosynthesis. In a recent study, the association of a long terminal repeat (LTR) to a Myb-like gene was found correlated to the red pigmentation in the flesh fruits of sweet orange cultivars. *Citrus* fruits are important also for their content of ascorbic acid. The gene transcription of key enzymes involved in the four known biosynthesis pathways of the vitamin C resulted up-regulated specifically in fruit, contributing to the

* Corresponding author: Jamila Bernardi. Istituto di Agronomia, Genetica e Coltivazioni Erbacee, Università Cattolica del Sacro Cuore, Piacenza, Italy E-mail: jamila.bernardi@unicatt.it.

high vitamin C accumulation in juice sacs. Moreover, new data related to the GalUR gene family in the citrus genome may suggest its involvement.

The expected variability within *Citrus* species is low, due to the origin by spontaneous mutation and vegetative propagation, leading to a narrow genetic basis. Sweet orange, lemon, lime and grapefruit, are characterized by high heterozygosis, but nearly all cultivars are similar, as they originate from a common ancestor hybrid. Single nucleotide polymorphisms (SNPs) identification performed on various accessions of *Citrus clementine* and *C. sinensis,* confirmed the higher heterozygosity of sweet orange respect to clementine; and the presence of very few SNPs linked to agronomical characteristics.

The development of next generation sequencing technologies will provide precise description of the genetic composition of citrus accessions and species. In particular, the availability of the citrus genome will permit to increase the opportunity identifying SNP markers to be used to develop citrus assay platforms for breeders. The further step will be to exploit both transcriptome and genome information to map the location of natural genetic variants that confer economically important traits mostly in the fruit.

Keywords: Anthocyanins, Vitamin C, Sweet orange, Molecular markers, Genome sequencing

INTRODUCTION

World production of citrus fruit has experienced a continuous growth. In the last decades total annual fresh and processed citrus fruit production was estimated at over 115 and 29 million tons, respectively, in the period 2010-2011 [1].

Citrus fruits are an important nutritional source for human health, contributing to a balanced diet and disease prevention. Among sweet oranges, in particular blood ones, have significant health-promoting properties, in addition with the high content of vitamin C and carotenoids [2-5]. These compounds, and mostly anthocyanins, contribute to protect against certain cancers, cardiovascular diseases [4-6], reduce oxidative stress in diabetic patients [7] and protect DNA against oxidative damage [8, 9]. A reduction of adipocytes development and weight gain in mice affected by obesity, when comparing blood orange juice with common one or water as a drink for mice, has been recently reported [10]. Among antioxidant properties, the ascorbate (ASC), also called vitamin C, is one of the most interesting compounds. The ASC content in citrus fruit juice sacs is 20–100 mg per 100 mL juice, which varies greatly depending on species or variety [11, 12].

It is widely known that ASC plays important roles not only in different plant development processes as antioxidant and enzymatic cofactor [13, 14], but also in maintaining human health, reducing risk of chronic diseases (such as cancer, cardiovascular disease and cataract), in the collagen formation, in normal bone development and in cancer treatment [15].

However, humans cannot synthesize their own ascorbic acid (AA) due to the absence of l-gulonolactone oxidase and ASC cannot be stored in the body either.

Despite the fact that citrus is a major crop in several countries, geneticists still have a limited understanding of the genome composition of the main important cultivars. The knowledge of the genome and its variability is of great importance to understand the origin of the cultivated species.

The genotyping, together with the availability of whole genome sequences of the most important cultivars, will help breeders to develop strategies for marker assisted selection (MAS). In particular, consumers are interested in traceability of the foods and an increase in their nutritional value.

CITRUS ORIGIN AND GENOME STRUCTURE

The most widely growing *Citrus* cultivars, including all sweet oranges, various satsuma, different clementines, and nearly all lemons, limes and grapefruit are bud sport selections that originate from spontaneous mutations in vegetative buds, while few derive from crosses. Despite the great number of citrus cultivars, they possess a very little genetic diversity within most of the major groups, with the exceptions of mandarins and pummelo [16].

Citrus breeding by hybridization is difficult because of the long generation time (generally 5 years or more), large space requirement for individual trees, and presence of nucellar embryony (a form of apomixis) existing in many cultivars [16]. Several of these challenges are being addressed by citrus breeders and geneticists, and new and promising tools to explore the citrus genome are coming to the aid.

With the exception of pummelo, citron and some mandarin species, the other species can be considered natural hybrids. Because of their origin, these species often share a common gene pool. The ancestry of major cultivar groups was revealed by sequencing [17] together with high density marker studies: most of the *Citrus* genomes are composed of large fragments derived from different ancestral taxa [18]. For example, sweet oranges derived from a backcross or more complex series of crosses involving mandarin and pummelo [17, 19, 20], grapefruit from pummelo × orange [21], and clementine from Willowleaf mandarin × sweet orange [22, 23] (Figure 1).

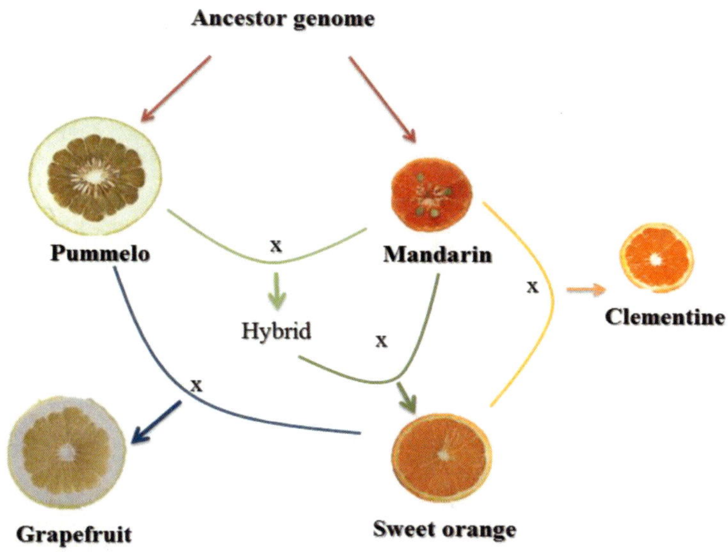

Figure 1. Proposed schematic representation of the origin of the most cultivated *Citrus* species based on molecular and sequencing data.

Despite the high heterozygosis, the variability within 'species' (e.g., *Citrus sinensis*, *C. paradisi*, and *C. limon*) is very low; the cultivars in these groups represent accumulated somatic mutations identified over centuries through on-tree or nucellar seedling mutations [16].

Most of the citrus are diploid with 2n=18 chromosomes and genome sizes of about 380 Mb [24]. Recently the genome sequence of a double haploid derived from sweet orange was published [17]. In addition, the International Citrus Genome Consortium has sequenced, assembled and annotated a clementine-derived haploid line that was retained in pathogen-free status, and which had already been propagated [25, 26]. Additional citrus sequencing projects already completed include a second sweet orange genome assembly produced from the clone 'Ridge Pineapple' [24], 11 varieties from Japan [27] and 150 varieties by a public-private consortium in Spain [28]. Because of the brief history of cultivation and the characteristics of its reproduction, the sweet orange genome sequence will serve as the primary reference genome for all citrus and related genera into the future and may provide a resource for the study of ancient genome traits of its ancestors, mandarin and pummelo [29]. The structure of the sweet orange genome is similar to that of Arabidopsis and rice, with a low level (20.5%) of repetitive elements, among which the class I LTR retrotransposons are predominant [17].

About 29 thousands protein-coding loci and 44 thousands transcripts were located along the nine sweet orange chromosomes. The gene transcripts have an average length of 1,817 bp, a mean coding sequence size of 1,255 bp and an average of 5.8 exons per gene [17].

Molecular Markers Used for Citrus Discrimination

The use of the entire *Citrus* genome as a reference and the resequencing of the main secondary species will be useful for deciphering the interspecific mosaic structure of species and cultivars. The polymorphism density identified in diploid sweet orange is 3.6 SNP/kb and 0.6 indels/kb [17]. The resulting estimations of within- and between-taxon differentiation is by now the result of polymorphism study with different nuclear markers such as SNP, simple sequence repeats (SSR), cleaved amplified polymorphic sequences (CAPS) and amplified fragment length polymorphism (AFLP). Amar et al. [30] assessed the informativeness and efficiency of three different molecular markers for genetic diversity among 24 *Citrus* and their relative species. Restriction fragment length polymorphisms (RFLPs), sequenced characterized amplified regions (SCARs), CAPS, SSRs, and SNPs are much more desirable for broad applications, and the citrus research community has been developing these resources over time [16]. Some of these markers were developed in absence of genome or transcriptome sequences, and as such they might be considered to be gene anonymous. Recently, the genome of Valencia orange was characterized for single nucleotide variations, small insertions and deletions by resequencing and alignment to the sequenced genome of sweet orange [28]. Two approaches are commonly used for high density genotyping. One consists of the use of array platforms, such as the GoldenGate SNP array, the other is the genotyping-by-sequencing method (GBS).

For instance, 1,456 SNPs, found heterozygous in clementine, were used to design a GoldenGate assay. The analysis of the ancestry of *Citrus* germplasm, found that most of the SNP markers (567), were useful to discriminate clementine varieties, but only few were found for pummelo (189), citron (99), and *C. micrantha* (17) [23]. In a more recent study [31], SNPs, surveyed by direct sequence comparison of the sequence tagged site (STS) fragment amplified from genomic DNA of cultivars representing the genetic diversity of citrus breeding in Japan, were used to develop a prototype multiplexed SNP genotyping GoldenGate. This high-throughput platform was then applied to a hybrid population of 88 progeny and 103 citrus accessions. A total of 351 SNPs (91%) could call different genotypes among the DNA samples, and a minimal marker set for cultivar identification of only seven markers was able to discriminate a subset of 98 accessions [31].

The major alternative to the GoldenGate SNP array is GBS, in which a defined subset of the genome is synthesized for each individual and then sequenced in multiplex using tags (barcodes) to identify reads derived from each individual [32]. The reduction of genome complexity is produced by digestion with restriction endonucleases, sometimes combined with PCR to produce short fragments, common to most individuals to be genotyped. However, restriction fragment polymorphisms or incomplete digestion of the template DNA can exclude specific sequences from the sequencing reactions, leading to missing data, imputed from the genotype of adjacent markers [32], to which it is necessary to add informatics costs. The initial cost-advantage of GBS methods is reduced for heterozygous species, such as citrus, because each fragment must be sequenced in considerable depth to ensure that both potential alleles at a locus are detected.

Another disadvantage of GBS consists of the targeting of genes that could be addressed by choosing methylation-sensitive restriction enzymes that will not cut frequently in the repetitive portion of the genome. Arrays can target genes of interest more precisely.

The revolution in sequencing technologies, including the sequencing of bacterial artificial chromosome (BAC) clones, BAC ends, and fairly extensive expressed sequence tag (EST) libraries for citrus accessions under multiple conditions, has produced a very substantial resource for high-throughput development, validation, and use of molecular markers for citrus linkage mapping. These markers are frequently based on EST sequences and therefore represent specific genes with known or predicted functions. A bioinformatics analysis was performed to find thousands of reliable SNPs to be further used in cultivar discrimination [33]. The results, obtained from validated data, emphasized the low genetic diversity of sweet orange and clementine, confirming also the high heterozygosity [33]. The used SNPs derived from ESTs had a poor ability to resolve the complexity of cultivar discrimination, but possess the potential to be used in studying *Citrus* phylogenetic relationships.

Furthermore, the problem in detecting *in silico* SNPs from ESTs was the high monomorphic rate encountered [29, 33].

FUNCTIONAL GENOMICS

EST collection is a valid tool to study the genetic diversity and includes a wide representation of sequences from many complementary DNA (cDNA) libraries derived from multiple reproductive (flowers, ovaries, fruits, seeds) and vegetative (roots, leaves, buds) organs and tissues (flesh, flavedo, abscission zones) at different developmental stages, challenged with biotic (*Phytophthora*, citrus tristeza virus, herbivory, *Penicillium*) and abiotic (salinity, iron deficiency, water deficit) agents, and hormonal treatments.

One of the first functional genomics projects in *Citrus* was performed by Forment et al. [34], in which 22,000 ESTs were collected from different tissues, developmental stages and stress conditions. Terol et al. [35] identified 13,000 putative unigenes with significant BLAST hits.

Further analyses and comparisons with Arabidopsis suggested the occurrence of citrus paralogues, putative conserved orthologues, single copy genes, duplication events, and increased number of genes for specific pathways.

In addition, Reis et al. [36] reported a huge EST sequencing effort. These data were collected in the CitEST Brazilian database [37] including more than 260,000 valid reads contained unigene sets from several citrus species, mainly sweet orange, mandarin and *Poncirus trifoliata*.

The microarray technology for transcript profiling in functional genomics was important in all plant systems and, in particular, in many agricultural crops. Among various tools, an Affymetrix array from public databases (HarvEST) is available. A recent work using the GeneChip array studied the transcriptional changes in tolerant and susceptible cultivars against biotic stress [38]. Additional projects used cDNA citrus microarrays or smaller custom arrays based on subtractive libraries.

Bernardi et al. [39] developed a specific microarray to support the analysis of the expression levels of genes known to be related to fruit ripening and anthocyanin accumulation. The custom chip was used to monitor expression levels of genes during fruit ripening in blood and common orange cultivars. The array included 301 probes derived from a subtracted SSH library [40], a cDNA–AFLP collection [41], and a set of regulatory genes from the HarvEST citrus database. SSH libraries were extensively used not only to find differentially expressed genes in pigmented and not pigmented cultivars [40], but also comparing juvenile and adult phase to find genes associated to flowering time [42].

Recently, RNA sequencing together with DNA sequencing were used to study the functional effects of the sweet orange heterozygosity at both the transcriptome and the whole-genome sequence level [17, 29]. Jiao et al. [29] demonstrated that there is a correlation between the expression level and the presence of SNPs and indels. In particular, most of the genes containing large deletions were weakly expressed and many genes (1,062) containing SNPs showed an allelic differential expression. Of these genes 150 and 55 were found originated from mandarin and pummelo, respectively, representing promising candidates to study the genetic basis of physiological traits and fruit quality of both ancestral and cultivated species [29].

Genes Involved in Anthocyanins Biosynthesis

In blood orange and its hybrids anthocyanins characterize fruit (flesh and rind), while in lemon and citron the red pigmentation is evident in some floral tissues and in young shoots and fruits [43]. The red pigments are synthesized via the flavonoid pathway, a branch of the phenylpropanoid ones, consisting of numerous enzymatic steps (Figure 2).

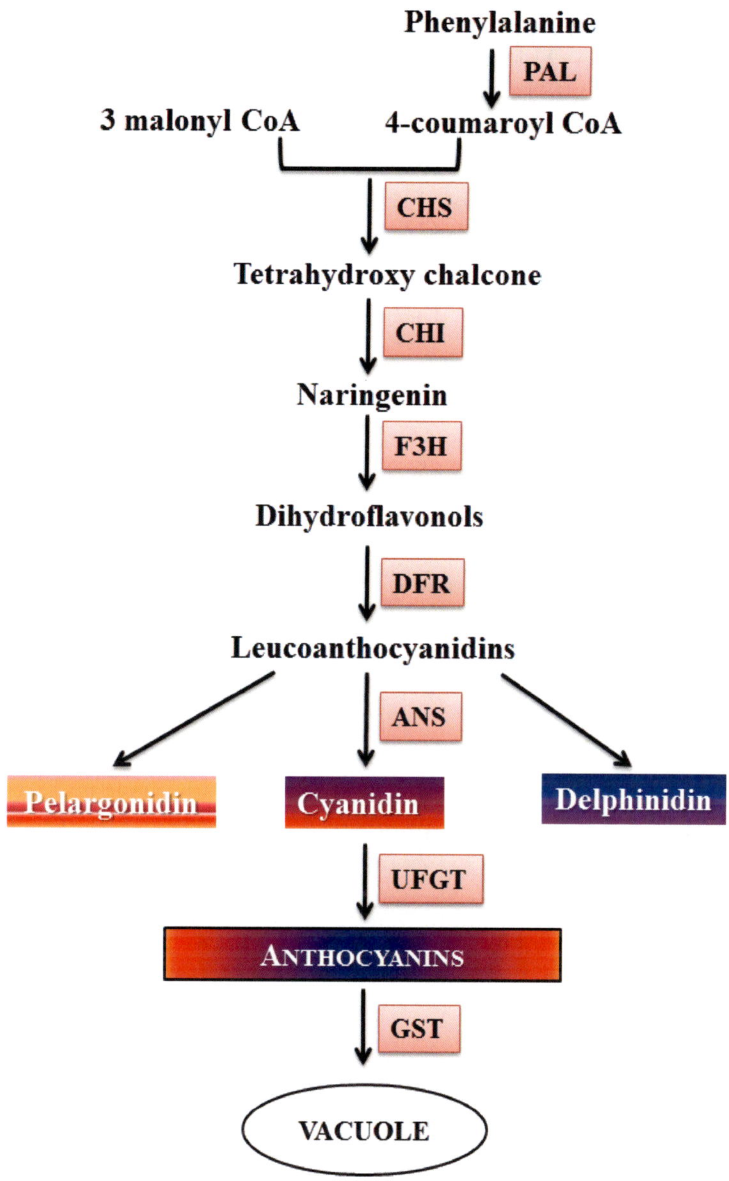

Figure 2. The anthocyanins biosynthetic pathway.

Abbreviations: PAL, phenylalanine ammonia lyase; CHS, chalcone synthase; CHI, chalcone isomerase; F3H, flavanone 3-hydroxylase; DFR, dyhydroflavonol reductase; ANS, anthocyanidin synthase; UFGT, UDP-glucose: flavonoid-3-O-glucosyltransferase; GST, glutathione S transferase.

In *C. sinensis* (L.) Osbeck structural genes coding for chalcone synthase (CHS), chalcone isomerase (CHI), flavanone 3-hydroxylase (F3H), dihydro-flavonol reductase (DFR), anthocyanidin synthase (ANS) and UDP-glucose: flavonoid-3-O-glucosyltransferase (UFGT) were characterized and cloned [44-48]. Cotroneo et al. [49] verified the transcription expression level of *CHS*, *ANS* and *UFGT* during the ripening through Real Time PCR, showing that in common oranges (Valencia), messenger RNAs (mRNAs) were detected at very low levels. Instead, in Moro cultivar (one of the most pigmented genotypes) there was a strict correlation between the transcript levels and the anthocyanin accumulation. The same genes were also compared in fruits of eleven different cultivars collected in a period in which the anthocyanin content was elevated. Generally pigmentation was correlated with the expression level of *CHS*, *ANS* and *UFGT* [49].

Anthocyanins are water-soluble compounds, synthesised in the cytoplasm and accumulated in the vacuoles. The phase of the vacuolarization is performed by the glutathione S transferase (GST), that otherwise protects cells by oxidative stress. GST gene families were firstly classified based on the exon/ intron structure of the genes, on sequence similarity and on amino acid residue conservation. Three distinct classes of plant *GSTs* were initially identified and indicated as I, II and III types *GST* genes. This classification schema has been refined [50] and six distinct classes have been characterized.

Phi (type I) and Tau (type III) classes are *GSTs* plant specific and they are the most representative classes in terms of number of sequences per class; Lambda, Theta, Zeta, Mapeg and dehydroascorbate reductase (*DHAR*) are less numerous, and they are in common with animals. Members of Phi class are otherwise involved in the vacuolarization of anthocyanins. In particular, a Phi class GST was isolated as a member taking part to the pigmentation of the flesh of blood orange fruits [40, 51]. Moreover, an *in silico* approach was used to collect and assemble all the ESTs coding for *GSTs* isolated in sweet orange, and this analysis was associated to a transcriptional approach for validation [52]. In particular, semiQuantitative RT-PCR analysis was performed to assess the expression levels of the *in silico* assembled mRNAs in different pigmented and not pigmented tissues in blood and common oranges, and to confirm the correspondence between the transcript isolated through a specific cDNA library and the tissue specificity evaluated through the *in silico* approach [52]. Spliced and unspliced forms have been previously described in literature mostly for *GST* Phi class, because they are responsible for the pigmentation of the fruit tissues [53]. RT-PCR analysis generates one band of the expected size in albedo, flavedo and flesh, while two amplicons of different size have been observed in leaves and ovary. The upper band corresponds to the unspliced transcript form (both the introns are retained), while the lower band is equivalent to the spliced transcript, generating the known protein product just described by [40] and [51].

Considering the genetic structure of genes coding enzymes involved in the anthocyanin pathway, there is a high similar sequence structure between blood and common oranges (Licciardello, personal communication), in addition to single nucleotide variations not associated to the phenotype.

Using different methodologies - Real time PCR [40, 48, 54], custom array [38] and Affymetrix GeneChip [55] - transcription profiles of Cadenera (common orange) and Moro (blood orange) cultivars were evaluated.

The down-regulation of the genes coding for the structural enzymes (*phenylalanine ammonia lyase*, *CHS*, *DFR*, *ANS*, *UFGT* and *GST*) of the bio-synthetic pathway was revealed in common orange, while an over-expression of all genes was detected in the pigmented cultivar.

The effect of low temperature on the anthocyanin synthesis has been documented [48]. In particular, the analysis of gene expression showed that the amount of transcripts quickly increased after 3-6 days of cold storage.

Moreover, the production of anthocyanin of 8 times higher than the level observed in the control sample, suggested a useful employ of cold storage to produce fruits with health-related attributes [56].

Regulation of Anthocyanin Biosynthesis

The similarity in the sequence structure of structural biosynthetic genes, associated to a different expression level between blood and common varieties, addressed researchers to investigate on regulatory genes involved in the control of pathway. These genes are characterized by transcription factors (TFs) controlling the different expression of the structural genes [57-60].

Tissues-specific regulation of structural genes is strictly correlated with combination of two different TF families: one is homolog to R2R3 domain of Myb proteins and the other to basic-Helix-Loop-Helix (bHLH) domain of Myc. These two families are involved in the regulation of the anthocyanin pathways, together with WD40-repeats proteins that have a role in assisting the process [57-60].

The regulation mechanism is presumably different in tissues characterized by the anthocyanin pigmentation, for instance rind and flesh.

Differences in the level or location of pigmentation were linked to transposon insertion in the promoter region or to the presence of loss-of function mutations in coding sequence of *Myb* genes [61-64].

Variation in pigment intensity or tissue specificity in plants is strictly dependent by the activity of the Myb TF [61-65]. Two different groups [66, 67] discovered new *Myb* genes involved in the control of the anthocyanin pathway. A large number of *Citrus* genes belonging to a previously unidentified *MYBA* gene family of *Vitis vinifera* was identified. It was the first documentation of highly homologous genes that regulate anthocyanin biosynthesis existing in taxonomically distant species such as citrus and grapevine. Even if PCR analysis confirmed the presence in *Citrus* of a homologous *Myb* sequence of *Vitis*, homology search on available genomic databases [16] did not confirm the existence of such sequence on citrus geno-me, needing further investigations [66].

The use of degenerate primers on R2R3 *Myb* genes of various species characterized by anthocyanins in different part of plants, allowed the isolation of a gene named *Ruby*, consisting of three exons and two introns. Its anthocyanin functional activity was evaluated with the expression under the control of the constitutive cauliflower mosaic virus (CaMV) 35S promoter in tobacco, where it resulted in visible purple-red pigmentation in undifferentiated callus and in developed tissues of regenerated plants [67]. The *Ruby* expression was detected in all pigmented tissues of blood orange fruits [67], and in young leaves and flower buds of lemon [68]. Moreover, the level of *Ruby* expression in different accessions of blood orange and in hybrids between clementine and Moro (OMO) and clementine and Tarocco (OTA) is directly correlated with the content of anthocyanin in flesh.

As showed in other plants, also in blood oranges it was elucidated that a *Myb*-like gene promoted stronger pigmentation in combination with *Myc*-like genes, suggesting some selectivity in the ability of the Ruby MYB protein to interact with different bHLH partners [67]. In sweet orange, Cultrone et al. [54] isolated and evaluated the gene structure of a *Myc*-

like gene, called *CsMyc2*, whose expression level was not well correlated with the anthocyanin synthesis. It was also confirmed by the no specific expression, when Ruby was combined with *CsMyc2*, probably because the latter gene was expressed at detectable levels in both common and blood oranges [67].

Considering of primary importance the development of a genetic marker for the presence of anthocyanin, and that the sequence analysis of *Ruby* revealed 100% nucleotide identity in the genetic structure on different blood and common oranges, the study of the upstream promoter region could help in the resolution of a possible genetic difference between pigmented and common accessions. Using a chromosome walking approach, Butelli et al. [67] discovered that, in pigmented varieties, this region was characterized by an insertion with high similarity with a LTR, that was absent in common varieties [67].

Moreover, in some cultivars, in association to the LTR, there was inserted also a retroelement, called Tcs1, showing the typical features of a Copia-like LTR retrotransposon. The insertion of retrotrasposons within or near transcriptionally active regions modifies the expression of the gene [69-71].

In *Vitis,* Kobayashi et al. [61] also reported that a retrotransposon-induced mutation in a homologue of *VlMybA*s, is associated with the loss of the pigmentation in white cultivars of *V. vinifera,* just the opposite to what happens in *Citrus.*

GENES INVOLVED IN ASCORBIC ACID METABOLISM

In addition to the importance of anthocyanins, citrus fruits are also known to be rich in vitamin C, a strong antioxidant agent. The vitamin C includes two bioactive forms: the reduced (l-ascorbic acid, AA) and the oxidized form (dehydroascorbate, DHA).

The vitamin C component and levels are due to the balance of its bio-synthesis, catabolism and recycling, whereas AA biosynthesis was considered the main source of vitamin C accumulation in plant cells [72]. In plants AA biosynthetic pathways consists of at least four distinct pathways known, including l-galactose (known as Smirnoff–Wheeler pathway), l-glucose pathway, galacturonic acid pathway, and myo-inositol pathway [73]. Among them, l-galactose pathway was considered the most important in high plants [73] (Figure 3).

This biosynthetic complex has been rather studied in fruit trees, such as kiwifruit [74], apple [75], peach [76], tomato [77, 78] and strawberry [79], while very poor information is currently available on AA synthesis in citrus.

Among all the genes, Yang et al. [80] investigated the expression profiles of six l-galactose pathway-related genes (*GMPase*, GDP-mannose pyro-phosphorylase; *GME*, GDP-mannose-3,5-epimerase; *GGP*, *GDP*, L-galactose-pyrophosphatase; *GPP*, L-galactose 1-P phosphatase; *GDH*, L-galactose de-hydrogenase; *GLDH*, L-galactono-1,4-lactone dehydrogenase) in association with the enzyme activities of ascorbate oxidase (*AO*), ascorbate peroxidase (*APX*), monodehydroascorbate reductase (*MDHAR*) and *DHAR*, as well as vitamin C content in pulps of sweet orange and mandarin fruits. These two citrus species, with obvious difference in vitamin C concentration (higher in orange fruits compared to mandarin) were analyzed during the ripening time. It is also known the (relative) importance of vitamin C in peel and leaf, in addition to the pulp [80].

AA contents highlighted very small differences considering total AA contents in peel or leaf of both species compared to pulp. The average of AA content in peel or leaf was evidently higher in satsuma mandarin than in orange. Four of six genes including *GME*, *GGP*, *GDH* and *GLDH* showed an increasing trend in sweet orange compared to mandarin. In particular the *GME* trend was confirmed to play a key role in the regulation of ASC biosynthesis in plants [81]. The overexpression of *GGP* was correlated to an increase in leaf AA [80, 82, 83], while *GDH* had no effect [84] and, as in kiwifruit, comparing genotypes with different ASC content, no obvious differences in gene expression were detected [74]. The role of *GLDH* in AA biosynthesis is controversial. No clear relationship between AA content and GLDH activity or gene expression was found in kiwifruit [74] and tomato [78] during fruit development and ripening. In citrus, gene expression results herein provided the hypothesis that higher expression of four genes (*GME*, *GGP*, *GDH* and *GLDH*) contributes at least partially to the higher ASC accumulation in orange pulp as compared with satsuma mandarin.

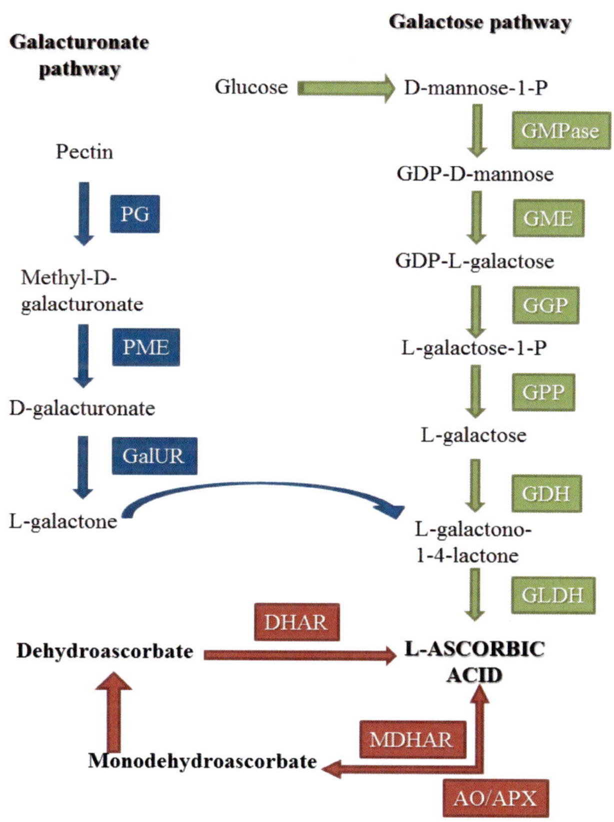

Figure 3. The two vitamin C pathways investigated in *Citrus*.

Abbreviations: PG, polygalacturonase, PME, pectin methyl esterase; GalUR, D-galacturonate reductase, GMPase, GDP-mannose pyrophosphorylase; GME, GDP-mannose-3,5-epimerase; GGP, GDP, L-galactose-pyrophosphatase; GPP, L-galactose 1-P phosphatase; GDH, L-galactose dehydrogenase; GLDH, L-galactono-1,4-lactone dehydrogenase; MDHAR monodehydroascorbate reductase; DHAR, dehydroascorbate reductase; AO, ascorbate oxidase; APX, ascorbate peroxidase.

In particular higher ASC contents in peel or leaf compared to pulp, in agreement with previous reports [11], may be attributable to the requirement of more antioxidants to counteract reactive oxidative species generated by stresses. Contrary to pulp, which is located in the inner part of the fruit, peel or leaves exposed outside are directly subjected to environmental stresses. Moreover glucose, that is the precursor of vitamin C [85], can also play an important signaling role in regulating gene expression of enzymes related to vitamin C metabolism [86]. Beneath this, fruit vitamin C content doesn't seem to be tightly linked to the primary metabolism and content of sugar [87].

Recently, in addition to the l-galactose pathway, some genes coding for the enzymes involved in the galacturonate pathway branch [17] were also evaluated. In particular, the gene encoding d-galacturonic acid reductase (*GalUR*) was investigated (Figure 3). Among the 18 *GalUR* paralogous genes found in the citrus genome, only the *GalUR*-12 was significantly upregulated in fruit, whereas the other did not show a similar expression pattern, supposing a diversification of gene transcription regulation in ASC biosynthesis [88]. *GalUR*-12 shares high sequence identity with the strawberry *GalUR* gene, which has been further tested for specific vitamin C production [88]. Considering these data it is possible to assume that *GalUR* may be the most important contributor to ASC accumulation in orange fruit.

CONCLUSION

The study of genes specifically involved in fruit development, in particular, related to antioxidant accumulation, were extensively discussed and the genome assembly seems to be the additional aid to the citrus geneticists to unravel the regulatory network of pigment-related pathways. Citrus breeders, otherwise, need to know precise information on the most important genes useful to develop improved cultivars. The large space and time requirements for citrus breeding can be reduced by MAS, which allows breeders to screen large populations of seedlings and select those predicted to have desirable traits prior to field planting [89]. The number of traits, for which markers have been identified, has increased rapidly in recent years and now includes nematode resistance [90], nucellar embryony [91], juvenility [92], and several morphological traits [93]. However, few of these studies focus on the fruit quality traits, that are critically important to select successful cultivars.

In addition, most of the markers are only known to be linked to a specific major-gene allele and may not correspond to quantitative trait loci, which can be selected in populations from other parents. The increasing information about the genetic architecture of *Citrus* genome will facilitate to find markers associated with fruit traits such as antioxidant components.

REFERENCES

[1] FAOSTAT, (2012). Food and Agriculture Organization of the United Nations Statistics - fresh and processed citrus fruit. Available at <http:// www.fao.org/fileadmin/ templates/est/COMM_MARKETS_MONITORING/Citrus/Documents/CITRUS_BUL LETIN_2012.pdf>. Accessed on December, 2013.

[2] Prior, R. L., Wu, X. L., (2006). Anthocyanins: Structural characteristics that result in unique metabolic patterns and biological activities. *Free Radic. Res.* 40, 1014–1028.

[3] Davies, K. M., (2007). Genetic modification of plant metabolism for human health benefits. *Mutat. Res.* 622, 122–137.

[4] De Pascual-Teresa, S., Moreno, D. A., García-Viguera, C., (2010). Flavanols and anthocyanins in cardiovascular health: A review of current evidence. *Int. J. Mol. Sci.* 11, 1679–1703.

[5] Paredes-López, O., Cervantes-Ceja, M. L., Vigna-Pérez, M., Hernández-Pérez, T., (2010). Berries: Improving human health and healthy aging, and promoting quality life. A review. *Plant Foods Hum. Nutr.* 65, 299–308.

[6] Toufektsian, M.-C., de Lorgeril, M., Nagy, N., Salen, P., Donati, M. B., Giordano, L., Mock, H. P., Peterek, S., Matros, A., Petroni, K., Pilu, R., Rotilio, D., Tonelli, C., de Leiris, J., Boucher, F., Martin, C., (2008). Chronic dietary intake of plant-derived anthocyanins protects the rat heart against ischemia-reperfusion injury. *J. Nutr.* 138, 747–752.

[7] Bonina, F. P., Leotta, C., Scalia, G., Puglia, C., Trombetta, D., Tringali, G., Roccazzello, A. M., Rapisarda, P., Saija, A., (2002). Evaluation of oxidative stress in diabetic patients after supplementation with a standardised red orange extract. *Diabetes Nutr. Metab.* 15, 14–19.

[8] Riso, P., Visioli, F., Gardana, C., Grande, S., Brusamolino, A., Galvano, F., Galvano, G., Porrini, M., (2005). Effects of blood orange juice intake on antioxidant bioavailability and on different markers related to oxidative stress. *J. Agric. Food Chem.* 53, 941–947.

[9] Guarnieri, S., Riso, P., Porrini, M., (2007). Orange juice vs. vitamin C: Effect on hydrogen peroxide-induced DNA damage in mononuclear blood cells. *Br. J. Nutr.* 97, 639–643.

[10] Titta, L., Trinei, M., Stendardo, M., Berniakovich, I., Petroni, K., Tonelli, C., Riso, P., Porrini, M., Minucci, S., Pelicci, P. G., Rapisarda, P., Reforgiato Recupero, G., Giorgio, M., (2010). Blood orange juice inhibits fat accumulation in mice. *Int. J. Obes.* 34, 578–588.

[11] Nagy, S., (1980). Vitamin C contents of citrus fruit and their products: a review. *J. Agric. Food Chem.* 28, 8-18.

[12] Lee, S. K., Kader, A. A., (2000). Preharvest and postharvest factors influencing vitamin C content of horticultural crops. *Postharvest Biol. Technol.* 20, 207–220.

[13] Olmos, E., Kiddle, G., Pellny, T. K., Kumar, S., Foyer, C. H., (2006). Modulation of plant morphology, root architecture, and cell structure by low vitamin C in Arabidopsis thaliana. *J. Exp. Bot.* 57, 1645–1655.

[14] Kotchoni, S. O., Larrimore, K. E., Mukherjee, M., Kempinski, C. F., Barth, C., (2009). Alterations in the endogenous ascorbic acid content affect flowering time in Arabidopsis. *Plant Physiol.* 149, 803–815.

[15] Sarkar, N., Srivastava, P. K., Dubey, V. K., (2009). Understanding the language of vitamin C. *Curr. Nutri. Food Sci.* 5, 53–55.

[16] Talon, M., Gmitter, F., (2008). Citrus genomics. *Intl. J. Plant Genomics* doi:10.1155/2008/528361.

[17] Xu, Q., Chen, L.-L., Ruan, X., Chen, D., Zhu, A., Chen, C., et al., (2013). The draft genome of sweet orange (*Citrus sinensis*). *Nature genet.* 45, 59–66.

[18] Garcia-Lor, A., Curk, F., Snoussi-Trifa, H., Morillon, R., Ancillo, G., Luro, F., Navarro, L., Ollitrault, P., (2013). A nuclear phylogenetic analysis: SNPs, indels and SSRs deliver new insights into the relation-ships in the "true citrus fruit trees" group (*Citrinae, Rutaceae*) and the origin of cultivated species. *Ann. Bot.* 111, 1-19.

[19] García-Lor, A., Luro, F., Navarro, L., Ollitrault, P., (2012). Comparative use of InDel and SSR markers in deciphering the interspecific structure of cultivated citrus genetic diversity: a perspective for genetic association studies. *Mol. Genet. Genomics* 287, 77–94.

[20] Ollitrault, P., Terol, J., Chen, C., Federici, C. T., Lotfy, S., Hippolyte, I., et al., (2012) A reference genetic map of C. clementina hort. ex Tan.; citrus evolution inferences from comparative mapping. *BMC Genomics* 13, 593.

[21] Gmitter, F. G., (1995). Origin, evolution and breeding of the grapefruit. *Plant Breed Rev.* 13, 345-363.

[22] Nicolosi, E., Deng, Z. N., Gentile, A., Malfa, S. L., Continella, G., Tribulato, E., (2000). Citrus phylogeny and genetic origin of important species as investigated by molecular markers. *Theor. Appl. Genet.* 100, 1155-1166.

[23] Ollitrault, P., Terol, J., Garcia-Lor, A., Bérard, A., Chauveau, A., Froeli-cher, Y., Belzile, C., Morillon, R., Navarro, L., Brunel, D., Talon, M., (2012). SNP mining in C. clementina BAC end sequences; transferability in the Citrus genus (Rutaceae), phylogenetic inferences and perspec-tives for genetic mapping. *BMC Genomics* 13, 13.

[24] Gmitter, F. G., Chen, C., Machado, M. A., Souza, A. A., Ollitrault, P., Froehlicher, Y., and Shimizu, T., (2012) Citrus genomics. *Tree Genet. Genomes* 8.

[25] Gbrowse Phytozome, Citrus clementina - JGI v1.0 (2014). Available at <http://www.phytozome.net/cgi-bin/gbrowse/clementine/>. Accessed on January, 2014.

[26] Aleza, P., Juárez, J., Hernández, M., Pina, J., Ollitrault, P., Navarro, L., (2009). Recovery and characterization of a Citrus clementina Hort. ex Tan. "Clemenules" haploid plant selected to establish the reference whole Citrus genome sequence. *BMC Plant Biol.* 9, 110.

[27] Shimizu, T., Yoshioka, T., Nagasaki, H., Kaminuma, E., Toyoda, A., Fujiyama, A., Nakamura, Y., (2012). Whole genome sequencing and mapping analysis for identifying polymorphism among 11 citrus varieties. In: *XII International Citrus Congress.* (Valencia, Spain), Oral Communication Abstract S03O03.

[28] Talon, M., Terol, J., Carbonell, J., Alonso, R., Ibañez, V., Tadeo, F. R., et al., (2013). Uncovering the Citrus genome and its applications. In: *Plant and Animal Genome Conference XXI.* (San Diego, CA), Poster Abstract W165.

[29] Jiao, W.-B., Huang, D., Xing, F., Hu, Y., Deng, X.-X., Xu, Q., Chen, L.-L., (2013). Genome-wide characterization and expression analysis of genetic variants in sweet orange. *Plant J.* 75, 954-964.

[30] Amar, M. H., Biswas, M. K., Zhang, Z., Guo, W.-W., (2011). Exploitation of SSR, SRAP and CAPS-SNP markers for genetic diversity of Citrus germplasm collection. *Scientia Hortic.* 128.

[31] Fujii, H., Shimada, T., Nonaka, K., Kita, M., Kuniga, T., Endo, T., Ikoma, Y., Omura, M., (2012). High-throughput genotyping in citrus accessions using an SNP genotyping array. *Tree Gen. Genomes* 9.

[32] Elshire, R., Glaubitz, J., Sun, Q., Poland, J., Kawamoto, K., Buckler, E., Mitchell, S., (2011). A robust, simple genotyping-by-sequencing (GBS) approach for high diversity species. *PloS One* 6, e19379.

[33] Bernardi, J., Mazza, R., Caruso, P., Recupero, G. R., Marocco, A., Licciardello, C., (2013). Use of an expressed sequence tag-based method for single nucleotide polymorphism identification and discrimination of Citrus species and cultivars. *Mol. Breed.* 31, 705-718.

[34] Forment, J., Gadea, J., Huerta, L., Abizanda, L., Agusti, J., Alamar, S., et al., (2005). Development of a citrus genome-wide EST collection and cDNA microarray as resources for genomic studies. *Plant Mol. Biol.* 57, 375–391.

[35] Terol, J., Conesa, A., Colmenero, J., Cercos, M., Tadeo, F., Agustí, J., et al., (2007). Analysis of 13000 unique Citrus clusters associated with fruit quality, production and salinity tolerance. *BMC Genomics* 8, 31.

[36] Reis, M. S., Takita, M. A., Palmieri, D. A., Machado, M. A., (2007). Bio-informatics for the Citrus EST project (CitEST). *Genet. Mol. Biol.* 3, 1024–1029.

[37] The Citrus EST Project (CitEST) (2007). Available at <http:// biotecnologia. centrodecitricultura.br/>. Accessed on January, 2014.

[38] Albrecht, U., Bowman, K., (2012). Transcriptional response of susceptible and tolerant citrus to infection with Candidatus Liberibacter asiaticus. *Plant Sci.*, 118–130.

[39] Bernardi, J., Licciardello, C., Russo, M., Chiusano, L., M., Carletti, G., Recupero, G., Marocco, A., (2010). Use of a custom array to study differentially expressed genes during blood orange (*Citrus sinensis* L. Osbeck) ripening. *J. Plant Physiol.* 167, 301–310.

[40] Licciardello, C., Russo, M. P., Vale', G., Recupero, R. G., (2008). Identification of differentially expressed genes in the flesh of blood and common oranges. *Tree Genet. Genomes* 4, 315-331.

[41] Marocco, A., Bortesi, A., Bertoli, A., Mazza, R., (2004). Gene transcription analysis during fruit ripening in sweet orange. *Proc. Int. Soc. Citriculture* 1, 188–191.

[42] Zhang, J.-Z., Ai, X.-Y., Sun, L.-M., Zhang, D.-L., Guo, W.-W., Deng, X.-X., Hu, C.-G., (2011). Molecular cloning and functional characterization of genes associated with flowering in citrus using an early-flowering trifoliate orange (*Poncirus trifoliata* L. Raf.) mutant. *Plant Mol. Biol.* 76, 187–204.[43] Reforgiato Recupero, G., Russo, G., (2009). Arancio, In: *Citrus: Trattato di Agrumicoltura,* eds. Edagricole, Milano: 95-101.

[44] Dixon, R. A., Palva, N. L., (1995). Stress-induced phenylpropanoid metabolism. *Plant Cell* 7, 1085-1097.

[45] Moriguchi, T., Kita, M., Tomono, Y., Endo-Inagaki, T., Omura, M., (1999). One type of chalcone synthase gene expressed during embryogenesis regulates the flavonoid accumulation in citrus cell cultures. *Plant Cell Physiol.* 40, 651-655.

[46] Reforgiato Recupero, G., Russo, M. P., Rapisarda, P., La Rosa, M., Guardo, M., Lo Piero, A. R., Petrone, G., (2000). Anthocyanin bio-synthesis in blood oranges. *Proc. Intl. Soc. Citricult.* 1, 681–682.

[47] Moriguchi, T., Kita, M., Tomono, Y., Endo-Inagaki, T., Omura, M., (2001). Gene expression in flavonoid biosynthesis: correlation with flavonoid accumulation in developing citrus fruit. *Physiol. Plant.* 111, 66-74.

[48] Lo Piero, A. R., Consoli, A., Puglisi, I., Orestano, G., Reforgiato Recupero, G., Petrone, G., (2005). Anthocyanin-less cultivars of sweet orange lack to express the UDP-glucose flavonoid 3-*O*-glucosyl transferase. *J. Plant Biochem. Biot.*. 14, 1-6.

[49] Cotroneo, P. S., Russo, M. P., Ciuni, M., Lo Piero, A. R., Reforgiato Recupero, G., (2006). Real time RT-PCR profiling of some of the anthocyanin biosynthetic genes during blood and common orange [*Citrus sinensis* (L.) Osbeck] fruit ripening). *J. Am. Soc. Hort. Sci.* 131, 537–543.

[50] Frova, C., (2003). The plant glutathione transferase gene family: genomic structure, functions, expression and evolution. *Physiol. Plant.* 119, 469–479.

[51] Lo Piero, A. R., Puglisi, I., Petrone, G., (2006). Gene isolation, analysis of expression and in vitro synthesis of glutathione s-transferase from orange fruit [*Citrus sinensis* L. (Osbeck)]. *J. Agric. Food Chem.* 54, 9227–9233.

[52] Licciardello, C., D'Agostino, N., Traini, A., Reforgiato Recupero, G., Frusciante, L., Chiusano, M. L. (2014). Characterization of the glutathione S-transferase gene family through ESTs and expression analyses within common and pigmented cultivars of *Citrus sinensis* (L.) Osbeck. *BMC Plant Biol.* 14:39.

[53] Licciardello, C., D'Agostino, N., Reforgiato Recupero, G., Chiusano, M. L. (2008). Evaluation of alternative splicing in the *Citrus sinensis* glutathione s transferase gene family. In: *Società Italiana Genetica Agraria Congress LII* (Padova-Italy). Oral Communication Abstract 1.06.

[54] Cultrone, A., Cotroneo, P. S., Reforgiato-Recupero, G., (2010). Cloning and molecular characterisation of R2R3-MYB and bHLHMYC transcription factors from Citrus sinensis. *Tree Genet. Genomes* 6, 101–112.

[55] Licciardello, C., D'Agostino, N., Russo, M. P., Reforgiato Recupero, G., Chiusano, M. L. (2007). Comparative analysis of expressed transcripts to investigate on tissue-specific genes. In: *Società Italiana Genetica Agraria Congress LI* (Riva del Garda-Italy). Poster Abstract D.80.

[56] Crifò, T., Petrone, G., Lo Cicero, L., Lo Piero, A. R., (2012). Short cold storage enhances the anthocyanin contents and level of transcripts related to their biosynthesis in blood oranges. *J. Agric. Food Chem.* 60, 476-481.

[57] Dooner, H. K., Robbins, T. P., Jorgensen, R. A., (1991). Genetic and developmental control of anthocyanin biosynthesis. *Annu. Rev. Genet.* 25, 173–199.

[58] Goodrich, J., Carpenter, R., Coen, E. S., (1992). A common gene regulates pigmentation pattern in diverse plant species. *Cell* 68, 955–964.

[59] Quattrocchio, F., Wing, J. F., Leppen, H. T. C., Mol, J. N. M., Koes, R. E., (1993). Regulatory genes controlling anthocyanin pigmentation are functionally conserved among plant species and have distinct sets of target genes. *Plant Cell* 5, 1497-1512.

[60] Procissi, A., Dolfini, S., Ronchi, A., Tonelli, C., (1997). Light-dependent spatial and temporal expression of pigment regulatory genes in developing maize seeds. *Plant Cell* 9, 1–12.

[61] Kobayashi, S., Goto-Yamamoto, N., Hirochika, H., (2004). Retrotransposon induced mutations in grape skin color. *Science* 304, 982.

[62] Schwinn, K., Venail, J., Shang, Y. J., Mackay, S., Alm, V., Butelli, E., Oyama, R., Bailey, P., Davies, K., Martin, C., (2006). A small family of MYB-regulatory genes controls floral pigmentation intensity and patterning in the genus Antirrhinum. *Plant Cell* 18, 831–851.

[63] Walker, A. R., Lee, E., Bogs, J., McDavid, D. A. J., Thomas, M. R., Robinson, S. P., (2007). White grapes arose through the mutation of two similar and adjacent regulatory genes. *Plant J.* 49, 772–785.

[64] Espley, R. V., Hellens, R. P., Putterill, J., Stevenson, D. E., Kutty-Amma, S., Allan, A. C., (2007). Red colouration in apple fruit is due to the activity of the MYB transcription factor, MdMYB10. *Plant J.* 49, 414–427.

[65] Takos, A. M., Jaffé, F. W., Jacob, S. R., Bogs, J., Robinson, S. P., Walker, A. R., (2006). Light-induced expression of a MYB gene regulates anthocyanin biosynthesis in red apples. *Plant Physiol.* 142, 1216–1232.

[66] Zhijian, T. L., Frederick, G., Grosser, J. W., Chen, C., Gray, D. J., (2011). Isolation and characterization of a novel anthocyanin-promoting MYBA gene family in Citrus. *Tree Genet. Genomes* 8, 675-685.

[67] Butelli, E., Licciardello, C., Zhang, Y., Liu, J., Mackay, S., Bailey, P., Reforgiato Recupero, G., Martin, C., (2012). Retrotransposons control fruit-specific, cold-dependent accumulation of anthocyanins in blood oranges. *Plant Cell* 24, 1242–1255.

[68] Licciardello, C., Butelli, E., Russo, M. P., Martin, C., Reforgiato Recupero, G. (2009). Isolation of genes controlling the anthocyanin bio-synthesis in *Citrus sinensis* L. Osbeck. In: *Società Italiana Genetica Agraria Congress LIII* (Torino-Italy). Poster Abstract 3.24.

[69] McClintock, B., (1984). The significance of responses of the genome to challenge. *Science* 226, 792–801.

[70] Feschotte, C., Jiang, N., Wessler, S. R., (2002). Plant transposable elements: where genetics meets genomics. *Nat. Rev. Genet.* 3, 329–341.

[71] Shapiro, J. A., (2005). Retrotransposons and regulatory suites. *Bioessays* 27, 122–125.

[72] Ishikawa, T., Dowdle, J., Smirnoff, N., (2006). Progress in manipulating ascorbic acid biosynthesis and accumulation in plants. *Physiol. Plantarum* 126, 343–355.

[73] Linster, C. L., Clarke, S. G., (2008). l-Ascorbate biosynthesis in higher plants: the role of VTC2. *Trends Plant Sci.* 13, 567–573.

[74] Bulley, S. M., Rassam, M., Hoser, D., Otto, W., Schunemann, N., Wright, M., MacRae, E., Gleave, A., Laing, W., (2009). Gene expre-ssion studies in kiwifruit and gene over-expression in Arabidopsis indicates that GDP-l-galactose guanyltransferase is a major control point of vitamin C biosynthesis. *J. Exp. Bot.* 60, 765–778.

[75] Li, M. J., Ma, F. W., Zhang, M., Pu, F., (2008). Distribution and meta-bolism of ascorbic acid in apple fruits (*Malus domestica* Borkh cv. Gala). *Plant Sci.* 174, 606–612.

[76] Imai, T., Ban, Y., Terakami, S., Yamamoto, T., Moriguchi, T., (2009). l-Ascorbate biosynthesis in peach: cloning of six l-galactose pathway-related genes and their expression during peach fruit development. *Physiol. Plantarum* 136, 139–149.

[77] Alhagdow, M., Mounet, F., Gilbert, L., Nunes-Nesi, A., Garcia, V., Just, D., et al., (2007). Silencing of the mitochondrial ascorbate synthesizing enzyme l-galactono-1,4-lactone dehydrogenase affects plant and fruit development in tomato. *Plant Physiol.* 145, 1408–1422.

[78] Ioannidi, E., Kalamaki, M. S., Engineer, C., Pateraki, I., Alexandrou, D., Mellidou, I., Giovannonni, J., Kanellis, A. K., (2009). Expression profiling of ascorbic acid-related genes during tomato fruit development and ripening and in response to stress conditions. *J. Exp. Bot.* 60, 663–678.

[79] Do Nascimento, J. R. O., Higuchi, B. K., Gomez, M., Oshiro, R. A., Lajolo, F. M., (2005). l-Ascorbate biosynthesis in strawberries: l-galac-tono-1,4-lactone dehydrogenase expression during fruit development and ripening. *Postharvest Biol. Technol.* 38, 34–42.

[80] Yang, X.-Y., Xie, J.-X., Wang, F.-F., Zhong, J., Liu, Y.-Z., Li, G.-H., Peng, S.-A., (2011). Comparison of ascorbate metabolism in fruits of two citrus species with obvious difference in ascorbate content in pulp. *J. Plant Physiol.* 168, 2196–2205.

[81] Gilbert, L., Alhagdow, M., Nunes-Nesi, A., Quemener, B., Guillon, F., Bouchet, B., et al., (2009). GDP-dmannose 3,5-epimerase (GME) plays a key role at the intersection of ascorbate and non-cellulosic cell-wall biosynthesis in tomato. *Plant J.* 60, 499–508.

[82] Dowdle, J., Ishikawa, T., Gatzek, S., Rolinski, S., Smirnoff, N., (2007). Two genes in Arabidopsis thaliana encoding GDP-l-galactose phosphorylase are required for ascorbate biosynthesis and seedling viability. *Plant J.* 52, 673–689.

[83] Laing, W. A., Wright, M. A., Cooney, J., Bulley, S. M., (2007). The missing step of the l-galactose pathway of ascorbate biosynthesis in plants, an l-galactose guanyltransferase, increases leaf ascorbate content. *Proc. Natl. Acad. Sci. US* 104, 9534–9539.

[84] Gatzek, S., Wheeler, G. L., Smirnoff, N., (2002). Antisense suppression of l-galactose dehydrogenase in Arabidopsis thaliana provides evidence for its role in ascorbate synthesis and reveals light modulated l-galactose synthesis. *Plant J.* 30, 541–553.

[85] Wheeler, G. L., Jones, M. A., Smirnoff, N., (1998). The biosynthetic pathway of vitamin C in higher plants. *Nature* 393, 365–369.

[86] Nishikawa, F., Kato, M., Hyodo, H., Ikoma, Y., Sugiura, M., Yano, M., (2005). Effect of sucrose on ascorbate level and expression of genes involved in the ascorbate biosynthesis and recycling pathway in harvested broccoli florets. *J. Exp. Bot.* 56, 65–72.

[87] Massot, C., Génard, M., Stevens, R., Gautier, H., (2010). Fluctuations in sugar content are not determinant in explaining variations in vitamin C in tomato fruit. *Plant Physiol. Biochem.* 48, 751–757.

[88] Agius, F., González-Lamothe, R., Caballero, J. L., Muñoz-Blanco, J., Botella, M. A., Valpuesta, V., (2003). Engineering increased vitamin C levels in plants by overexpression of a D-galacturonic acid reductase. *Nat. Biotechnol.* 21, 177–181.

[89] Roose, M. L., Close, T. J., (2008). Genomics of Citrus, a major fruit crop of tropical and subtropical regions. In: *Genomics of Tropical Crop Plants,* P. H. Moore and R. Ming, eds. (Springer), pp. 187-200.

[90] Xu, X., Deng, Z., Zheng, Q., Chen, C., Gmitter, F., (2009). Developing specific markers and improving genetic mapping for a major locus Tyr1 of citrus nematode resistance. *Mol. Plant Breed.* 7, 497-504.

[91] Kepiro, J. L., Roose, M. L., (2010). AFLP markers closely linked to a major gene essential for nucellar embryony (apomixis) in Citrus maxima × Poncirus trifoliata. *Tree Genet. Genomes* 6, 1-11.

[92] Gulsen, O., Uzun, A., Seday, U., Kafa, G., (2011). QTL analysis and regression model for estimating fruit setting in young Citrus trees based on molecular markers. *Sci. Hortic.* 130, 418-424.

[93] Sahin-Cevik, M., Moore, G. A., (2012). Quantitative trait loci analysis of morphological traits in Citrus. *Plant Biotechnol. Rep.* 6, 47-57.

In: Citrus
Editor: Khizar Hayat

ISBN: 978-1-63117-985-3

Chapter 3

CITRUS FLAVONOIDS: THEIR BIOSYNTHESIS, FUNCTIONS AND GENETIC IMPROVEMENT

Sabaz Ali Khan**, Rafiq Ahmad, Saeed Ahmad Asad and Muhammad Shahzad
Department of Environmental Sciences, COMSATS University, Abbottabad, Pakistan

ABSTRACT

Citrus is the genus of the *Rutaceae* family and is one of the world's most important fruit crops. The common citrus fruits are mandarin, pummelo, sweet orange, sour orange, lime, citron, lemon, and grapefruit. Citrus fruits are eaten as fresh, processed into juices and are also added to different dishes and beverages. These are rich in certain phytonutrients called as phytochemicals that are vital in both health promotion and disease prevention.

Among these phytochemicals, flavonoids are abundantly found in citrus. Flavonoids can exercise their antioxidant activity in several ways, e.g. as antiradical, as anti-lipoperoxidaters and as metal chelaters. There are several enzymes involved in flavonoids biosynthesis.

Flavanone-3-hydroxylase is a key enzyme acting at the flavanone branch point and synthesizes dihydrokaempferol and dihydroquercetin. Flavonol synthase, is a 2-oxoglutarate-dependent dioxygenase and catalyzes the conversion of natural dihydroflavonols, i.e., dihydrokaempferol, to the corresponding flavonols. Dihydroflavonol 4-reductase is a pivotal enzyme of the flavonoid biosynthesis and reduced dihydroflavonols. Dihydroflavonols are the direct precursors for the formation of leucoanthocyanidins and anthocyanins. The leucoanthocyanidin oxygenase enzyme also known as leucoanthocyanidin dioxygenase and anthocyanidin synthase is an oxoglutarate-dependent oxygenase and catalyses the conversion of leucoanthocyanidin to anthocyanidin, an essential step in the formation of colored metabolites in anthocyanins biosynthesis.

---

* Corresponding author: Sabaz Ali Khan. Department of Environmental Sciences, COMSATS University, 22060 Abbottabad, Pakistan. E-mail: sabzktk@yahoo.com; sabaz@ciit.net.pk.

On the genetic level, several putative glucosyltransferase clones have been obtained from citrus. Glucosyltransferases (GTs) are involved in the flavonone biosynthesis, which is the major group of flavonoids found in citrus. So far, seven different GTs have been analyzed in citrus through various techniques, such as designing degenerate primers against the signature PSPG box, analyzing candidate sequences and walking out to obtain full-length clones and mining expressed sequence tags. The results clearly indicate that the putative GTs were not constitutively expressed and there were varying degrees of GTs expression among different tissues and stages of development.

Keywords: Citrus flavonoids, Flavonone, Antioxidant activity, Human diseases, Biosynthesis of flavonoids, Genetic improvement

INTRODUCTION

Citrus is the genus of flowering plants of the *Rutaceae* family and is an important fruit crop with a total world production of 11.65 million metric tons [1]. China, Nigeria and Colombia are the major citrus producers with a 56.1 % combined production of the world (Figure 1). The common citrus fruits are mandarin, pummelo, sweet orange, sour orange, lime, citron, lemon, and grapefruit. Citrus fruits are eaten as fresh, processed into juices and are also added to different dishes and beverages [2]. The literature record of citrus domestication and cultivation history dates back to 2100 BC [3, 4].

It is considered to have originated from the Malay Archipelago and Southeast Asia, occurring from Northern India to China and in the South through Malaysia, the East Indies and the Philippines [2]. Citrus are diploids having nine pairs of chromosomes (2n = 2x = 18), although polyploids have also been reported, and are vegetatively propagated.

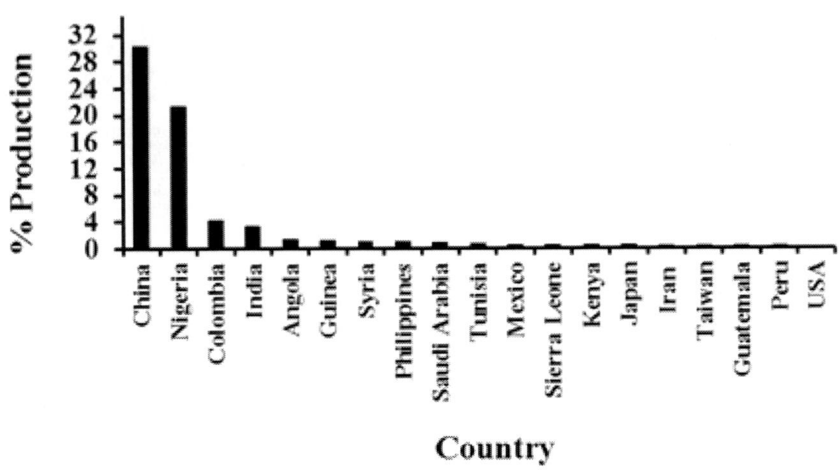

Figure 1. Production (%) of citrus fruits in the leading citrus growing countries (FAOSTAT, 2011).

Citrus fruits are well known for their fragrance and this is partly because of flavonoids and limonoids in their peels [5]. These are rich in certain phyto-nutrients called as phytochemicals that are vital in both health promotion and disease prevention [6]. Citrus contains a number of antioxidants such as beta-carotene, ascorbic acid, terpenoids, alkaloids, beta-sitosterol, carotene, flavonoids, flavone glycosides, and rutin [7].

Epidemiological studies have shown an inverse relationship between dietary flavonoids intake and cardiovascular diseases [8]. It is found that the possible beneficial effects are due, not only to the high amounts of vitamins and minerals, but also due to the antioxidant properties of flavonoids [8].

Citrus breeding is very slow as well as difficult by conventional methods, because of an extended juvenile period, large tree size, polyembryony, high heterozygosity and self-incompatibility.

Many citrus species are outcrossing and it can take 10 years or even longer for a citrus plant to give fruits since its first cross [9, 10].

Further, the most important commercial types, sweet orange and grapefruit, are not true species, but rather complex hybrids which cannot be easily reconstituted [9, 10].

Citrus genome size is, however, relatively small with a C value estimated as 0.6 picogram per haploid DNA content [11], equivalent to approximately 367 Mb, which is about three times the size of the *Arabidopsis* genome (see the International Citrus Genome/Genomics Consortium home page, ICGC).

Thus, alternative methods of plant improvement such as the use of genetic transformation to improve existing varieties of citrus are very attractive to those concerned with citrus improvement. Gene cloning and genetic transformation allows the significant characteristics associated with important citrus types to be maintained, while adding one or a few new favorable traits [12, 13]. Additionally, it may be possible to suppress unfavorable traits using these techniques [14]. The citrus fruit palatability and health value can be improved by manipulating the flavonoid biosynthetic pathway, leading to altered levels and/or types of flavonoids that may be more health beneficial.

The Different Types of Citrus Flavonoids

Many studies are carried out on the thousands of phytochemicals that may have important physiological effects. Phytochemicals can be defined as substances found in edible fruits and vegetables that may exhibit a potential for modulating the human metabolism in a manner favorable for the prevention of chronic and degenerative diseases. An increased consumption of fruit and vegetables may protect against degenerative pathologies, such as cancer and atherosclerosis [8, 15].

Citrus fruits are the principal source of such important nutrients and they contain vitamin C, folate, dietary fiber and flavonoids, which are suggested to be responsible for the prevention of cancer and degenerative diseases [16].

The class of flavonoids comprises of at least 6000 molecules, divided into subgroups: flavanones, flavones, flavonols, leucoanthocyanidins, anthocyanins and isoflavonoids. These are abundant in flowers, fruits and leaves and have a diverse set of functions [17].

Citrus fruits are a rich source of flavanones, which is one of the flavonoid groups, and are naturally synthesized in the fruit and involved in the prevention of many human diseases [18, 19]. Some of them are tasteless, others are responsible for the bitterness of some citrus species [20, 21], and are present in the glycoside or aglycone forms. Among the aglycone forms, narin-genin and hesperetin are the most important flavanones, while among the glycoside forms, two types are classified: neohesperidosides and rutinosides [22, 23]. Neohesperidosides flavanones (naringin, neohesperidin and neoeriocitrin) consist of a flavanone with neohesperidose (rhamnosyl-a-1, 2 glucose) and they have a bitter taste, while rutinosides flavanones (hesperidin, narirutin and didymin) have a flavanone and a disaccharide residue e.g. rutinose (ramnosyl-a-1, 6 glucose) and they are tasteless.

Flavanones are usually present in diglycoside form, conferring the typical taste to the citrus fruits [23].

Only little difference in the glycosylated flavonoids amounts was found in lemon juice extracted from several cultivars [24]. Eriocitrin, 6, 8-di-C-β-glycosyldiosmin and 6-C-β-glycosyldiosmin are particularly abundant in lemon and lime, while they are almost absent in other citrus fruits.

Flavones is another important group and can be found in all parts of the plants, above and below ground level, in vegetative and generative organs [25]. Flavones are especially isolated from essential oil of citrus fruits (in the flavedo) and are also identified in juice [26]. The main flavones in citrus are diosmin, apigenin, luteolin, diosmetin, and tangeretin.

Flavonols are also an important class of flavonoids and they exhibit anti-inflammatory and antitumoral properties, free radical scavenging, alteration of the mitotic cycle in tumor cells, gene expression modification, and anti-angiogenesis activities [27]. Quercetin, Quercetin-3-glucoside, quercetin-galactoside, quercetin-xyloside, quercetin-rhamnoside, quercetin-arabinoside, and rutin are the important flavonols.

The leucoanthocyanidins are the precursors for catechins and proantho-cyanidins, which are involved in food and feed quality of plant products [28]. They are also direct precursors of one of the most conspicuous flavonoid class, the anthocyanins [29], which has a wide range of functions.

Isoflavonoids are structurally distinct from other flavonoid classes in that they contain a C15 skeleton based on 1, 2-diphenylpropane. The biological activities of isoflavonoids are quite diverse, including antimicrobial, estrogenic and insecticidal features [30].

Anthocyanins group constitutes the coloring compounds of flowers and fruits, but sometimes also of leaves, buds and roots [31].

They are mainly in the epicarp, but they also color the mesocarp of oranges and perform various functions such as attraction of pollinators and seed dispersers, UV light damage protection, plant defense against pathogen attack, and are strong antioxidants. The anthocyanin content is strongly dependent on the level of maturation.

Catechins, leucoanthocyanin and proanthocyanins are not citrus fruit specific compounds because they are also found in other fruits and vegetables, while other flavonoids are only found in citrus. Flavonoids types and amount greatly varies among different plant species and even within species. For example, in grapefruit, which is considered a fairly homogeneous citrus group, the major types of flavonoids differ between different varieties and selections [32-34].

DISTRIBUTION AND ACCUMULATION OF FLAVONOIDS IN CITRUS

Flavonoids are present in dietary fruits and vegetables [23]. The 7-O-glycosylflavanones are the most abundant flavonoids in all citrus fruits [35]. The citrus peels are richer in flavonoids than are the seeds e.g., glycosidic flavonoids are widely found in peel [36]. The lemon seed mainly contains eriocitrin and hesperidin, while the peel is rich in neoeriocitrin, naringin and neohesperidin. Moreover, the glycosylated flavanone concentrations are different; neoeriocitrin and naringin have similar concentrations in peel while, in seed, eriocitrin is 40 times more abundant than naringin [37]. Bitter orange is a very rich source of neohesperidin and naringin and these compounds can be used in the production of sweeteners. Since a citrus fruit is peeled, peel and seeds are not used. It is necessary to consider these by-products as natural antioxidants in foods [38]. For example, the peels of pummelo contribute 30% of the fruit weight and yet it has been dumped without recognizing the possible nutritional value of the peels. Recently, a spectrophotometric analysis performed to evaluate the flavonoid activity of pummelo peels on the fish tissues showed a reduction in peroxide value indicating the inhibition of lipid peroxidation [39].

Among the neohesperidoside flavanones, naringin, neohesperidin and neoeriocitrin, are mainly present in bergamot, grapefruit and bitter orange juices. Among rutinoside flavanones, hesperidin, narirutin and didymin, are present in bergamot, orange, mandarin and lemon juices [40]. Flavanone chemical structures are specific for every species, which renders them as markers of adulteration in commercial juices [41, 42]. Amounts of flavanon glycosides differ in citrus, e.g., lemon is rich in eriocitrin and hesperidin while the other citrus fruits have smaller amounts of glycosylated naringin [37, 36]. Flavanone glycosyl compositions of peels and seeds are quite different than those of juices. Naringin has been found in lemon peel and seed and in mandarin seed, but it is not present in the juices of these fruits [42]. Naringin is never present in sweet orange juice, but only in bitter orange, and its presence is therefore used to detect adulteration [41]. Flavones and flavonols have also been found in citrus, but in low concentrations, and are studied to evaluate their antioxidant ability. For example, two C-glucosylflavones i.e. 6, 8-di-C-β-glycosyldiosmin and 6-C-β-glycosyldiosmin have been isolated from the peel of lemon fruit [24].

Citrus species accumulate comparatively large quantities of flavanone glycosides in their leaves and fruits as compared to other tissues [37].

In bitter citrus, naringin is found as most abundant component among the major flavonoids, with rhoifolin also present in relatively large amounts. Of the total 23.36 ± 11.39 mg/g dry weight flavonoids, naringin was 11.342 ± 6.90 mg/g dry weight [37]. In addition to naringin and rhoifolin, narirutin, neohesperidin, isorhoifolin, naringin-6-malonate conjugate, neodiosmin and poncerin were also quantitated. Bocco et al. demonstrated that naringin and rhoifolin were around 70% and narirutin and isorhoifolin was about 15% of the total flavonoids found in bitter citrus [37].

Researchers found that the levels of flavonoids were higher in the flavedo, the peels, than in the juices [43] and therefore more investigations are needed on these materials that are commonly considered as wastes.

Some citrus species, such as sweet orange and mandarin, contain only rutinosides, while others, such as pummelo has only flavanone neohesperidosides [44]. There are a number of citrus hybrids, such as grapefruit and sour orange that contain both bitter neohesperidosides and tasteless rutinosides. Although in most plants secondary metabolites, including flavonoids, tend to accumulate primarily in mature tissues and organs [45, 46], in citrus the largest amounts of flavonoids are produced in young, actively growing tissues [47]. Synthesis of the flavanone glycosides in citrus is highly regulated. They are primarily synthesized in rapidly growing young leaves and fruits, where they may comprise large percentages of the fresh and dry weights of the organs [32, 47, 48]. For example, the bitter tasting neohesperidoside naringin can constitutes up to 70% of the dry weight of a young grapefruit [49]. During cell elongation and subsequent maturation of leaves and fruit, flavonoids production slows down or stops; consequently, flavonoid concentrations are lower in these organs as a result of dilution effects. Even though the largest quantities of naringin are present in juvenile grapefruit tissues, the mature, edible fruit and juice of this citrus type still contain relatively large amounts of naringin [18, 20, 33].

Health Beneficial Effects of Citrus Flavonoids

Flavonoids are secondary metabolites in plants that influence growth, development and responses to environmental stresses and thus are biologically and agriculturally important [45, 46]. They may protect plants exposed to biotic or abiotic stresses such as infections, wounding, UV irradiation, ozone, pollutants and other hostile environmental conditions due to their antioxidant and free radical scavenging properties [50]. Some other flavonoids are currently used as drugs or dietary supplements to cure or prevent various diseases and in particular some of these compounds seem to be efficient in preventing and inhibiting various types of cancers and inflammatory and thrombogenic diseases [51-53]. These same characteristics have more recently made flavonoids of interest to scientists, medical personnel and consumers for the potential medicinal benefits derived from their consumption [45, 50].

Flavonoid constituents in citrus profoundly affect fruit and juice taste [49, 54, 55], and also the human health. For example, naringin, as well as other citrus flavonoids, are of great interest to those in the food and pharmaceutical industries because of their demonstrated antioxidant, anti-inflammatory, antiulcer and cholesterol-lowering effects, as well as their possible beneficial effects on several chronic conditions [45].

Flavonoids are powerful antioxidants against free radicals, because they act as "radical-scavengers". This activity is attributed to their hydrogen-donating ability. The phenolic groups of flavonoids serve as a source of a readily available "H" atoms such that the subsequent radicals produced can be delocalized over the flavonoid structure [56]. The chemical nature of flavonoids depends on structural class, degree of hydroxylation, other substitutions and conjugations and the degree of polymerization [57].

Three parameters are tested to report whether a flavonoid is antioxidant or not? These are: (a) the rate constant (k) with different types of radicals, (b) decay kinetics and stability of the aroxyl radical, and (c) the stoichiometry of the radical-scavenging reaction.

According to kinetic studies of aroxyl radical formation and decomposition reactions, the antioxidant capacity of a flavonoid is linked to its particular chemical structure. Three structural groups are important for the evaluation of their antioxidant capacity [58]: (A) the orthodihydroxy (catechol) structure in the B-ring, which confers greater stability to aroxyl radicals, possibly through hydrogen bonding, and which participates in electron dislocation

(B) the 2, 3-double bond, in conjugation with a 4-oxo function, responsible for electron dislocation from the B-ring and (C) the presence of both 3-(a)-and 5-(b)-hydroxyl groups.

Obviously, the flavonoid antioxidant capacity is linked to a combination of these chemicals and structural elements [56].

The antiradical activity of several citrus flavonoids, in comparison with the superoxide anion, has been studied using many methods and with different structural correlations [59].

This activity is influenced by the flavonoids concentration in the reaction environment, increasing from zero to the maximum, or determining the auto-oxidation of the flavonoids itself. The common structural element is the configuration of the C-ring with the 3-hydroxyl group that activates the double bond at position 2 and 3. When the concentration of the antioxidant is below 100 μM, the presence of the hydroxyl groups in the B-ring is important for the antiradical activity. Kaempferol, for example, has no activity against the superoxide ion at 10 μM, but only has in the range 60–100 μM. The absence of the hydroxyl group at position 3 in flavanones and flavones decreases their antioxidant ability [60]. The double bond at position 2, 3 makes the structure more reactive, for this reason, apigenin is a moderate antioxidant compound, while naringenin has no activity against the superoxide ion. Moreover, it has been reported that the corresponding 3-O-glucosides are more active than being their aglycones [61].

In a recent study, flavonoids (flavanols, flavanones and flavonols) were isolated from citrus mandarin and citrus mandarin pomace and were tested for their antioxidant activity [62, 63]. Other authors have determined the anti-oxidant capacity of the polyphenols, anthocyanins, hydroxycinnamic acids and ascorbic acid contained in juices of some varieties of pigmented oranges (Moro, Sanguinella, Tarocco and Washington) [64]. All examined orange juices showed an antioxidant capacity due to total phenol amounts and their ability to interact with the bio-membrane. The phenolic compositions, the ascorbic acid contents and the antioxidant activities of fresh Sicilian orange juices from pigmented (Moro, Tarocco and Sanguinella) and non-pigmented (Oval, Valencia and Navel) varieties of orange have been analyzed [65]. The antioxidative activities of flavonoids in lemon fruit have been studied using linoleic acid autoxidation, the liposome oxidation system, and the low-density lipoprotein (LDL) oxidation system [24]. Citrus flavonoids have an anti-oxidant action in a hydrophilic environment while, in a lipophilic environment, some molecules (neohesperidin, hesperetin, didymin and isosakuranetin) show a reduced antioxidant capacity, and others (naringin, narirutin, naringenin, neoeriocitrin, heridictyol) invert their behaviour, becoming prooxidants [66].

The protective role of flavonoids in living systems is mostly due to their antioxidant potential, which is related to transfer of reactive oxygen species (ROS), chelation of metal catalysts, activation of antioxidant enzymes and inhibition of certain types of oxidases and colon cancer [67].

The above considerations reflected the existence of clear scientific evidence that certain flavonoids possess antioxidant properties with synergistic and protective effects on vitamin C.

Flavonoids also have the potential to stimulate the immune system, induce protective enzymes in the liver or block damage to genetic material. At present, there is overwhelming evidence to indicate that free radicals cause oxidative damage to lipids, proteins, and nucleic acids. Free radicals may lie at the heart of the etiology or natural history of a number of diseases, including cancer and atherosclerosis [68]. Therefore, antioxidants, which can neutralize free radicals become the central importance in the prevention of these diseases.

Meanwhile, flavonoids can protect humans against cardiovascular diseases by reducing the oxidation of low-density lipoprotein [44]. Plant flavonoids may also reduce the risk of thrombosis by inhibiting platelet aggregation and adhesion. Although, flavonoids inhibit platelet aggregation by mediating in other enzyme systems, their direct antioxidant properties also participate in their antithrombotic action [68].

THE FLAVONOIDS BIOSYNTHESIS AND RELATED ENZYMES IN CITRUS

The flavonoid biosynthetic pathway in citrus is similar to those of other plant species [35]. Flavanones are the flavonoids that accumulate most abundantly in citrus species, which is unusual in other plants [49, 54, 55].

These are important for citrus taste in the glycosylated form, in which a disaccharide is attached to the aglycone through the C-7 hydroxyl group.

Several enzymes are involved in the biosynthesis of flavonoids in citrus plants, these are Phenylalanine ammonialyase (PAL), Cinnamate 4-hydroxyla-se (C4H), 4-coumarate:CoA ligase (4CL), Chalcone synthase (CHS), Chalcone isomerase (CHI), Flavone synthase I, II (FNSI, FNSII), Flavanone-3-hydro-xylase (F3H), Flavonol synthase (FLS), Dihydroflavonol 4-reductase (DFR), Leucoanthocyanidin oxygenase enzyme (LDOX), Isoflavone synthase (IFS) and Isoflavone reductase (IFR) (Table 1). Phenylalanine ammonialyase is a key enzyme in the phenylpropanoid pathway [39] and is responsible for the non-oxidative deamination of the amino acid L-Phenylalanine forming trans-cinammate and ammonium ion.

PAL has been extensively studied because of its importance in plant stress responses, tissue wounding, protection against UV radiation, low temperature, levels of nitrogen, phosphate and iron [69], pathogenic attack and ethylene response [70]. C4H is an oxireductase enzyme that synthesizes the second step of phenylpropanoid pathway by the incorporation of one atom of oxygen to a transcinnamate molecule in the presence of NADPH, H^+, O_2 and a heme group as a cofactor, generating one molecule of 4-hydroxycinnamate, NADP and H_2O. 4CL converts 4-coumarate (or *p*-coumaric acid) to 4-coumaroyl-CoA in the presence of ATP. Enzymatic assays utilizing *Arabidopsis thaliana* proteins determined that 4CL enzyme might also use cinnamic, caffeic, ferulic, 5-hydroxyferulic and sinapic acids as substrate, converting them to their corresponding CoA thiol esters [71]. Chalcone synthase is an acyltransferase enzyme that catalyses the condensation of 4-coumaroyl-CoA to the first flavonoid naringenin chalcone, in the presence of three molecules of malonyl-CoA. Higher plants evolved two completely independent enzyme systems to catalyze flavone synthesis using the same substrates. Both enzymes never occur side by side in the same organism: only in *Apiaceae* family, soluble 2-oxoglutarate and Fe^{2+} dependent dioxygenase, flavone synthase I (FNS I) is present. Flavanone-3-hydroxylase (F3H), is a key enzyme acting at the flavanone branch point and is the first in the flavonol pathway, converting the flavanones (2S)-naringenin and (2S)-eriodictyol to (2R,3R)-dihydrokaempferol and (2R,3R)-dihydroquercetin, respectively [72].

Table 1. Enzymes involved in the biosynthesis of citrus flavonoids

Enzyme	Function/Pathway	References
Phenylalanine ammonialyase (PAL)	Phenylpropanoid pathway	[76]
Cinnamate 4-hydroxylase (C4H)	Phenylpropanoid pathway	[77]
4-coumarate:CoA ligase (4Cl)	Converts 4-coumarate to 4-coumaroyl-CoA	[78]
Chalcone synthase (CHS)	Catalyses the condensation of 4-coumaroyl-CoA to the first flavonoid naringenin chalcone	[79]
Chalcone isomerase (CHI)	Flavanone biosynthesis	[80]
Flavone synthase I, II (FNSI, FNSII)	Flavones synthesis	[81]
Flavanone-3-hydroxylase (F3H)	Flavonol pathway	[82]
Flavonol synthase (FLS)	Flavonol pathway	[83]
Dihydroflavonol 4-reductase (DFR)	Flavonoid biosynthesis	[84]
Leucoanthocyanidin oxygenase enzyme (LDOX)	Anthocyanin biosynthesis	[85]
Isoflavone synthase (IFS) and Isoflavone reductase (IFR)	Isoflavone pathway	[86]

Flavonol synthase, one of the main enzymes of the flavonol biosynthesis, is a 2-oxoglutarate-dependent dioxygenase and catalyzes the conversion of natural (2R,3R)-dihydroflavonols, i.e., dihydrokaempferol, to the corresponding flavonols [73]. Dihydroflavonol 4-reductase is a pivotal enzyme of the flavonoid biosynthesis and belongs to the short chain dehydrogenase/reductase or DFR superfamily [74]. Dihydroflavonols are the direct precursors for the flavonols branching and for the formation of flavan 3, 4-diols (leucoanthocya-nidins) and anthocyanin production. Reduction of dihydroflavonols at position 4, catalyzed by DFR, leads to flavan-2, 3 trans-3,4-cis diols (leucopelargonidin) intermediates in anthocyanidin formation [75]. The leucoanthocyanidin oxygenase enzyme (LDOX) also known as leucoanthocyanidin dioxygenase and anthocyanidin synthase is an oxoglutarate-dependent oxygenase and catalyzes the conversion of leucoanthocyanidin to anthocyanidin, an essential step in the formation of colored metabolites in anthocyanin biosynthesis.

Isoflavone synthase is the first enzyme in the isoflavone pathway and converts flavanone substrates into isoflavone products.

Genetic Improvement of Citrus Flavonoids

In citrus, producing bitter flavonone-7-neohesperidosides, the compounds, the genes and enzymes that are responsible for their production are most extensively produced in young, rapidly growing tissues, including seedlings, young flushes of mature trees, flowers and young fruits [21, 32, 47, 48].

These compounds are still found in mature tissues of leaves and fruits, but in smaller amounts per tissue volume because of dilution as the organs grow. Naringin, one of the flavanone neohesperidosides, is by far the most abundant compound in grapefruit [54]. Although some 'tartness' is a desirable specific character of grapefruit taste, excessive bitterness decreases grapefruit consumption and its commercial value [51, 52].

Thus, to increase consumer consumption, it might be advantageous to produce grapefruit plants or it products with decreased bitter flavanone levels. For this purpose, juice debittering processes exist, but they may also remove non-bitter flavonoids and other important compounds such as vitamin C [87].

In citrus, glucosyltransferases (GTs) catalyze the transfer of sugars from high energy sugar donors to other substrates. Several different secondary product GTs exist in the tissues of grapefruit, making it a model plant for studying their structure and function.

Expression patterns of seven putative secondary product GTs were studied during grapefruit growth and development by quantifying mRNA expression levels in the roots, stems, leaves, flowers, and mature fruit to establish whether the genes are expressed constitutively or if one or more could be expressed in a tissue specific manner and/or developmentally regulated [88]. Six growth stages were defined from which RNA was extracted, and expression levels were quantified by standardized densitometry of gene-specific RT-PCR products. Results showed that there were varying degrees of putative glucosyl-transferase (PGT) expression in different tissues and at different development-tal stages. These results have advanced the knowledge of dynamics of expre-ssion and potential regulation of secondary metabolism in citrus [88].

There are two sugars transferring enzymes involved in the synthesis of naringin from naringenin, a flavanone-specific 7-O glucosyltransferase (GT) that "captures" the naringenin and adds a glucose [89], and a rhamnosyl-transferase enzyme that attaches a rhamnose to the glucose [21, 90].

Also limonoid UDP-glucosyltransferase has been reported to catalyze the conversion of limonoid aglycones to limonoid 17-O-glucosides [91]. A limo-noid glucosyltransferase isolated and purified from the albedo tissue of citrus was found to glucosylatelimonoate A-ring monolactone (non-bitter) to produce limonoate A-ring monolactone 17-O-glucoside. Glucosylation of limonoate A-ring monolactone prevents lactonization and thus prevents formation of limonin. While limonin, limonoate A-ring monolactone, and limonoate 17-O-glucoside are present in fruit tissues and juices [92], relative levels of these different compounds vary in different citrus species. Thus, the issue of delayed bitterness in juice (conversion of the non-bitter limonoate A-ring monolactone to the bitter limonin via acid-mediated ring closure) differs by species [93]. Attempts have been made towards understanding the regulation of secondary metabolism in grapefruit with special emphasis on secondary product GTs as well as elucidating grapefruit GT clone structure and function.

Identifying tissue and developmental expression patterns for each putative glucosyltransferase (PGT) gene is an important aspect for improving our understanding of secondary metabolism in citrus [88].

Several putative secondary product glucosyltransferase (PGT) clones have been obtained from citrus young leaf tissue by a variety of approaches. These include designing degenerate primers against the signature PSPG box, analyzing candidate sequences and walking out to obtain full-length clones [94], expressed sequence tag (EST) mining of a directionally-cloned grapefruit leaf cDNA library [95], searching the limited citrus sequence data for PSPG box signature sequences and designing primers to search for similar clones in grapefruit [96], and other bioinformatic approaches. These PGT clones were assigned as PGT 1–4, PGT 5/6, and PGT 7–8 in order of their discovery. PGT 1 was previously characterized as not being a flavonoid GT [95], while, functional characterization of PGT 2 and 3 is ongoing. Evidence suggests that PGT 4 does not use a flavonoid as a glucose acceptor and PGT 5/6 is so named because while contigs obtained through gene-walking they have greater than 90% homology.

PGT 7 has been shown to be a flavonol 3-O-GT through bio-chemical analysis [96]. PGT 8 has 98% homology to a clone from *Citrus unshiu*, protein expressed from this clone was shown to have lim-GT activity. PGT8 also has 100% homology to a Marsh grapefruit clone annotated to be a lim-GT, although biochemical analyses were not performed (unpublished data).

The results clearly indicate that the putative GTs were not constitutively expressed and that there were varying degrees of PGT expression between different tissues and stages of the development. While levels of bitter naringin and limonin in different grapefruit tissues have been well-studied [32, 47], the levels of flavonol-3-O-glycosides are not as well-studied. Still, it is possible that flavonol-3-glycoside synthesis in grapefruit roots may have a role in interaction with other organisms as has been observed for other plants [97].

These results suggest that PGT 3 and PGT 4 play a significant role in secondary metabolism in grapefruit roots.

Expression of PGT 2–7 was also variable in stem tissue at various stages of development. It is readily apparent that the flavonol-specific 3-O-GT (PGT 7) gene was expressed at the highest levels in all stems with its highest level of expression (130%). There was a general trend of increasing PGT expression as the stems developed and entered a growth phase and then decreased as stems became increasingly lignified; this suggests a change in secondary metabolic activity during this process.

As the young seedling develops and grows, the stem is exposed to more sunlight suggesting that UV protection of the tissues may be an important consideration. It should be noted that naringin and limonin concentrations decrease with maturity of tissues and may indicate a general trend for metabolism of some secondary products in citrus [47].

Grapefruit leaves have been shown to be metabolically very active and to synthesize high levels of naringin and limonin [47, 92]. This suggests that secondary metabolism in general may be more active in young leaf tissue.

Although a comprehensive study of secondary metabolites in developing leaf tissues has not been conducted to date, some groups have reported composition of metabolites in leaves and other tissues [55, 32].

It is clear from the results that PGT 2–7 are not constitutively expressed and each shows its own dynamic expression in the youngest leaves at different developmental stages. The flavonol-specific 3-O-GT continues to be expressed in young leaves from all stages, PGT 2, however, is expressed more strongly in the youngest leaves from stage 5 plants (120%), PGT 4 expression is greatest in the first true leaves produced by seedlings (57%), and PGT 3 expression occurs throughout with higher levels of gene expression of 96% in the youngest leaves.

In contrast, expression in older, mature leaves showed a different pattern with a general trend of lower PGT expression except for significant expression of the PGT 3 gene in older cotyledons. Although the specific metabolic functions of all these PGTs are not yet known, previous studies have shown that grapefruit leaves are not as metabolically active as they grow older and tend to accumulate a waxy coating [47, 89]. The central flavonoid biosynthetic genes CHS, CHI, and F3H from *C. unshiu* are also known to conform to this expression pattern [98].

As functions of more of the putative GTs become known through biochemical characterization, possible points of gene regulation may be identified and related back to secondary metabolism. The expression pattern of Lim-GT was tested in the albedo and leaf tissue of five different citrus species from 60–210 days after flowering [93]. They were able to detect expression in leaves of all species at 180–210 days after flowering. To date, limonoid glucosides have not been reported in grapefruit vegetative tissues and this is consistent with the undetectable transcription levels of PGT 8 in the leaves, stems, and roots of Duncan grapefruit.

Expression of PGT 2–7 genes in fully developed flowers is also reported. For this purpose, RNA was extracted from the whole flower. The flavonol-specific 3-O-GT coded for PGT 7 was found to be dominantly expressed (66%) in flowers as compared to the other putative GTs, although expression of PGT 2 and PGT 3 was also detected. This is not surprising as flavonols and flavonol glycosides are typically found in white flowers [99]. Flavonoids have been shown to have roles in pollen development and fertility in some species, and may be a possible physiological function for some of these GTs in flower tissues.

While lim-GT has been isolated and biochemically characterized from orange and pummelo albedo tissue [91], it should be noted that expression levels were relatively low in mature Duncan grapefruit albedo tissue, although detectable with greater PCR amplification. lim-GT expression was detected in albedo tissues of Marsh grapefruit [93].

Quercetin 3-O-glucoside has been detected in combination of fruit extracts from different citrus varieties [100]. This suggests that *C. paradisi* PGT 7 (flavonol-3-O-GT) may be active in citrus fruit tissues consistent with the expression data. PGT 2 was expressed in Duncan flavedo and may be involved in glucosylation of flavedo-specific metabolites such as simple terpenoids. PGT 3 was the only GT expressed in quantifiable levels in all fruit tissues, with highest levels in segment membranes. Because of the predominant expression in the juice vesicles, this gene and its ultimate secondary metabolite glycoside product may be of interest in terms of human nutrition. PGT 3's potential involvement in the production of glycosides that influence taste characteristics, such as the well-known bitter flavonoid diglycoside, naringin, is also of potential interest in terms of commercial application. However, it should be noted that the fruit's secondary product accumulation appears to be a highly dynamic process and it is yet to be clearly established if glycosylated secondary metabolites, such as naringin, are synthesized at their site of accumulation and/or produced in other tissues and transported to other tissues for storage. An effort was made to alter the types and levels of flavanone neo-hesperidosides in citrus, where an *Agrobacterium*-mediated genetic transformation approach was employed [37].

Grapefruit epicotyl stem segments were transformed with sense and antisense constructs of the target genes chalcone synthase (CHS) and chalcone isomerase (CHI), whose products catalyze the first two steps in the flavonoid biosynthetic pathway. Transformation with each of the individual constructs led to a different and unpredictable combination of viability, phenotypic change, transgene steady-state expression and alteration in flavonoid content in the resulting transgenic plants. Therefore, further research efforts are needed in this regard to optimize the transformation conditions for obtaining more desired results.

CONCLUSION

Flavanones are the dominant group of flavonoids in citrus and beyond their effect on citrus flavor, they have been implicated as important dietary components with a role in maintaining healthy blood vessels and bones, as cancer and mutagenesis-suppressing agents and as anti-allergic, anti-inflammatory and anti-microbial compounds [101, 102, 103].

The sensation of bitterness in citrus products emanates from different causes.

The bitterness caused by flavanone-glycosides, often referred as 'primary' bitterness, is common only to the bitter citrus species such as grapefruit; bitter orange; pummelo and should not be confused with the bitterness caused by the triterpene limonin that occurs in both bitter and non-bitter species [92].

Limonin-based bitterness is often referred to as' delayed' bitterness as much of the limonin in intact citrus fruit tissues occurs as a tasteless precursor, limonoate A-ring monolactone [92].

Compositional studies on the profile of flavonoids affecting the so-called 'primary bitterness' in various citrus species have established that the bitter species contain mostly flavanone neohesperidosides which are bitter; e.g. naringin while the non-bitter species contain mostly flavanone rutinosides, which are tasteless [104].

The key flavor-determining step of citrus flavanone-glycoside bio-synthesis is catalyzed by rhamnosyltransferases; 1, 2 rhamnosyltransferases (1,2RhaT) catalyze the biosynthesis of the bitter neohesperidosides, while 1,6 rhamnosyltransferases (1,6 RhaT) catalyze the biosynthesis of the tasteless rutinosides. Phylogenetic analysis of the flavonoid glycosyltransferase gene family places Cm1, 2RhaT on a separate gene cluster together with the only other functionally characterized flavonoid-glucoside rhamnosyl transferase gene, suggesting a common evolutionary origin for rhamnosyltransferases specializing in glycosylation of the sugar moieties of flavonoid glucosides.

Developmental studies on the accumulation of flavanone-glycosides in citrus and the corresponding glycosyltransferase enzyme activities show that flavanone-glycosides are synthesized in large quantities only in young tissue (leaves, flowers and fruits), and are later diluted in fruit to their final concentration during the process of development and ripening [47, 90].

Glycosyltransferases involved in plant secondary metabolism are a large group of enzymes classified as glycosyltransferase family 1 [105]. Flavonoid glycosyltransferases have been studied in many species, and a growing number of genes have been isolated and functionally characterized [105].

Naringin, a flavanone diglycoside, is one of the main compounds that produces bitterness in the leaves and fruit tissues of grapefruit. It accounts for up to 40–70% of the dry weight of very young fruit and leaf tissue [47].

Naringin synthesis tends to be highest in very young leaves which have a higher rate of metabolism due to growth demands than older leaves [47]. Naringin concentration is also higher in young developing fruits compared to mature fruits [47, 106].

The flavonoid biosynthetic pathways are attractive targets for metabolic engineering, to modulate a variety of plant characteristics [107, 108].

In this context, isolation of the gene Cm1, 2 RhaT provides a new tool to manipulate fruit flavor and health-benefiting value. The potential of metabolic engineering for the production of commercially desirable plant flavonoids has also been demonstrated in microorganisms [109]. However, full realization of this potential will require the use of plant genes encoding various modification enzymes such as flavonoid glucosyl and rhamnosyltransferases.

There is potential to engineer citrus plants that could yield fruit with enhanced taste.

REFERENCES

[1] FAOSTAT., (2011). Statistical databases agriculture data, agricultural production, major food and agricultural commodities and producers. Food and Agriculture Organization of the United Nations.<http:// faostat3.fao.org/faostat-gateway/go/to/download/Q/QC/E> Accessed on 18 February, 2014.

[2] Gmitter, F. G., Chen, J. C., Rao, M. N., Soneji, J. R., (2007). Citrus Fruits. In: C. Kole (Ed.). *Genome Mapping and Molecular Breeding in Plants, Fruits and Nuts,* Vol. 4. Springer-Verlag Berlin Heidelberg. pp. 265-279.

[3] Webber, H. J., (1967). History and development of the citrus industry. In: Reuther, W., Webber, H. J., Batchelor, L. D., (eds.). *The Citrus Industry,* Vol. 1 (rev.). Univ. of California Press. pp. 1–39.

[4] Scora, R. W., (1988). Biochemistry, taxonomy and evolution of modern cultivated citrus. In: Goren, R., Mendel, K., (eds.) Citriculture. *Proc. Intl. Soc. Citricult.* pp. 227–289.

[5] Zarina, Z., Tan, S. Y., (2013). Determination of flavonoids in *Citrus grandis* (Pomelo) peels and their inhibition activity on lipid peroxidation in fish tissue. *Inter. Food Res. J.* 20, 313-317.

[6] Okwu, D. E., (2004). Phytochemicals and vitamin content of indigenous species of South Eastern Nigeria. *J. Agric. Food Chem.* 6, 30-37.

[7] Hayat, K., Abbas, S., Jia, C., Xia, S., Zhang, X., (2011). Comparative study on phenolic compounds and antioxidant activity of feutrell's early and kinnow peel extracts. *J. Food Biochem.* 35, 454-471.

[8] Hertog, M. G., Hollman, P. C. H., Katan, M. B., Kromhout, D., (1993). Dietary antioxidant flavonoids and risk of coronary heart disease. *Lancet.* 342, 1007-11.

[9] Moore, G. A., (2001). Oranges and lemons: clues to the taxonomy of citrus from molecular markers. *Trends. Gen.* 17, 536-40.

[10] Stover, E., Castle, W., Chao, C. T., (2005). Trends in US sweet orange, grapefruit and mandarin-type cultivars. *Hort. Technol.* 15, 501-506.

[11] Guerra, M. S., (1984). Cytogenetics of *Rutaceae*. II. Nuclear DNA content. *Caryologia*, 37, 219-226.

[12] Gutiérrez-E, M. A., Luth, D., Moore, G. A., (1997). Factors affecting the *Agrobacterium*-mediated transformation in Citrus and production of sour orange (*Citrus aurantium* L.) plants expressing the coat protein gene of *Citrus tristeza* virus. *Plant. Cell. Rep.* 16, 745-753.

[13] Luth, D., Moore, G., (1999). Transgenic grapefruit plants obtained by *Agrobacterium tumefaciens*-mediated transformation. *Plant. Cell. Tissue. Organ. Cult.* 57, 219-222.

[14] Jorgensen, R. A., Cluster, P. D., English, J., Que, Q., Napoli, C. A., (1996). Chalcone synthase cosuppression phenotypes in petunia flowers: comparison of sense vs.

antisense constructs and single copy vs. complex T - DNA. *Plant. Mol. Biol.* 31, 957-973.

[15] Keys, A., (1995). Mediterranean diet and public health: Personal reflections. *Am. J. Clin. Nut.* 61, 1321-1323.

[16] Ejaz, S., Ejaz, A., Matsuda, K., Chae, W. L., (2006). Lemonoids as cancer chemo protective agents. *J. Sci. Food. Agri.* 86, 339-345.

[17] Harborne, J. B., Williams, C. A., (2000). Advances in flavonoid research since 1992. *Phytochem.* 55, 481-504.

[18] Nogata, Y., Sakamoto, K., Shiratsuchi, H., Ishii, T., Yano, M., Ohta, H., (2006). Flavonoid composition of fruit tissues of citrus species. *Biosci. Biotechnol. Biochem.* 70, 178-192.

[19] Yao, L. H., Jiang, Y. M., Shi, J., Tomas-Barberan, F. A., Datta, N., Singanusong, R., (2004). Flavonoids in food and their health benefits. *Plant. Foods. Hum. Nutr.* 59, 113-122.

[20] Holdena, J. M., Bhagwata, S. A., Haytowitza, D. B., Gebhardta, S. E., Dwyerb, J. T., Petersonb, J., Beechera, G. R., Eldridgec, A. L., Balentined, D., (2005). Development of a database of critically evalua-ted flavonoids data: Application of USDA'^{s} data equality evaluation system. *J. Food. Compost. Anal.* 18, 829-844.

[21] Frydman, A., Weisshaus, O., Bar-Peled, M., Huhman, D. V., Sumner, L. W., Martin, F. R., Lewinsohn, E., Fluhr, R., Gressel, J., Eyal, Y., (2004). Citrus fruit bitter flavours: isolation and functional characterization of the gene *Cm1, 2rhaT* encoding a1, 2 rhamnosyltransferase, a key enzyme in the biosynthesis of the bitter flavonoids of citrus. *Plant. J.* 40, 88-100.

[22] Gionfriddo, F., Postorino, E., Bovalo, F., (1996). I flavanoni glucosidici nel succo di bergamotto. *Essenze - Derivati agrumari.* 66, 404-416.

[23] Macheix, J. J., Fleuriet, A., Billot, J., (1990). The main phenolics of fruits. In: *Fruit Phenolics.* Boca Raton, FL: CRC Press. pp. 1-103.

[24] Miyake, Y., Yamamoto, K., Morimitsu, Y., Osawa, T., (1998). Characteristics of antioxidative flavonoid glycosides in lemon fruit. *Food. Sci. Technol. Intl.* 4, 48-53.

[25] Markens, S., Forkmann, G., (1999). Cloning and expression of flavone synthase II from Gerbera hybrids. *Plant. J.* 20, 611-618.

[26] Robards, K., Antolovich, M., (1997). Analytical chemistry of fruit bio-flavonoids. *Analyst.* 122, 12R-34R.

[27] Hayashi, A., Gillen, A. C., Lott, J. R., (2000). Effects of daily oral administration of quercetin Chalcone and modified citrus pectin on implanted colon-25 tumor growth in balb-c mice. *Altern. Med. Rev.* 5, 546-452.

[28] Martensa, S., Teerib, T., Forkmann, G., (2002). Heterologous expression of dihyroflavonol 4-reductases from various plants. *FEBS. Letts.* 531, 453-458.

[29] Sibhatu, M. B., (2003). Cloning and sequencing of *glucosyltransferase* (*GT*) genes from grapefruit (*Citrus paradisi*) seedlings; searching for 7-O-GT. *PhD thesis*, East Tennessee State University, Tennessee.

[30] Tahara, S., Ibrahim, R. K., (1995). Phenylated Isoflavonoids- An update. *Phytochem.* 38, 1073-1094.

[31] Herrman, K., (1976). Flavonols and flavonones in food plants: A review. *J. Food Technol.* 11, 433-448.

[32] Berhow, M. A., Tisserat, B., Kanes, K., Vandercook, C. E., (1998). Survey of phenolic compounds in citrus. *USDA, ARs, Technical Bulletin no. 1856*, US Government printing office, Washington DC.

[33] Peterson, J. J., Beecher, G. R., Bhagwat, S. A., Dwyer, J. T., Gebhardt, S. E., Haytowitz, D. B., Holden, J. M., (2006). Flavonones in grapefruit, lemons and limes: a compilation and review of the data from the analytical literature. *J. Food. Compo. Annals.* 19, 574-580.

[34] Rouseff, R. L., Martin, S. F.,Youtsey, C. O., (1987). Quantitative survey of narirutin, naringin, hesperidin and neohesperidin in citrus. *J. Agri. Food. Chem.* 35, 1027-1030.

[35] Lewinsohn, E., Britsch, L., Mazur, Y., Gressel, J., (1989). Flavanone glycosides biosynthesis in Citrus-Chalcone synthase, UDP-glucose: flavanone-7-0-glucosyltransferase activities in cell-free extracts. *Plant. Physiol.* 91, 1323-1328.

[36] Yusof, S., Mohd Ghazali, H., Swee King, G., (1990). Naringin content in local citrus fruits. *Food. Chem.* 37, 113-121.

[37] Bocco, A., Cuvelier, M. E., Richard, H., Berset, C., (1998). Antioxidant activity and phenolic composition of citrus peel and seed extracts. *J. Agri. Food Chem.* 46, 2123-2129.

[38] Kroyer, G., (1986). Über die antioxidative aktivitat von zitrusfruchtscha-len (antioxidative activity of citrus peels). *Zeitschrift. Fur. Ernaehrung-swiss.* 25, 63-69.

[39] Zarina, Z., Tan, S. Y., (2013). Determination of flavonoids in *Citrus grandis* peels and their inhibition activity on lipid peroxidation in fish tissue. *Intl. Food. Res. J.* 20, 313-317.

[40] Horowitz, R. M., (1986). Taste effects of flavonoids. *Prog. Clin. Biol. Res.* 213, 163-175.

[41] Mouly, P., Arzouyan, C. R., Gaydou, E. M., Estienne, J. M., (1994). Differentiation of citrus juices by factorial discriminant analysis using liquid chromatography of flavonone glycosides. *J. Agri. Food. Chem.* 42, 70-79.

[42] Ooghe, W. C., Detavernier, C. M., (1997). Detection of the addition of Citrus reticulate and hybrids to *Citrus sinensis* by flavonoids. *J. Agri. Food Chem.* 45, 1633-1637.

[43] Zhang, M., Duan, C., Zang, Y., Huang, Z., Liu, G., (2011). The flavonoid composition of flavedo and juice from the pummel cultivar (*Citrus grandis* (L.) Osbeck) and the grapefruit cultivar (*Citrus paradise*) from China. *Food. Chem.* 129, 1530-1536.

[44] Kawaii, S., Tomono, T., Katase, E., Ogawa, K., Yano, M., (1999). Quantification of flavonoid constituents in Citrus fruits. *J. Agri. Food. Chem.* 47, 313-318.

[45] Ververidis, F., Transtas, E., Douglas, C., Vollmer, G., Kretzschmar, G., Panopoulos, N., (2007a). Biotechnology of flavonoids and other phenyl-propanoid-derived natural products. Part 1: Chemical diversity, impacts on plant biology and human health. *Biotechnol. J.* 2, 1214-1234.

[46] Ververidis, F., Transtas, E., Douglas, C., Vollmer, G., Kretzschmar, G., Panopoulos, N., (2007b). Biotechnology of flavonoids and other phenyl-propanoid-derived natural products. Part 11: reconstruction of multi-enzyme pathways in plants and microbes. *Biotechnol. J.* 2, 1234-1249.

[47] Jourdan, P. S., McIntosh, C. A., Mansell, R. L., (1985). Naringin levels in citrus tissues. II Quantitative distribution of naringin in *Citrus paradise* Macfad. *Plant. Physiol.* 77, 903-08.

[48] Castillo, J., Benevente, O., Del Rio, J. A., (1993). Hesperitin 7-O- glucoside and pruning in Citrus species (*C. aurantium and C. paradise*). A study of their quantitative distribution in immature fruits and as immediate precursors of neohesperidin and naringin in *C. aurantium*. *J. Agri. Food Chem.* 41, 1920-1924.

[49] Kesterson, J. W., Hendrickson, R., (1953). Naringin, a bitter principle of grapefruit. *Fla. Agri. Exp. Sta. Bull.* 511.

[50] Korkina, L. G., (2007). Phenylpropanoid as naturally occurring antioxidants: from plant defense to human health. *Cell. Mol. Biol.* 53, 15-25.

[51] Drewnowski, A., Gomez-Carneros, C., (2000). Bitter taste phytonutrients and the consumer: a review. *Am. J. Clin. Nutr.* 72, 1424-1435.

[52] Drewnowski, A., Henderson, S. A., Shore, A. B., (1997). The taste responses to naringin, a flavonoid and the acceptance of grapefruit juices are related to genetic sensitivity to the 6n-propylthouracil. *Am. J. Clin. Nutr.* 66, 391-397.

[53] Wilcox, L. J., Borradaile, N. M., Huff, M. W., (1999). Antiantherogenic properties of naringenin, a citrus flavonoid. *Cardio. Drug. Rev.* 17, 160-178.

[54] Horowitz, R. M., Gentili, B., (1969). Taste and structure in phenolic glycosides. *J. Agri. Food. Chem.* 17, 696-700.

[55] Horowitz, R. M., Gentili, B., (1977). Flavonoids constituents of citrus. In: Nagy, S., Shaw, P. E., Vedhuis, M. K., (Eds.). *Citrus Science and Technology*. Westport, CT, AVI Publishing. pp. 397-426.

[56] Di Majo, D., Giammanco, M., La Guardia, M., Tripoli, E., Giammanco, S., Finotti, E., (2005). Flavonones in Citrus fruit: structure-antioxidant activity relationships. *Food. Res. Intl.* 38: 1161-1166.

[57] Calabro`, M. L., Galtieri, V., Cutroneo, P., Tommasini, S., Ficarra, P., Ficarra, R., (2004). Study of the extraction procedure by experimental design and validation of an LC method for determination of flavonoids in *Citrus bergamia* juice. *J. Pharma. Biomed. Anal.* 35, 349-363.

[58] Bors, W., Heller, W., Michel, C., Saran, M., (1990a). Radical chemistry of flavonoids antioxidant. In: Emerit (editor). *Antioxidants in therapy and preventive medicine*. Plenum press. pp. 165-170.

[59] Darmon, N., Ferrandiz, V., Canal, M. T., Mitjavilla, S., (1990). Activite antiradicallaire de flavonoies vis-à-vis de I anion superexide et du radical hyroxyle. *Liaison-Grupe. Polyphen. Bull.* 15, 158-162.

[60] Sichel, G., Corsaro, C., Scalia, M., Di Bilio, A. J., Bonomo, R., (1991). In vitro scavenger activity of some flavonoids and melanins against O^{2-}. *Free. Rad. Biol. Med.* 11, 1-8.

[61] Pincemail, J., Deby, C., Lion, Y., Braguet, P., Hans, P., Drien, K., (1986). Role of flavonoids in lipoperoxidation and radicular reactions. In: Farkas, L., Gabor, M., Kallay, F. (Edn.). Flavonoids and bioflavonoids. *Proceedings of the 7th Hungarian bioflavonoid symposium*, Szeged, Hungary. Elsevier Science, New York. pp. 423-36.

[62] Hayat, K., Zhang, X., Chen, H., Xia, S., Jia, C., Zhong, F., (2010a). Liberation and separation of phenolic compounds from citrus mandarin peels by microwave heating and its effect on antioxidant activity. *Sep. Puri. Technol.* 73, 371-376.

[63] Hayat, K., Zhang, X., Farooq, U., Abbas, S., Xia, S., Jia, C., Zhong, F., Zhang, J., (2010b). Effect of microwave treatment on phenolic content and antioxidant activity of citrus mandarin pomace. *Food Chem.* 123, 423-429.

[64] Hayat, K., Hussain, S., Abbas, S., Farooq, U., Ding, B., Xia, S., Jia, C., Zhang, X., Xia, W., (2009). Optimized microwave-assisted extraction of phenolic acids from citrus mandarin peels and evaluation of antioxidant activity *in vitro*. *Sep. Puri. Technol.* 70, 63-70.

[65] Proteggente, A. R., Saija, A., De Pasquale, A., Rice Evans, C., (2003). The compositional characterization and antioxidant activity of fresh juices from Sicilian sweet orange varieties. *Free. Rad. Res.* 37, 681-687.

[66] Finotti, E., Di Majo, D., (2003). Influence of solvents on the antioxidant property of flavonoids. *Die. Nahrung.* 47, 186-187.

[67] Chidambara, M. K. N., Kim, J., Vikram, A., Patil, B. S., (2012). Differential inhibition of human colon cancer cells by structurally similar flavonoids of citrus. *Food. Chem.* 132, 27-34.

[68] Hung, D. J., Ku, S. C., Tsan, C. C., Chuan, L. H., (2010). Antioxidant potentials of buntan pumelo (*Citrus grandis* Osbeck) and its ethanolic and acetified fermentation products. *Food. Chem.* 118, 554-458.

[69] Dixon, R. A., Paiva, N. L., (1995). Stress induced phenylpropanoid metabolism. *Plant. Cell.* 7, 1085-1097.

[70] Marcos, J. F., González-Candelas, L., Zacarías, L., (2005). Involvement of ethylene biosynthesis and perception in susceptibility of citrus fruits to *Penicillium digitatum* infection and the accumulation of defense related mRNAs. *J. Exp. Bot.* 56, 2183-2193.

[71] Costa, M. A., Bedgar, D. L., Moinuddin, S. G. A., Kin, K. W., Cardenas, C. L., Cochrane, F. C., Shockey, J. M., Helms, G. L., Amakura, Y., Takahashi, H., (2005). Characterization in vitro and in vivo of the putative multigene 4-coumarate: CoA ligase network in *Arabodopsis*: Syringyl lignin and sinapate/sinapyl alcohol derivative formation. *Phyto-chem.* 66: 2072-2091.

[72] Pelt, J. L., Downes, W. A., Schoborg, R. W., McIntosh, C. A., (2003). Flavonone 3-hydroxylase expression in *Citrus paradisi* and *Petunia hybrida* seedlings. *Phytochem.* 64, 435- 444.

[73] Wellmann, F., Lukacin, R., Moriguchi, T., Britsch, L., Schiltz, E., Matern, U., (2002). Functional expression and mutational analysis of flavonol synthase from *Citrus unshie. Eur. J. Biotechnol. Plant. Physiol.* 126, 485-493.

[74] Shimada, N., Sasaki, R., Sato, S., Kaneko, T., Tabata, S., Aoki, T., Ayabe, S., (2003). A comprehensive analysis of six dihydroflavonol 4-reductases encoded by a gene cluster of the *Lotus japonicus* genome. *J. Exp. Bot.* 56, 2573-2585.

[75] Heller, W., Forkmann, G., (1993). Biosynthesis of flavonoids. In: Harborne, J. B., (editor) *The flavonoids: Advances in Research since 1986*. Chapman and Hall, London. pp. 499-35.

[76] Ritter, H., Schulz, G. E., (2004). Structural basis for the entrance into the phenylpropanoid metabolism catalyzed by phenylalanine ammonialyase. *Plant Cell.* 16, 3426-3436.

[77] Mizutani, M., Ohta, D., Sato, R., (1997). Isolation of a cDNA and a genomic clone encoding cinnamate 4-hydroxylase from *Arabidopsis* and its expression manner in planta. *Plant Physiol.* 113, 755-763.

[78] Costa, M. A., Bedgar, D. L., Moinuddin, S. G. A., Kin, K. W., Cardenas, C. L., Cochrane, F. C., Shockey, J. M., Helms, G. L., Amakura, Y., Takahashi, H., et al. (2005). Characterization in vitro and in vivo of the putative multi gene 4-coumarate:

CoA ligase network in *Arabidopsis*: Syringyl lignin and sinapate/sinapyl alcohol derivative formation. *Phyto-chemistry*. 66, 2072-2091.
[79] Claudot, A. C., Ernst, D., Sandermann, H., Drouet, A., (1999). Cloning and characterization of two members of chalcone synthase gene family from walnut. *Plant Physiol. Biochem.* 37, 721-730.
[80] Weisshaar, B., Jenkins, G. I., (1998). Phenylpropanoid biosynthesis and its regulation. *Curr. Opin. Plant Biol.* 1, 251-257.
[81] Martens, S., Mithofer, A., (2005). Flavones and flavone synthases. *Phytochemistry* 66, 2399-2407.
[82] Pelt, J. L., Downes, W. A., Schoborg, R. W., McIntosh, C. A., (2003). Flavanone 3-hydroxylase expression in *Citrus paradisi* and Petunia hybrid seedlings. *Phytochemistry*. 64, 435-444.
[83] Wellmann, F., Lukacin, R., Moriguchi, T., Britsch, L., Schiltz, E., Matern, U., (2002). Functional expression and mutational analysis of flavonol synthase from *Citrus unshiu*. *Eur. J. Biochem*. 269, 4134-4142.
[84] Shimada, N., Sasaki, R., Sato, S., Kaneko, T., Tabata, S., Aoki, T., Ayabe, S., (2005). A comprehensive analysis of six dihydroflavonol 4-reductases encoded by a gene cluster of the *Lotus japonicas* genome. *J. Exp. Bot.* 56, 2573-2585.
[85] Saito, K., Kobayashi, M., Gong, Z., Tanaka, Y., Yamazaki, M., (1999). Direct evidence for anthocyanidin synthase as a 2-oxoglutarate-depen-dent oxygenase; molecular cloning and functional expression of cDNA from a red form of *Perilla frutescens*. *Plant J.* 17, 181-189.
[86] Jung, W., Yu, O., Lau, S. C., Okeefe, D., Odell, J., Fader, G., McGonigle, B., (2000). Identification and expression of isoflavone synthase, the key enzyme for biosynthesis of isoflavones in legumes. *Nat. Biotechnol.* 18, 208-212.
[87] Ferreira, L., Afonso, C., Vila-Real, H., Alfaia, A., Ribeiro, M. H. L., (2008). Evaluation of the effect of high pressure on naringin hydrolysis in grapefruit juice with naringinase immobilized in calcium alginate beads. *Food. Technol. Biotechnol*. 46, 146-50.
[88] Jala, J. D., Daniel, K. O., Cecilia, A. M., (2011). Secondary product glucosyltransferase and putative glucosyltransferase expression during *Citrus paradisi* (c.v. Duncan) growth and development. *Phytochem.* 72, 1732-38.
[89] McIntosh, C. A., Mansell, R. L., (1990). Biosynthesis of naringin in *Citrus paradisi:* UDP-glucosyltransferase activity in grapefruit seed-lings. *Phytochem.* 29, 1533-1538.
[90] Bar-Peled, M., Fluhr, R., Gressel, J., (1993). Juvenile-specific localization and accumulation of a rhamnosyltransferase and its bitter flavonoid in foliage, flowers and young citrus fruits. *Plant. Physiol.* 103, 1377-1384.
[91] Karim, M. R., Hashinaga, F., (2002). Isolation and characterization of a limonoid glucosyltransferase from pummel albedo tissue. *Food. Chem.* 76, 431-436.
[92] McIntosh, C. A., Mansell, R. L., (1997). Three dimentional analysis of limonin limonoate A- ring monolactone and naringin in the fruit of three varieties of *Citrus paradisi*. *J. Agri. Food Chem.* 45, 2876-2883.
[93] Zaare-Nahandi, F., Hosseinkhani, S., Zamani, Z., AsadiAbkenar, A., Omidbaigi, R., (2008). Delayed expression of limonoid UDP- glucosyl-transferase makes delayed bitterness in citrus. *Biochem. Biophys. Res. Comm.* 371, 59-62.
[94] RoySarkar, T., Strong, C. L., Sibhatu, M. B., Pike, L. M., McIntosh, C. A., (2007). Cloning expression, and characterization of a putative flavonoid glucosyltransferase

from grape fruit leave. In: Nikolau, B. J., Wurtele, E. S. (Eds.). *Concepts in Plant Metabolomics*. Springer. pp. 247-57.

[95] RoySarkar, T., (2004). cDNA cloning, expression and characterization of a putative glucosyltransferase (GT) from grapefruit leaves. *East Tennessee State University Master's Thesis*.

[96] Owens, D. K., McIntosh, C. A., (2011). Biosynthesis and function of citrus glycosylated flavonoids. *Rec. Adv. Phytochem*. 41, 67-95.

[97] Subramanian, S., Stacey, G., Yu, O., (2007). Distinct crucial roles of flavonoids during legume nodulation. *Trends. Plant. Sci.* 12, 282-285.

[98] Moriguchi, T., Kita, M., Tomano, Y., Endo, T., Omura, M., (2001). Gene expression in flavonoid biosynthesis: correlation with flavonoid accumulation in developing citrus fruit. *Physiol. Plant.* 111, 66-74.

[99] Mol, J., Grotewold, E., Koes, R., (1998). How genes paint flowers and seeds. *Trends. Plant. Sci.* 3, 212-17.

[100] Bilbao, M., Andres-Lacueva, C., Jauregui, O., Lamuela-Raventos, R., (2007). Determination of flavonoids in a citrus fruit extract by LC-DAD and LC-MS. *Food. Chem*. 101, 1742-1747.

[101] Rouseff, R. L., Naim, M., (2000). Citrus flavour stability. In: Ho, C. T., Risch, S. J. (Eds.). *Flavor Chemistry: Industrial and Academic Research*. American Chemical Society, Washington DC. pp. 101-122.[102] Manthey, J. A., Guthrie, N., (2002). Antiproliferative activities of citrus flavonoids against six human cancer cell lines. *J. Agri. Food Chem*. 50, 5837-5843.

[103] Ballester, A. R., Teresa, L. M., de Vos, R. C. H., Bovy, A. G., Gonzalez-Candelas, L., (2013). Citrus phenylpropanoids and defence against pathogens. Part I: Metabolic profiling in elicited fruits. *Food Chem.* 136, 178-185.

[104] Rousseff, R. L., Martin, S. F., Youtsey, C. O., (1987). Quantitative survey of narirutin, naringin, heperidin and neohesperidin in citrus. *J. Agri. Food Chem.* 35, 1027-1030.

[105] Vogt, T., Jones, P., (2000). Glycosyltransferases in plant natural product synthesis: characterization of a supergene family. *Trends. Plant. Sci*. 5, 380-386.

[106] Albach, R. F., Juarez, A. T., Lime, B. J., (1969). Time of Naringin production in grapefruit. *J. Am. Soc. Hort. Sci.* 94, 605-609.

[107] Forkmann, G., Martens, S., (2001). Metabolic engineering and applications of flavonoids. *Curr. Opin. Biotechnol.* 12, 155-160.108. Ballester, A. R., Lafuente, M. T., Forment, J., Gadea, J., de Vos, R. C. H., Bovy, A. G., Gonzalez-Candelas, L., (2011). Transcriptomic profiling of citrus fruit peel tissues reveals fundamental effects of phenylpropanoids and ethylene on induced resistance. *Mol. Plant Pathol.* 12, 879-897.

[109] Hwang, E. I., Kaneko, M., Ohnishi, Y., Horinouchi, S., (2003). Production of plant-specific flavanones by *Escherichia coli* containing an artificial gene cluster. *Appl. Environ. Microbiol.* 69, 2699-3006.

In: Citrus
Editor: Khizar Hayat

ISBN: 978-1-63117-985-3

Chapter 4

ADVANCES IN STUDY OF CAROTENOIDS IN CITRUS FRUIT

Xiangyu Liu[1], Juan Li[2] and Jiezhong Chen[1*]
[1]College of Horticulture, South China Agricultural University, Guangzhou, China
[2]Department of Horticulture, Zhongkai University of Agriculture and Engineering, Guangzhou, China

ABSTRACT

Carotenoids, which are a class of important natural pigments, endow plants with yellow, orange and red color, and play crucial functions in photosynthesis and synthesis of abscisic acid. In addition, carotenoids are closely related to human health. Recent studies suggest that carotenoids are not only the precursor of vitamin A, but also play important roles in antioxidant capacity, human immunity improvement and cancer prevention. Citrus is rich in bioactive compounds and has been an excellent source of carotenoids for humans and other animals. So, putting effort into the research and development of citrus carotenoids is worthwhile. In this article we reviewed the composition, biosynthesis and regulation of carotenoids in citrus fruit, and the various biological functions such as the antioxidant property, light protective effects and anticancer effect.

Keywords: Citrus, Carotenoids, Biosynthesis, Regulation, Biological activities

INTRODUCTION

Citrus is one of the world's major fruit crops and has been loved by people for its aesthetic appearance, delicious taste and high nutritional value. Citrus is now grown in more than 140 countries in the world and occupies a very important position in the international trade of agricultural products [1]. Nutrition and health care is an eternal theme for humans,

* Corresponding author address: College of Horticulture, South China Agricultural University, Guangzhou, 510642, China; E-mail: cjzlxb@scau.edu.cn.

and fruit nutrition and safety is also a major focus of human society in the twenty-first century. A large number of epidemiological studies suggested that citrus fruit could be conducive to prevention of cancer [2,3], cataracts [4], age-related macular degeneration [5], and osteoporosis [6,7]. This is mainly due to many bioactive compounds in citrus fruit, including vitamin C, flavonoids, carotenoids, limonin and others.

Carotenoids are a large class of lipophilic pigments, synthesized through the isoprenoid pathway in all photosynthetic organisms and many non-photosynthetic bacteria and fungi. Carotenoids generally consist of eight isoprene units that joined together to form a 40-carbon isoprenoid. The most obvious feature of the carotenoid molecule is the long polyene chain, which may extend from 3 to 15 conjugated double bonds [8]. In nature, more than 700 carotenoids have been identified and are usually divided into two groups, carotenes that only consist of hydrocarbon structure, and xanthophylls, which contain oxygen atoms in the structure.

In plants, carotenoids are mainly distributed in the chloroplasts and chromoplasts. Carotenoids are essential components for photosynthesis, and play an important role in protecting photosynthetic organs and preventing photooxidation damage [9, 10]. Carotenoids endow plants with brilliant colors ranging from yellow to red, to attract insects, birds and other animals to pollination and seed dispersal [9]. Carotenoids can be metabolized to plant hormones and abscisic acid (ABA) in plants [11], and precursors of vitamin A in humans and animals [12]. In addition, carotenoids also play an important role in human health, such as free radical quenching, human immunity enhancement, prevention of cancer [8]. Therefore, seeking plant resources, which are rich in carotenoids, exploring carotenoids synthesis, metabolic and regulation mechanism, and improving the content in plant edible tissues have been the focus of concern in plant research. Citrus are rich in carotenoid composition with approximately 115 carotenoids, including geometric isomers [13,14]. Citrus is not only an important source for human uptake of carotenoids; it is also a good material for plant carotenoid metabolism and regulation research.

The Biosynthesis of Carotenoids In Citrus

Carotenoids are synthesized in plastids and the main chain synthesis is the same in higher plants [15-18]. The pathway of carotenoid biosynthesis in plants is illustrated in Figure 1. The five-carbon (C5) compound isopentenyl diphosphate (IPP), which is synthesized from glyceraldehyde-3-phosphate and pyruvate via the methylerythritol phosphate (MEP) pathway, is reversibly catalyzed to form its allylic isomer dimethylallyl phosphate (DMAPP) by IPP isomerase (IPPI) [8]. Subsequent step-by-step condensations of DMAPP and three molecules of IPP result in the immediate precursor of carotenoids, geranylgeranyl pyrophosphate (GGPP; C20) by geranylgeranyl diphosphate synthase (GGPS). The first committed step in carotenoid biosynthesis is the head-to-head condensation of two molecules of GGPP to form colorless phytoene (C40) by phytoene synthase (PSY) [19]. Then a series of conjugated carbon carbon double bonds are introduced into phytoene to generate all-trans lycopene and the enzymes responsible for the series of desaturation reactions are phytoene desaturase (PDS), ζ-carotene desaturase (ZDS) and carotene isomerase (CRTISO) [17,20]. Cyclization of lycopene is a crucial branching point in the pathway. Lycopene β-cyclase (LCYb) can introduce two β-rings into lycopene to form β-carotene, while lycopene ε-cyclase (LCYe) only introduces one ε-ring to yield δ-carotene and then to yield α-carotene with the addition of one β-ring catalyzed by LCYb [21]. Hydroxylation of α-carotene results in the formation of lutein via α-cryptoxanthin catalyzed by ε-ring hydroxylase (CRTLe) and β-ring hydroxylase (CRTLb) [22,23]. Hydroxylation of β-carotene leads to the formation of zeaxanthin via β-cryptoxanthin catalyzed by CRTLb and then to form violaxanthin via antheraxanthin by zeaxanthin epoxidase (ZEP) [24]. Violaxanthin can be converted to neoxanthin by neoxanthin synthase (NXS) [25,26]. Finally, neoxanthin is cleaved to yield abscisic acid (ABA) by 9-cis-epoxycarotenoid dioxygenase (NCED) [27].

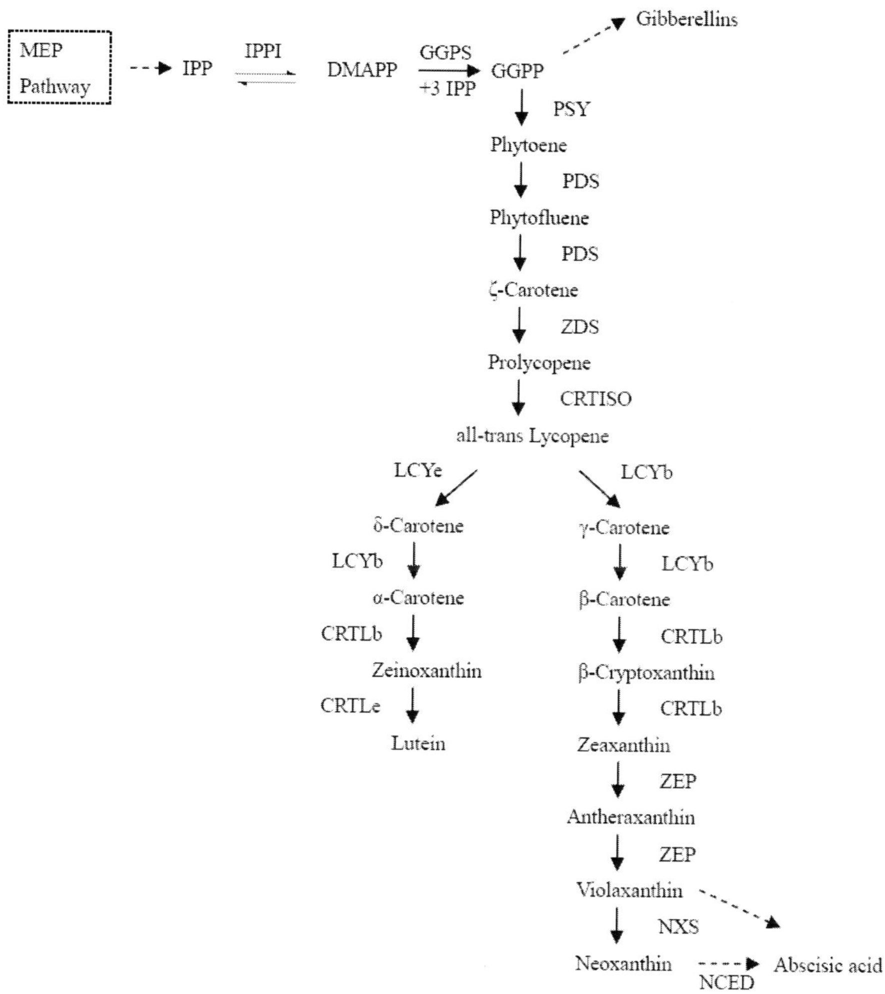

Figure 1. The carotenoid biosynthetic pathway in citrus. MEP, methylerythritol phosphate; IPP, isopentenyl diphosphate; DMAPP, dimethylallyl diphosphate; GGPP, geranylgeranyl diphosphate; IPPI, IPP isomerase; GGPP, geranylgeranyl diphosphate; GGPS, geranyl diphosphate synthase; PSY, phytoene synthase; PDS, phytoene desaturase; ZDS, ζ-carotene desaturase; CRTISO, carotene isomerase; LCYe, ε-cyclase; LCYb, β-cyclase; CRTLb, β-ring hydroxylase; CRTLe, ε-ring hydroxylase; ZEP, zeaxanthin epoxidase; NXS, neoxanthin synthase; NCED, 9-cis-epoxycarotenoid dioxygenase.

CAROTENOID ACCUMULATION IN CITRUS

Compared with model plants, tomato and Arabidopsis, research of citrus carotenoids started relatively late, but it gradually caused widespread concern and achieved gratifying progress in recent years. For example, studies on carotenoid content and composition in citrus fruit have been conducted extensively and carotenoid metabolic profiling in different species or varieties is also established [28-30]. All genes that encode key enzymes in the pathway of citrus carotenoid biosynthesis have been cloned and the expressions of these genes are analyzed during fruit development [31-34]. Some citrus carotenoid mutants have been explored and the related mechanism is also preliminarily studied [35-37].

The composition and content of carotenoids in citrus fruit are influenced by many factors, such as geographical origin [38], cultivation conditions [28] and types [39,40], in which it varies greatly among different species or varieties. Studies showed that violaxanthin, lutein, zeaxanthin and β-cryptoxanthin are the major carotenoids in fruits of Satsuma mandarin (*Citrus unshiu* Marc.) and sweet orange (*Citrus sinensis* Osbeck), accounting for about 80% of total carotenoids [18,35]. Satsuma mandarin fruits mainly accumulated β-cryptoxanthin, while sweet orange fruits predominantly accumulated violaxanthin isomers, (9-cis)-violaxanthin [41]. Melendez-Martinez [42] also established that violaxanthin [mainly (9-cis)-violaxanthin], antheraxanthin [mainly (9-cis)-antheraxanthin], zeaxanthin, mutatoxanthin, and β-cryptoxanthin are the major carotenoids in juices from Valencia oranges.

Carotenoid compositions in 25 citrus genotypes have been analyzed and it was found that variability in carotenoid compositions was more interspecific than intraspecific and three major basic taxa of citrus could be differentiated according to it: *Citrus reticulata* (mandarins) accumulated both cis-violaxanthin and β-cryptoxanthin, and that *Citrus medica* (citrons) accumulated β-cryptoxanthin without cis-violaxanthin, while *Citrus maxima* (pummelos) only accumulated cis-violaxanthin and with lack of β-cryptoxanthin [26].

Tao [43] analyzed the carotenoid contents of 53 citrus varieties and reported that lutein, zeaxanthin and β-cryptoxanthin were major carotenoids in both peel and pulp, but with low β-carotene and very low α-carotene. In general, carotenoid contents were highest in mandarins, followed by sweet orange, lemon, and lowest in pummelo. Lutein, zeaxanthin and β-cryptoxanthin in peel were about 2.5-15 times higher as that in pulp and thus the peel was the principal location for the carotenoid stock in citrus fruit [43]. Lycopene, which accounts for more than half of total carotenoids in ripe tomato fruits [44], is absent in common citrus fruits, and only a few cultivars were reported to accumulate lycopene up to now, such as 'Cara Cara' navel orange and some red grapefruit varieties [29,39,45]. In addition, citrus fruits also accumulate some specific carotenoids, such as β-citraurin, β-citraurinene and β-apo-8'-carotenal [28], and the β-citraurin is also the main reason due to which the Clementine and Dancy tangerine fruits appear reddish in color [46].

Carotenoid compositions also change during citrus fruit development. Study found that α-carotene, β-carotene and lutein were major carotenoids in immature fruit peel of Satsuma mandarin, and no detection of β-cryptoxanthin and zeaxanthin; but in the ripe fruits, α-carotene, β carotene could hardly be detected and lutein, zeaxanthin and especially β-cryptoxanthin became the major carotenoids in peel [31]. Lee [41] studied the developmental patterns of carotenoids in Hamlin, Earlygold and Budd Blood sweet orange juices and uncovered that a dramatic increase occurred in β-cryptoxanthin, α-cryptoxanthin and zeaxanthin at the late stage of maturation, and lutein showed an obvious decrease, while the amount of α-carotene, β-carotene and antheraxanthin changed a little.

Regulation of Carotenoid Metabolism in Citrus Fruit

Transcriptional Regulation

Carotenoid metabolism, which is a branch of the isoprenoid metabolic pathway in plants, is very complex and affected by various environmental factors and development processes. However, the regulation of carotenoid metabolism at the gene level is poorly understood. The first reported gene involved plant carotenoid metabolism was *pTOM5* that was received from the tomato in 1987 [47], and then confirmed to be phytoene synthase gene a few years later. From the analysis of GenBank log, the first gene related to citrus carotenoid metabolism is the gene of capsanthin/capsorubin synthase, which was isolated in 1999 [48] and was later proved to be highly homologous to neoxanthin synthase. But now, the whole genome sequencing of orange and mandarin has been completed internationally, and genes of key enzymes in the citrus carotenoids metabolic pathway have also been found and annotated [49].

Carotenoid biosynthesis in the fruit of plants is predominantly regulated by fruit development. During tomato fruit ripening, chloroplast was transformed to form chromoplast and carotenoid content increased 10-15 times, in which the lycopene content increased about 300 times [50]. After veraison of tomato fruit, *PSY* gene expression increased by 10-20 times, and *PDS* expression increased nearly 3 times while *LCYb* and *LCYe* expressions were significantly decreased [51,52]. Tomato color mutants have been valuable in elucidating regulatory mechanisms during fruit ripening. In tomato *Delta* mutant, *LCYe* expression increased markedly and resulted in large accumulation of δ-carotene [52], while in the *Beta* mutant, high transcripts levels of *LCYb* gene led to large accumulation of β-carotene [53], suggesting that the accumulation of carotenoids could be greatly regulated at the transcription level in tomato fruit.

In citrus both up- and down-regulation of transcription of carotenoid genes have been found. For example, *PSY* gene expression increased along with fruit development in the peel and pulp of the Satsuma mandarin and to the maximum level in the latest stage [31, 32]. The *PDS* transcript in the pulp was at a low level in the young fruit and it increased towards maturation like *PSY*; but in the peel, in contrast to *PSY*, the level of the *PDS* transcript remained constant after an increase in July, indicating non-coordinate regulation of *PDS* and *PSY* in the peel [54]. During the ripening of citrus fruit, expressions of *PDS*, *ZDS*, *LCYb* and *ZEP* genes markedly increased while *LCYe* expression disappeared, showing that the carotenoid accumulation in citrus fruit resulted from interactions of these gene expressions [18]. Alquezar [37] have isolated two *LCYb* genes from orange fruit, named *Csβ-LCY1* and *Csβ-LCY2*, and confirmed that expression of *Csβ-LCY1* was at low levels and remained relatively constant during fruit ripening; while *Csβ-LCY2* showed a chromoplast-specific expression and marked increase in both peel and pulp along with fruit ripening, in parallel with the accumulation of β,β-xanthophylls. In addition, in the 'Star Ruby' red grapefruit (*Citrus paradisi* cv. Star Ruby), accumulation of lycopene during maturation was associated with a substantial reduction in the expression of *β-LCY2* and *β-CHX* genes with respect to Navel oranges.

Environmental Regulation

Carotenoid accumulation in citrus fruit is greatly affected by the growth environment and agronomic measures. Sufficient light is necessary for carotenoid synthesis. Red grapefruit cultivated in long-day districts accumulated more lycopene [55]. Bagging could decrease the carotenoid content in 'Hongshigan' citrus (*C.reticulata* × *C.sinensis*), which mainly inhibits the accumulation of β-cryptoxanthin [55]. A modest increase in light intensity can effectively improve soluble sugar and carotenoids content in citrus fruit, and reduce the accumulation of organic acids [56,57]. Light quality also affects carotenoid metabolism of citrus. Red light irradiation could accelerate the red color development in postharvest citrus fruit, and increase total carotenoids content [58].

High temperature causes serious degradation of carotenoids in citrus peel, especially for β-cryptoxanthin [59]. An early study reported that the optimal temperature for carotenoid accumulation in flavedo was 15 – 25°C and that an ethylene treatment at these temperatures noticeably accelerated carotenoid accumulation in the flavedo of citrus fruit [60]. Recent research also found that storage at 20°C rapidly increased the carotenoid content in flavedo and maintained the content in juice sacs. In contrast, storage at 5 and 30°C gradually decreased the content in juice sacs [61]. The sugar content of fruit also affects carotenoid synthesis. Iglesias [62] showed that supplement of exogenous sucrose promoted carotenoid accumulation in citrus peel, and meanwhile carbohydrate starvation stress created by defoliation inhibited carotenoid accumulation, suggesting that plenty of sugar accumulation is the basis for carotenoid synthesis.

Chemical Regulation

It was found that preharvest treatment with exogenous gibberellin (GA) could inhibit the chlorophyll degradation and carotenoid biosynthesis, and delay the fruit coloring in persimmon fruit, which mainly inhibited the synthesis of β-cryptoxanthin in fruit [63]. Abscisic acid (ABA) plays an important role in carotenoid synthesis. Richardson and Cowan [64] found that ABA content in late-colored navel orange was higher than that in the early-colored variety, and they inferred that ABA content might not be conducive to the carotenoid synthesis. Application of exogenous ABA also inhibited carotenoid accumulation in navel orange [65]. Application of ethylene for citrus fruit coloration has been around for a long time, which could promote the chlorophyll degradation and carotenoids appearance. But debates have continued whether ethylene could influence the carotenoid metabolism. Steward [66] revealed that ethylene could induce the accumulation of β-cryptoxanthin and β-citraurin in Robinson navel orange peel, promoting the orange or orange red color. Methyl jasmonate (MeJA) can promote the chlorophyll degradation and β-carotene accumulation. After 4 hours of treatment with MeJA on Golden Delicious apple at 25°C, degradation of chlorophyll and lutein accelerated significantly and β-carotene increased 2 times over control treatment [67].

Application of MeJA on strawberry in vitro could accelerate the degradation of fruit chlorophyll, and β-carotene increased slightly [68].

Application of 2-(4-chlorophenylthio-)-triethylamine hydrochloride (CPTA) to induce lycopene accumulation is the most successful example of carotenoids regulation. Coggins [69] first found this phenomenon, and then Hsu [70] compared the inducing effects of different ethyl amine compounds on lycopene accumulation, and later these compounds proved to be inhibitors of lycopene cyclase [71]. 2-(4-methyl-phenoxy) triethylamine (MPTA), the analogue of CPTA, could also induce the accumulation of lycopene, but the increased accumulation didn't lead to a corresponding reduction in β-cryptoxanthin and zeaxanthin that were transformed from lycopene, and total carotenoids also increased compared with the control [72], implying that MPTA may activate some steps of carotenoid biosynthesis process.

Research on plant carotenoid metabolism related to mineral elements is seldom involved. Study showed that Mn^{2+} was indispensable to GGPP synthase activity, and meanwhile Mn^{2+} was also the key factor that led GGPP to carotenoid metabolism or other isoprenoid metabolism [73]. So Mn^{2+} plays a very important link of plant carotenoid metabolism. In addition, when phosphorus content in citrus peel was high, carotenoid content was also high and coloring improved, suggesting a high relationship between phosphorus and carotenoid accumulation [74].

Biological Activities of Carotenoids

Carotenoids reveal various biological functions, especially in relation to human health and their roles as biological antioxidants. In general, the major value of carotenoids in human nutrition is their role as provitamin A, but recently more and more studies support that their capacity of quenching singlet oxygen and acting as free radical scavengers and antioxidants *in vivo* can provide additional health benefits. Therefore their roles as biological antioxidants and as regulators of the immune system have been the subject of intense scrutiny.

Provitamin A Activity

Vitamin A deficiency is one of most serious deficiency diseases in the world and affects an estimated 250 million children under 5 years of age [75]. Serving as precursors for vitamin A, has been the best-established function of carotenoids. But it is restricted to some carotenoids with β-ring end groups, such as β-carotene, zeaxanthin and β-cryptoxanthin, in which β-carotene is believed to be the most important for animal and human nutrition. Almost 40 years ago, these carotenoids were reported to be cleaved by an intestinal 15-15'-dioxygenase to form retinoids when ingested in the diet [76]. Retinoids such as retinol (vitamin A), retinal (the main visual pigment), and retinoic acid (which controls morphogenesis) play important functions as visual pigments and signaling molecules. Furthermore, it has been known that high doses of β-carotene are nontoxic and did not result in any vitamin A toxicity on clinical treatment [77]. The β-carotene is also widely used to prevent or cure various diseases, which are caused by vitamin A deficiency, such as xerophthalmia, night blindness, and age-related diseases of the eyes such as cataract and macular degeneration (AMD) [78,79]

Antioxidant / Pro-Oxidant Properties

The free radical theory indicates that many diseases and aging of the human body are related to the damage effect of the free radical. Therefore, removing excess oxygen free radicals in the body is conducive to prevent diseases and delay aging. Besides the antioxidant enzyme, non-enzymatic antioxidants also play a role in free radical scavenging, and carotenoid is just one of non-enzymatic antioxidants. It has long been found that carotenoids were effective at quenching the high-energy states, both triplet and singlet that might occur in photosynthesis [80]. At sufficient concentrations, carotenoids could protect lipids from peroxidative damage *in vitro* [81]. Lorenzo reported that β-cryptoxanthin could repair the oxidant-induced DNA damage caused by free radicals [82].

Specifically, β-carotene exhibits a good radical-trapping antioxidant property only at partial pressures of oxygen, significantly less than 150 torr, the pressure of oxygen in normal air; and at higher oxygen pressures, β-carotene loses its antioxidant activity and shows a pro-oxidant effect, particularly at relatively high concentrations [83]. Similar oxygen-pressure-dependent behaviors also exist in other carotenoids. Zhang and Omaye [84] also revealed that β-carotene with low pressure conditions can effectively inhibit DNA strand breaking caused by the AAPH free radicals; while the pro-oxidant effect of β-carotene was significant at high O_2 tension and it caused supercoiled DNA to completely breakdown to circular and linear forms. So, it should be noted that in certain high-risk groups (e.g. smokers) there could be adverse effects of high doses of carotenoids, perhaps because of their pro-oxidant properties [85].

Immunological Competence and Cancer Prevention

The earlier research on the effects of carotenoids on the immune function mostly focused on β-carotene. Seifter [86] reported a marked stimulatory action of β-carotene on the growth of the thymus gland and a large increase in the number of thymic small lymphocytes. Bendich [87] pointed out that β-carotene could enhance T and B lymphocyte proliferative responses, stimulate effector T cell functions, and enhance macrophage, cytotoxic T cell and natural killer cell tumoricidal capacities, as well as increase the production of certain interleukins. Similar effects of β-carotene on proliferation of lymphocyte cells were also demonstrated in rat, pig and cattle [88]. For the human body, β-carotene can increase the number of helper T cells and T-lymphocyte cells, and enhance natural killer cell activity [89]. In terms of enhancing cellular immunity and humoral immune response, some non-provitamin A carotenoids are more effective than β-carotene, such as lutein, lycopene, astaxanthin and canthaxanthin [88].

β-carotene may reduce the risk of some cancers. Mice fed with β-carotene had augmented tumor immunity against syngeneic fibrosarcoma cells [90]. Higher β-carotene consumption was associated with a lower risk of breast cancer in case-control studies [91]. *In vitro*, β-carotene also inhibited the growth of MCF-7 and Hs578T while lycopene inhibited MCF-7 and MDA-MB-231 human breast cancer cells [92]. In addition, some experimental animal studies have shown that α-carotene had higher activity than β-carotene in suppressing tumorigenesis in the skin, lung, liver and colorectum [93,94].

Increasing research supports that high lycopene intake or tissue levels are related to decreased prostate cancer incidence [2,95]. For example, lycopene could lead to about a 30–40% decrease in the risk of developing prostate cancer, especially advanced prostate cancer [2]. Subjects that took lycopene for 3 weeks had smaller tumors, less involvement of the surgical margins and less diffuse involvement of the prostate by pre-cancerous high-grade prostatic intraepithelial neoplasia [96]. An *in vitro* study also showed that lycopene in the growth medium reduced the proliferation of prostate cancer cells [97]. Furthermore, lycopene was also reported to be associated with a lower risk of breast cancer [92,98].

Lutein is an important nutrient for prevention of cancer [3]. A 10-year study following 120,000 U.S. men and women found that a significant reduction in lung cancer occurred in patients with the highest intake of lutein and zeaxanthin [99]. Another survey based on 20 South Pacific Island populations uncovered that a markedly lower incidence rate of lung cancer was observed among Fijians, who digest more lutein daily than inhabitants of other South Pacific region [100]. Slattery [101] used dietary data to show that lutein was inversely associated with colon cancer in both men and women. Canthaxanthin can also suppress the proliferation of human colon cancer cells [102], and proved to be effective in inhibiting both oral and colon carcinogenesis in rats [103]. However, there are also some studies or cases that show no association between intake of carotenoids and cancers risk [104,105].

The mechanisms of cancer prevention by carotenoids are proposed as followed: the antioxidant effect, to prevent oxidative damage; interference with growth factors, to inhibit the proliferation of cancer cells; increasing gap junctional intercellular communication, to make the cancer cells affected by the surrounding environment; enhancing immune function; regulation of cellular proliferation, cell cycle progression and apoptotic signaling, to induce apoptosis of cancer cells [106,107].

Light Protective Effects

Carotenoids can protect the eyes and skin from light-induced damage. Age-related diseases of the eye such as cataract and macular degeneration (AMD) are common problems in the world. Much research suggests that carotenoids can reduce the incidence of these diseases.

The concentration of β-carotene and α-tocopherol in blood serum were inversely associated with the incidence of cataracts [4]. The macula of the eye contains two carotenoids: lutein and zeaxanthin [108]. The two carotenoids could protect retina from light-induced damage through absorption of blue light, and protect the optic nerve from free radical damage by quenching singlet oxygen formed in the photoreceptors.

In addition, clinical study suggests that enough antioxidants from the food can reduce the occurrence of skin burn, inflammation, immune suppression and even the cell canceration in strong light [109]. Lycopene, β-carotene or lutein could lower UV-induced lipid peroxidation of human skin fibroblast cells *in vitro* [110].

Carotenoids and Bone Homeostasis

Carotenoids have great effects on prevention and treatment of osteoporosis and it may be an osteogenic factor in preventing osteoporosis in human subjects [6]. Among various carotenoids, β-cryptoxanthin has been found to have huge stimulatory effects on bone calcification and osteoblastic bone formation, and large inhibitory effects on osteoclastic bone resorption in vitro [111]. Through inducing apoptosis and enhancing intercellular communication, β-cryptoxanthin affects the gene expression of various proteins that are related to osteoblastic bone formation and resorption, to improve the bone health [7].

The Application of Carotenoids

Food Colorant

Carotenoids present natural colors from yellow to red and are conducive to human health due to its lots of biological activities. They are very excellent food colorant, and widely used in lactic acid drink, ice cream, seasoning and fruit wine. In addition, Carotenoids can be also used as tablet pigments in the pharmaceutical industry [112].

Nutritional Supplements

Data from a variety of media showed that the global market of total carotenoids was estimated at over $700 million in 1999, and that nutritional supplement products accounted for about 15%; the number had increased to $935 million by 2005, in which the proportion of nutritional supplements rose to nearly 30% [113]. At present, materials of carotenoid products are mainly astaxanthin, β-carotene, lutein, lycopene, canthaxanthin, annatto and zeaxanthin. Among them, astaxanthin, β-carotene, canthaxanthin and lutein occupy 85% of market share. And yet 4 types of carotenoids are most widely used in nutritional supplements: β-carotene, lutein, lycopene and canthaxanthin [113]. As mentioned above, β-carotene, lutein and lycopene have many healthcare functions and they are also the main carotenoids in human serum. In contrast, astaxanthin and canthaxanthin are limited in nutritional supplements. Nutritional supplements of carotenoids can present in various forms, such as liquid, tablet and capsule [114].

Feed Additive

Egg yolk color is one of the important indexes to measure the quality of eggs and directly affects the prices and market competitiveness. Consumers generally prefer the eggs with higher yolk color. Egg yolk contains abundant carotenoids and its color depends on the content and composition of carotenoids [115]. For egg-laying poultry intake of exogenous carotenoids can enhance egg yolk color significantly. So carotenoids are widely used as a feed additive in egg-laying poultry [115]. Furthermore, from the coloring function, more carotenoids are used in aquatic feed. Carotene, lutein, astaxanthin and zeaxanthin are primary pigments in the skin of aquatic animals. Dietary carotenoids play a very important role in keeping the skin and muscle color of fish, for carotenoids deposit as original or other transformed forms *in vivo* after absorption. Feeding the fish with astaxanthin and canthaxanthin could significantly increase carotenoids content in muscle and improve the skin color, of which astaxanthin has better effect [116].

In general, lycopene is widely used in health care products due to its powerful ability of quenching active oxygen species. Lutein is mainly used for the egg yolk coloring and it is the fastest-growing one in the international market in recent years. Now astaxanthin is mainly used as feed additive in aquaculture, for example used in salmon and trout farming to make meat bright in color. The traditional use of canthaxanthin is to make the egg yolk ruddy, but now it is mostly used in aquaculture. Taken together, the main application of carotenoid materials is as a food additive and the food additive market is relatively small; there are only β-carotene and annatto. Carotenoids used as nutritional supplements and health care are emerging items and will develop greatly in the future.

Strategies for Improving Carotenoids Composition and Content in Citrus

Varietal Breeding

All along, people are motivated to breed crops to achieve better quality or higher yield. Citrus breeding has made great progress by pursuing higher yields and better fruit quality in decades past. So, varietal breeding (such as sport selection) is an available strategy for the improvement of carotenoids in citrus. To date, many citrus mutants related to color change have been found and served as a new germplasm; the well-known ones are some red mutants that accumulate lycopene in pulp [29,39]. As we know lycopene is absent in common citrus fruit, and only a few cultivars with red pulp can accumulate it. These color mutants are excellent materials for the purposes of both research and application. Citrus cultivars with pink or red pulp can be found in grapefruit, sweet orange, and occasionally in lemon, such as 'Cara Cara' navel orange (*C. sinensis* L. Osbeck), 'Hong Anliu' sweet orange, 'Star Ruby' grapefruit (*C. paradisi* Macf.), 'Ruby Red' grapefruit and 'Hirado Buntan' pummelo (*Citrus grandis* L. Osbeck). Lycopene and β-carotene were the main pigments that cause the red variation in citrus and the low level of lycopene led to pink pulp compared with high content in red pulp [29, 39, 43]. There is a significant correlation between the concentrations of lycopene and β-carotene in these cultivars, and they are synthesized in the pulp itself rather than acquired via transport from other tissues [29]. But the studies on the mechanism of lycopene accumulation in fruits of mutant are still at the initial stages. Recently, Alquezar [37] isolated a chromoplast-specific expression LCYb gene *Csβ-LCY2*, and during fruit maturation there was a substantial reduction in the expression of *Csβ-LCY2* in 'Star Ruby' red grapefruit with respect to Navel orange.

In addition, there are also some reports about color variation in citrus peel. Rodrigo [35] found a novel mutant Pinalate, which was derived from the Navelate orange, and its peel color was yellow instead of the typical bright orange. In Pinalate, linear carotenoids (phytoene, phytofluene and ζ-carotene) are massively accumulated, while 98% of the carotenoids are xanthophylls and apocarotenoids in the Navelate flavedo tissue (colored part of the skin) [35]. A citrus spontaneous mutant, *navel negra*, has been reported and it produced fruits with an abnormal brown-colored flavedo instead of the bright orange coloration, due to the change of ripening-related chlorophyll (Chl) degradation [117].

Genetic Engineering of Carotenoid Metabolism

Due to the identification of biosynthesis genes of carotenoids, it provides valuable genetic resources for the application of gene engineering to change the carotenoid compositions and improve the carotenoid content in plants. As the research progresses, it would be possible to regulate the carotenoid biosynthesis through gene engineering in a faster and targeted manner in citrus.

Improving the Rate-Limiting Step

In recent years, enhancing the yield of carotenoids in plant has achieved success through improving the key limiting steps in carotenoid biosynthesis by gene engineering [118]. As mentioned above, the first committed step in the process of carotenoid biosynthesis is the formation of colorless phytoene from the condensation of two molecules GGPP catalyzed by phytoene synthase (PSY), a rate-limiting enzyme in carotenoid biosynthesis in canola and tomato plants, which has been confirmed. Therefore, the *PSY* gene attracts much attention and has been extensively studied in carotenoid genetic engineering. Research found that PSY occurred as three isozymic patterns in maize and rice, respectively encoded by *PSY1*, *PSY2* and *PSY3* genes [119,120]. *PSY1* is necessary for carotenoid formation in corn seed, and *PSY2* is crucial for the carotenoid synthesis in leaf, while *PSY3* plays a very important role in carotenoid synthesis in root and abscisic acid generation under stress [119,120]. Overexpression of *PSY-1* gene can improve carotenoid content in transgenic tomato plants, but at the same time it leads to a shortage of gibberellin and makes the plant dwarf as the endogenous GGPP molecules are consumed excessively [121]. The data suggested that dwarfism was a consequence of metabolic competition for the common carotenoid and GA precursor GGPP, channeling it into carotenoids and away from GA synthesis. In order to overcome the detrimental effects of *PSY-1* overexpression, the bacterial phytoene synthase gene (*crtB*) was introduced under the control of a ripening-specific promoter [122]. The overexpression of *PSY* successfully increased the carotenoids content in ripening fruit without dwarfism, as the pool of GGPP in ripe fruit is greater than that in green tissues and GA synthesis is no longer required.

The transformation of the Hongkong kumquat (*Fortunella hindsii* Swingle) with the *PSY* gene from the ‘Cara Cara’ navel orange has been studied and it had a 2.5-fold average increase of phytoene in transgenic plants; and lycopene, β-carotene, and β-cryptoxanthin in transgenic fruits were also markedly increased, which made kumquats change color from yellow to orange [123]. Some implications are also given based on the findings that the increase of phytoene content provides sufficient substrate for β-carotene and β-cryptoxanthin synthesis and leads to a relatively high level accumulation [123].

Furthermore, it should be understood that a famous example that people may benefit from carotenoid genetic engineering is 'Golden Rice', genetically modified rice that produces β-carotene. Rice endosperm lacks provitamin A and other carotenoids, but GGPP could be formed in the endosperm [124]. Therefore, in order to enable the metabolism of GGPP to carotenoids, three biosynthetic genes, the daffodil *PSY* and *LCYb* genes and bacterial phytoene desaturase genes (*crtI*) were co-transformed into rice. The endosperm of resulting transformants contained lutein, zeaxanthin, β-carotene and α-carotene in varying proportions, and the carotenoid level in the transgenic endosperm was estimated at 1.6 μg/g [125]. It is estimated that in order to supply the RDA of provitamin A in an average rice meal (300 g), 2.0 μg/g of β-carotene must be present in endosperm and the level would seem to be attainable.

Improving the Branching Point

LYCb and LYCe are the key enzymes of branching point of carotenoid biosynthesis in plants. The formation of α-carotene requires the action of two enzymes LCYe and LCYb, whereas LCYb converts lycopene into β-carotene in two steps. Adjusting the relative expression levels between these two enzymes in plants could change the carotenoid accumulation. The content of β-carotene in tomato fruit was increased by 3.8 times due to the transformation of the *LYCb* gene [126]. Dharmapuri [127] overexpressed the *LYCb* under the control of the fruit-specific promoter in tomato and found that β-carotene increased by 12 times in fruits of the transformants and the transgenes, and the phenotypes were inherited in a dominant Mendelian fashion. Carotenoid levels were also upregulated by suppression of *LCYe*. In potato, tuber-specific silencing of *LCYe* increased the total carotenoid level in tubers up to 2.5-fold and β-carotene level up to 14-fold [128].

Productions of ketocarotenoid have been successfully achieved in plants by introduction of the β-carotene ketolase gene from microorganism. Ketocarotenoids, such as canthaxanthin and astaxanthin, are produced by some algae and cyanobacteria but are rare in plants [129]. A β-carotene ketolase gene isolated from the alga was introduced into carrot and it revealed that up to 70% of total carotenoids were converted to novel ketocarotenoids, in which astaxanthin, adonirubin, and canthaxanthin were most prevalent, followed by echinenone, adonixanthin and β-cryptoxanthin [130]. A transgenic potato line accumulating zeaxanthin because of inactivated zeaxanthin epoxidase was re-transformed with the β-carotene ketolase gene (*crtO*) from the cyanobacterium [131]. Transgenic plants expressing *crtO* constitutively accumulated echinenone, 3'-hydroxyechinenone, and 4-ketozeaxanthin together with astaxanthin in tubers. The newly formed ketocarotenoids comprised approximately 10–12% of the total carotenoids in leaves and tubers. The above results show that specific expression of branching point genes could offer certain contribution to the change of plant carotenoid accumulation.

In addition, increasing the content of corresponding endogenous precursors can be another feasible measure to improve the carotenoid accumulation. For example, overexpression of 1-deoxy-D-xylulose 5-phosphate synthase (DXS) could add the intermediate 1-deoxy-D-xylulose 5-phosphate (DXP), and then increase the available IPP source. In Arabidopsis, the transgenic plants that over express *DXS* gene significantly increase the content of related substance in carotenoid metabolism pathway, in which tocopherol is 2 times the normal level, and ABA is 4 times while total carotenoids are close to 1.5 times the normal level [132].

Conclusion

Up to now, the carotenoid biosynthetic pathway has been made clear and carotenoid compositions in citrus were also analyzed. At the same time, some key genes are also identified and studied at the level of transcription. But many issues have yet to be addressed in detail. For example, there is less study on the regulation of carotenoid metabolism in citrus, mainly reflected in no identified transcription factors that influence carotenoid formation and few means to regulate the carotenoid accumulation. The application of gene engineering and proteomic study are also insufficient in citrus. Hopefully, finishing the whole genome sequencing of citrus will close the gap with model plants, and make it easy to understand the regulatory mechanisms in the carotenoid pathway and the transgenic strategy to modify carotenoid content and composition. In addition, attention to varietal breeding and exploring natural mutants that relate to alterations of carotenoid content and compositions is worthy of study.

References

[1] Liu, Y.Q., Heying, E., Tanumihardjo, S.A., (2012). History, global distribution, and nutritional importance of citrus fruits. *Compre. Rev. Food Sci. Food Saf.* 11, 530-545.
[2] Giovannucci, E., Rimm, E.B., Liu, Y., Stampfer, M.J., Willett, W.C., (2002). A prospective study of tomato products, lycopene, and prostate cancer risk. *J. Natl. Cancer Inst.* 94, 391-398.
[3] Khachik, F., Beecher, G., Smith J., (2004). Lutein, lycopene, and their oxidative metabolites in chemoprevention of cancer. *J. Cell. Biochem.* 59, 236-246.
[4] Knekt, P., Heliövaara, M., Rissanen, A., Aromaa, A., Aaran, R., (1992). Serum antioxidant vitamins and risk of cataracts. *Bri. Med.* 305, 1392-1394.
[5] Zhou, H., Zhao, X., Johnson, E.J., Lim, A., Sun, E., Yu, J., Zhang, Y., Liu, X., Snellingen, T., Shang F., Liu, N., (2011). Serum carotenoids and risks of age-related macular degeneration in a Chinese population sample. *Invest. Ophthalmol. Vis. Sci.* 52, 4338-4344.
[6] Yamaguchi, M., Igarashi, A., Uchiyama, S., Morita, S., Sugawara, K., Sumida, T., (2004). Prolonged intake of juice (*Citrus Unshiu*) reinforced with β-crypthoxanthin has an effect on circulating bone biochemical markers in normal individuals. *J. Health Sci.* 50, 619-624.
[7] Yamaguchi, M., Uchiyama, S., (2008). Combination of β-cryptoxanthin and zinc has potent effects on apoptotic cell death and suppression of bone resorption-related gene expression in osteoclastic cells. *Int. J. Mol. Med.* 22, 221-228.

[8] Fraser, P.D., Bramley, P. M., (2004). The biosynthesis and nutritional uses of carotenoids. *Prog. Lipid Res.* 43, 228-265.

[9] Bartley, G.E., Scolnik, P.A., (1995). Plant carotenoids, pigments for photoprotection visual attraction and human health. *Plant Cell* 7, 1027-1038.

[10] Tracewell, C.A., Vrettos, J.S., Bautista, J.A., Frank, H.A., Brudvig, G.W., (2001). Carotenoid photooxidation in photosystem II. *Arch. Biochem. Biophys.* 385, 61-69.

[11] Schwartz, S.H., Qin, X., Zeevaart, J.A.D., (2003). Elucidation of the indirect pathway of abscisic acid biosynthesis by mutants, genes and enzymes. *Plant Physiol.* 131, 1591-1601.

[12] Von Lintig, J., Wyss, A., (2001). Molecular analysis of vitamin A formation, cloning and characterization of β-carotene 15, 15'-dioxygenase. *Arch. Biochem. Biophys.* 385, 47-52.

[13] Rouseff, R., Raley, L., Hofsommer, H., (1996). Application of diode array detection with a C-30 reversed phase column for the separation and identification of saponified orange juice carotenoids. *J. Agric. Food. Chem.* 44, 2176-2181.

[14] Meléndez-Martínez, A.J., Britton, G., Vicario, I.M., Heredia, F.J., (2005). Color and carotenoid profile of Spanish Valencia late ultrafrozen orange juices. *Food Res. Int.* 38, 931-936.

[15] Hirschberg, J., (2001).Carotenoid biosynthesis in flowering plants. *Curr. OPin. Plant Biol.* 4, 210-218.

[16] Sandmann, G., (2001). Carotenoid biosynthesis and biotechnological application. *Arch. Biochem. Biophys.* 385, 4-12.

[17] Isaacson, T., Ronen, G., Zamir, D., Hirschberg, J., (2002). Cloning of tangerine from tomato reveals a carotenoid isomerase essential for the production of β-carotene and xanthophylls in plants. *Plant Cell.* 14, 333-342.

[18] Kato, M., Ikoma,Y., Matsumoto, H., Sugiura, M., Hyodo, H., Yano, M., (2004). Accumulation of carotenoids and expression of carotenoid biosynthetic genes during maturation in citrus fruit. *Plant Physiol.* 134, 824-827.

[19] Kato, M., (2012). Mechanism of carotenoid accumulation in citrus fruit. *J. Japan. Soc. Hort. Sci.* 81, 219-233.

[20] Park, H., Kreunen, S.S., Cuttriss, A. J., DellaPenna, D., Pogson, B.J., (2002). Identification of the carotenoid isomerase provides insight into carotenoid biosynthesis, prolamellar body formation, and photomorphogenesis. *Plant Cell* 14, 321-332.

[21] Cunningham, F.X., Pogson, B., Sun, Z.R., McDonald, K.A., DellaPenna, D., Gantt, E., (1996). Functional analysis of the beta and epsilon lycopene cyclase enzymes of Arabidopsis reveals a mechanism for control of cyclic carotenoid formation. *Plant Cell.* 8, 1613-1626.

[22] Tian, A., Musetti, V., Kim, J.M., Magallanes-Lundback, M., DellaPenna, D., (2004). The *Arabidopsis LUT1* locus encodes a member of the cytochrome P450 family that is required for carotenoid ε-ring hydroxylation activity. *Proc. Natl. Acad. Sci. USA*. 101, 402-407.

[23] Kim, J., DellaPenna, D., (2006). Defining the primary route for lutein synthesis in plants, the role of Arabidopsis carotenoid β-ring hydroxylase CYP97A3. *Proc. Natl. Acad. Sci. USA*. 103, 3474-3479.

[24] DellaPenna, D., Pogson, B., (2006). Vitamin synthesis in plants, tocopherols and carotenoids. *Annu. Rev. Plant Biol.* 57, 11-38.

[25] Bouvier, F., D'Harlingue, A., Backhaus, R.A., Kumagai, M.H., Camara, B., (2000). Identification of neoxanthin synthase as a carotenoid cyclase paralog. *Eur. J. Biochem.* 267, 6346-6352.
[26] Fanciullino, A. L., Dhuique-Mayer, C., Luro, F., Cassanova, J., Morillon, R., Ollitrault, P., (2006). Carotenoid diversity in cultivated citrus is highly influenced by genetic factors. *J. Agric. Food. Chem.* 55, 7405-7417
[27] Kato, M., Matsumoto, H., Ikoma, Y., Okuda, H., Yano, M., (2006). The role of carotenoid cleavage dioxygenases in the regulation of carotenoid profiles during maturation in citrus fruit. *J. Exp. Bot.* 57, 2153-2164.
[28] Gross, J., Bazak, H., Blumenfeld, A., Ben-Arie, R., (1984). Changes in chlorophyll and carotenoid pigments in the peel of 'Triumph' persimmon (*Diospyros kaki L.*) induced by pre-harvest gibberellin (GA3) treatment. *Sci. Hort.* 24, 305-314.
[29] Xu, J., Tao, N., Liu, Q., Deng, X., (2006). Presence of diverse ratios of lycopene/β-carotene in five pink or red-fleshed citrus cultivars. *Sci. Hortic.* 108, 181-184
[30] Matsumoto, H., Ikoma, Y., Kato, M., Kuniga, T., Nakajima, N., Yoshida, T., (2007). Quantification of carotenoids in citrus fruit by LC-MS and comparison of patterns of seasonal changes for carotenoids among citrus varieties. *J. Agric. Food. Chem.* 55, 2356-2368.
[31] Ikoma, Y., Komatsu, A., Kita, M., Ogawa, K., Omura, M., Yano, M., Moriguchi, T., (2001). Expression of a phytoene synthase gene and characteristic carotenoid accumulation during citrus fruit development. *Physiol. Plant* 111, 232-238.
[32] Kim, I.J., Ko, K.C., Kim, C.S., Chung, W.I., (200l). Isolation and expression patterns of a cDNA encoding phytoene synthase in Citrus. *J. Plant Physiol.* 158, 795-800
[33] Kim, I.J., Ko, K.C., Kim, C.S., Chung, W.I., (200l). Isolation and characterization of cDNAs encoding β-carotene hydroxylase in Citrus. *Plant Sci.* 161, 1005-1010.
[34] Costa, M., Otoni, W., Moore, G., (2002). An evaluation of factors affecting the efficiency of Agrobacterium-mediated transformation of Citrus paradisi (Macf.) and production of transgenic plants containing carotenoid biosynthetic genes. *Plant Cell Rep.* 21, 365-373.
[35] Rodrigo, M. J., Mareos, J.F., Alférez, F., Mallent, M.D., Zacarías, L., (2003). Characterization of Pinalate, a novel Citrus sinensis mutant with a fruit-specific alteration that results in yellow pigmentation and decreased ABA content. *J. Exp. Bot.* 54, 727-738.
[36] Liu, Q., Xu, J., Liu, Y., Zhao, X., Deng, X., Guo, L., Gu, J., (2007). A novel bud mutation that confers abnormal patterns of lycopene accumulation in sweet orange fruit (*Citrus sinensis* L. Osbeck). *J. Exp. Bot.* 58, 4161-4171.
[37] Alquézar, B., Zacarías, L., Rodrigo, M.J., (2009). Molecular and functional characterization of a novel chromoplast-specific lycopene β-cyclase from Citrus and its relation to lycopene accumulation. *J. Exp. Bot.* 60, 1783-1797.
[38] Mouly, P.P., Gaydou, E.M., Lapierre, L., Corsetti, J., (1999). Differentiation of several geographical origins in single-strength Valencia orange juices using quantitative comparison of carotenoid profiles. *J. Agric. Food. Chem.* 47, 4038-4045.
[39] Lee, H. S., (200l). Characterization of carotenoids in juice of red navel orange (Cara Cara). *J. Agric. Food. Chem.* 49, 2563-2568.

[40] Dhuique-Mayer, C., Caris-Veyrat, C., Ollitrault, P., Curk, F., Amiot, M.J., (2005). Varietal and interspecific influence on micronutrient contents in citrus from the Mediterranean area. *J. Agric. Food. Chem.* 53, 2140-2145.

[41] Lee, HS., Castle, W.S., (2001). Seasonal changes of carotenoid pigments and color in Hamlin, Earlygold, and Budd blood orange juices. *J. Agric. Food. Chem.*49, 877-882.

[42] Melendez-Martínez, A.J., Vicario, I., Heredia, F., (2007). Review, analysis of carotenoids in orange juice. *J. Food Compos. Anal.* 20, 638-649.

[43] Tao, J., Zhang, S.L., Xu, J.G., Liu, C.R., (2003). Analysis of major carotenoid composition and its content in citrus fruit. *Sci. Agric. Sin.* 36, 1202-1208. (in Chinese)

[44] Burns, J., Fraser, P.D., Bramley, P.M., (2003). Identification and quantification of carotenoids, tocopherols and chlorophylls in commonly consumed fruits and vegetables. *Phytochemistry* 62, 939-947.

[45] Lee, H.S., Coates, G.A., (2002). Characterization of color fade during frozen storage of red grapefruit juice concentrates. *J. Agric. Food. Chem.* 50, 3988-3991.

[46] Curl, A.L., (1965). The Occurrence of beta-Citraurin and of beta-Apo-8′-Carotenal in the Peels of California Tangerines and Oranges. *J.Food. Sci.* 30, 13-18.

[47] Ray, J.A., Bird, C.R., Maunders, M., Grierson, D., (1987). Sequence of pTOM5, a ripening related cDNA from tomato. *Nucl. Acids Res.* 24, 10587.

[48] Xu, C., Chen, D., Zhang, S., (2001). Molecular cloning of full length capsanthin/capsorubin synthase homologous gene from orange. *J. Exp. Biol.* 34, 147-150. (in Chinese)

[49] Orange (*Citrus sinensis*) Genome Annotation Project, (2013). Available at <http://citrus.hzau.edu.cn/orange/>. Accessed on October, 2013.

[50] Fraser, P. D., Truesdale, M. R., Bird, C.R., Schuch, W., Bramley, P.M., (1994). Carotenoid biosynthesis during tomato fruit development (Evidence for tissue-specific gene expression). *Plant Physiol.* 105, 405-413.

[51] Giuliano, G., Bartley, G. E., Scolnik, P. A., (1993). Regulation of carotenoid biosynthesis during tomato development. *Plant Cell* 5, 379-387.

[52] Ronen, G., Cohen, M., Zamir, D., Hirschberg, J., (1999). Regulation of carotenoid biosynthesis during tomato fruit development, expression of the gene for lycopene epsilon-cyclase is down-regulated during ripening and is elevated in the mutant *Delta. Plant J.* 17, 341-351.

[53] Ronen, G., Carmel, G.L., Zamir, D., Hirschberg, J., (2000). An alternative pathway to β-carotene formation in plant chromoplasts discovered by map-based cloning of Beta and old-gold color mutations in tomato. *Proc. Natl. Acad. Sci. USA.* 97, 11102-11107.

[54] Kita, M., Komatsu, A., Omura, M., Yano, M., Ikoma, Y., Moriguehi, T., (2001). Cloning and expression of CitPDS1, a gene encoding phytoene desaturase in citrus. *Biosci. Biotechnol. Bioche.* 65, 1424-1428.

[55] Bower, J., Kleynhans, S., Rabe, E., (1991). Color evaluation of pigmented grapefruit. *Citrus J.* 1, 36-38.

[56] Tao, J., Zhang, S.L., An, X.M., Zhao, Z.Z., (2003). Effects of light on carotenoid biosynthesis and color formation of citrus fruit peel. *Chin. J. Appl. Ecol.* 14, 1833-1836. (in Chinese)

[57] Chen, J., Zhang S., Zhang, L., Zhao, Z., Xu, J., (2002). Fruit photosynthesis and assimilate translocation and partitioning : Their characteristics and role in sugar

accumulation in developing Citrus unshiu fruit. *Acta Botanica Sinica* 44, 158-163. (in Chinese)

[58] Ohishi, H., Watanabe, J., Kadoya, K., (1996). Effect of red light irradiation on skin coloration and carotenoid composition of stored "Miyauchi" iyo (*Citrus iyo* hort. ex Tanaka) tangor fruit. *Bull. Exp. Farm CoH. Agr.* 17, 33-37.

[59] Sun, M., Pan, S., Hu, J., Fu, H., Xu, X., (2008). Study on effect of environment on stability of citrus peel carotenoid. *Food Science* 29, 127-129. (in Chinese)

[60] Wheaton, T.A., Stewart, I., (1973). Optimum temperature and ethylene concentrations for postharvest development of carotenoid pigments in citrus. *J. Ame. Soc. Hortic. Sci.* 98, 337-340.

[61] Matsumoto, H., Ikoma, Y., Kato, M., Nakajima, N., Hasegawa, Y., (2009). Effect of Postharvest Temperature and Ethylene on Carotenoid Accumulation in the Flavedo and Juice Sacs of Satsuma Mandarin (Citrus unshiu Marc.) Fruit. *J. Agric. Food. Chem.* 57, 4724-4732.

[62] Iglesias, D.J., Tadeo, F.R., Legaz, F., Primo-Millo, E., Talon, M., (2001). In vivo sucrose stimulation of colour change in citrus fruit epi-carps, Interactions between nutritional and hormonal signals. *Physiol. Plant* 112, 244-250.

[63] Gross, J., (1987). Carotenoids. Pigments in Fruits. Academic Press, London.

[64] Richardson, G.R., Cowan, A.K., (1995). Abscisic acid content of citrus flavedo in relation to colour development. *J. Hortic. Sci.* 70, 769-773.

[65] Wang, G., Xia, X., (2005). Effects of exogenous ABA and GA3 on dominant pigment contents in peel of sweet orange. *Plant Physiol. Commun.* 41, 168-170. (in Chinese)

[66] Steward, I., Wheaton, T.A., (1972). Carotenoids in citrus, Their accumulation induced by ethylene. *J. Agric. Food. Chem.* 20, 448-449.

[67] Perez, A.G., Sanz, C., Richardson, D.G., Olías, J.M., (1993). Methyl jasmonate vapor promotes β-carotene synthesis and chlorophyll degradation in Golden Delicious apple peel. *J. Plant Growth Regul.* 12, 163-167.

[68] Perez, A.G., Sanz, C., Olías, R., Olías, J.M., (1997). Effect of methyl jasmonate on in vitro strawberry ripening. *J. Agric. Food. Chem.* 45, 3733-3737.

[69] Coggins, C.W., Henning, G.L., Yokoyama, H., (1970). Lycopene, accumulation induced by 2-(4-chlorophenylthio-)-triethylamine hydrochloride. *Science* 168, 1589-1590.

[70] Hsu, W.J., Poling, S.M., DeBenedict, C., Rudash, C., Yokoyama, H., (1975). Chemical inducers of carotenogenesis. *J. Agric. Food. Chem.* 23, 831-834.

[71] Bouvier, F., D'Harlingue, A., Camara, B., (1997). Molecular analysis of carotenoid cyclase inhibition. *Arch. Biochem. Biophys.* 346, 53-64.

[72] Tao, J., Zhang, S., Zhang, L., (2002). Effect of MPTA on carotenoid biosynthesis in the peel of citrus fruit. *J. Plant Physiol. Mol. Biol.* 28, 46-50. (in Chinese)

[73] Dogbo, O., Laferriere, A., D'Harlingue, A., Camara, B., (1988). Carotenoid biosynthesis, Isolation and characterization of a bifunctional enzyme catalyzing the synthesis of phytoene. *Proc. Natl. Acad. Sci. USA*. 85, 7054-7058.

[74] Yao, Q., Li, D., Ishii, T., (1999). Influence of VA mycorrhiza on juice components and rind colour of citrus fruit. *J. Fruit Sci.* 16, 38-42. (in Chinese)

[75] World Health Organization, (2013). Available at <http://www.who.int/nutrition/topics /vad/en/index.html>. Accessed on October, 2013.

[76] Olson, J.A., Hayaishi, O., (1965). The enzymatic cleavage of beta-carotene into vitamin A by soluble enzymes of rat liver and intestine. *Proc. Natl. Acad. Sci.* 54, 1364-1370.
[77] Mathews-Roth, M.M., (1989). Beta-carotene, clinical aspects. *New Protect. Roles Sel. Nutr.* 22, 17-38.
[78] Sommer, A., West, K.P., (1996).Vitamin A deficiency: health, survival, and vision. Oxford Univ. Press, New York.
[79] Cooper, D.A., (2004). Carotenoids in health and disease: recent scientific evaluations, research recommendations and the consumer. *J. Nutr.* 134, 221–224.
[80] Fujimori, E., Livingston, R., (1957). Interactions of chlorophyll in its triplet state with oxyen, carotene, etc. *Nature* 180, 1036-1038.
[81] Handelman, G.J., (1996). Carotenoids as scavengers of active oxygen species. In, Cadenas E, Packer L, eds. Handbook of antioxidants. New York, Marcel Dekker.
[82] Lorenzo, Y., Azqueta, A., Luna, L., Bonilla, F., Domínguez, G., Collins, A.R, (2009). The carotenoid β-cryptoxanthin stimulates the repair of DNA oxidation damage in addition to acting as an antioxidant in human cells. *Carcinogenesis* 30, 308-314.
[83] Burton, G.W., Ingold, K.U., (1984). Beta-carotene, an unusual type of lipid antioxidant. *Science* 224, 569-573.
[84] Zhang, P., Omaye, S., (2001). DNA strand breakage and oxygen tension, effects of [beta]-carotene, [alpha]-tocopherol and ascorbic acid. *Food. Chem. Toxicol.* 39, 239-246.
[85] Palozza, P., Calviello, G., Bartoli, G.M., (1995). Prooxidant activity of β-carotene under 100% oxygen pressure in rat liver microsomes. *Free Rad. Biol. Med.* 19, 887-892.
[86] Seifter, E., Rettura, G., Levenson, S.M., (1981). Carotenoids and cell-mediated immune responses. In, The Quality of Foods and Beverages, Chemistry and Technology (Charalambois, G. & Inglett, G., eds.) Vol. 2, Academic Press, New York.
[87] Bendich, A., (1991). β-Carotene and the immune response. *Pro. Nutr. Soe.* 50, 263-274.
[88] Chew, B.P., Park, J.S., (2004). Carotenoid action on the immune response. *J. Nutr.* 134, 257-261.
[89] McDevitt, T.M., Tchao, R., Harrison, E.H., Morel D.W., (2005). Carotenoids normally present in serum inhibit proliferation and induce differentiation of a human monocyte/macrophage cell line (U937). *J. Nutr.* 135, 160-164.
[90] Tomita, Y., Himeno, K., Nomoto, K., Endo, H., Hirohata, T., (1987). Augmentation of tumor immunity against syngeneic tumors in mice by β-carotene. *J. Natl. Cancer Inst.* 78, 679-681.
[91] Clavel-Chapelon, F., Niravong, M., Joseph, R.R., (1997). Diet and breast cancer, review of the epidemiologic literature. *Cancer Detect. Prev.* 21, 426-440.
[92] Prakash, P., Russell, R.M., Krinsky, N.I., (2001). In vitro inhibition of proliferation of estrogen-dependent and estrogen-independent human breast cancer cells treated with carotenoids or retinoids. *J. Nutr.* 131, 1574-1580.
[93] Murakoshi, M., Nishino, H., Satomi, Y., Takayasu, J., Hasegawa, T., Tokuda, H., Iwashima, A., Okuzumi, J., Okabe, H., Kitano, H., Iwasaki, R., (1992). Potent preventive action of α-carotene against carcinogenesis, Spontaneous liver carcinogenesis and promoting stage of lung and skin carcinogenesis in mice are suppressed more effectively by α-carotene than by β-carotene. *Cancer Res.* 52, 6583-6587.

[94] Narisawa, T., Fukaura, Y., Hasebe, M., Ito, M., Aizawa, R., Murakoshi, M., Uemura, S., Khachik, F., Nishino, H., (1996). Inhibitory effects of natural carotenoids, α-carotene, β-carotene, lycopene and lutein, on colonic aberrant crypt foci formation in rats. *Cancer Lett.* 107, 137-142.

[95] Chen, L., Stacewicz-Sapuntzakis, M., Duncan, C., Sharifi, R., Ghosh, L., Breemen, R., Ashton, D., Bowen P.E., (2001). Oxidative DNA Damage in Prostate Cancer Patients Consuming Tomato Sauce-Based Entrees as a Whole-Food Intervention. *J. Natl. Cancer Inst.* 93, 1872-1879.

[96] Kucuk, O., Sarkar, F.H., Sakr, W., Djuric, Z., Pollak, M.N., Khachik, F., Li, Y.W., Banerjee, M., Grignon, D., Bertram, J.S., Crissman, J.D., Pontes, E.J., Wood, D.P., (2001). Phase II randomized clinical trial of lycopene supplementation before radical prostatectomy. *Cancer Epidemiol. Biomark. Prev.* 10, 861-868.

[97] Kim, L., Rao, A.V., Rao, L.G., (2002). Effect of lycopene on prostate LNCaP cancer cells in culture. *J. Med. Food* 5, 181-187.

[98] Nahum, A., Hirsch, K., Danilenko, M., Watts, C.K.W., Prall, O.W.J., Levy, J., Sharoni, Y., (2001). Lycopene inhibition of cell cycle progression in breast and endometrial cancer cells is associated with reduction in cyclin D levels and retention of p27(Kip1) in the cyclin E-cdk2 complexes. *Oncogene* 20, 3428-3436.

[99] Michaud, D.S., Feskanich, D., Rimm, E.B., Colditz, G.A., Speizer, F.E., Willett, W.C., Giovannucci, E., (2000). Intake of specific carotenoids and risk of lung cancer in 2 prospective US cohorts. *Am. J. Clin. Nutr.* 72, 990-997.

[100] Marchand, L.L., Hankin, J.H., Bach, F., Kolonel, L.N., Wilkens, L.R., Stacewicz-Sapuntzakis, M., Bowen, P.E., Beecher, G.R., Laudon, F., Baque, P., Daniel, R., Seruvatu, L., Henderson, B.E., (1995). An ecological study of diet and lung cancer in the South Pacific. *Int. J. Cancer* 63, 18-23.

[101] Slattery, M.L., Benson, J., Curtin, K., Khe-Ni, M., Schaeffer, D., Potter, J.D., (2000). Carotenoids and colon cancer. *Am. J. Clin. Nutr.* 71, 575–82.

[102] Onogi, N., Okuno, M., Matsushima-Nishiwaki, R., Fukutomi, Y., Moriwaki, H., Muto, Y., Kojima, S., (1998). Antiproliferative effect of carotenoids on human colon cancer cells without conversion to retinoic acid. *Nutr. Cancer* 32, 20-24.

[103] Tanaka, T., Kawamori, T., Ohnishi, M., Makita, H., Mori, H., Satoh, K., Hara, A., (1995). Suppression of azoxymethane-induced rat colon carcinogenesis by dietary administration of naturally occurring xanthophylls astaxanthin and canthaxanthin during the postinitiation phase. *Carcinogenesis*16, 2957-2963.

[104] Cohen, L.A., Zhao, Z., Pittman, B., Khachik, F., (1999). Effect of dietary lycopene on -methylnitrosourea-induced mammary tumorigenesis. *Nutr. Cancer* 34, 153-159.

[105] Terry, P., Jain, M., Miller, A.B., Howe, G.R., Rohan, T.E., (2002). Dietary intake of folic acid and colorectal cancer risk in a cohort of women. *Nutr. Cancer* 42, 167-172.

[106] Tanaka, T., Shnimizu, M., Moriwaki, H., (2012). Cancer chemoprevention by carotenoids. *Molecules* 17, 3202-3242.

[107] Palozza, P., Serini, S., Calvielio, G., (2006). Carotenoids as modulators of intracellular signaling pathways. *Curr. Signal Transd. T.* 1, 325-335

[108] Bone, R., Landrumb, J., Friedes, L., Gomez, C.M., Kilburn, M.D., Menendez, E., Vidal, I., Wang, W., (1997). Distribution of lutein and zeaxanthin stereoisomers in the human retina. *Exp. Eye Res.* 64, 211-218.

[109] Sies, H., Stahl, W., (2004). Nutritional protection against skin damage from sunlight. *Annu. Rev. Nutr.* 24, 173-200.

[110] Eichler, O., Sies, H., Stahl, W., (2002). Divergent optimum levels of lycopene, β-carotene and lutein protecting against UVB irradiation in human fibroblasts. *Photochem. Photobiol.* 75, 503-506.

[111] Yamaguchi, M., (2012). Role of carotenoid β-cryptoxanthin in bone homeostasis. *J. Biomed. Sci.* 19, 36.

[112] Allam, K.V., Kumar, G.P., (2011). Colorants-the cosmetics for the pharmaceutical dosage forms. *Int. J. Pharm. Pharm. Sci.* 3, 13-21.

[113] Britton, G., Liaaen-Jensen, S., Pfander, H., (2007). Carotenoids, Natural Functions. Vol. 4. Bosel, Birkhauser, 23-24.

[114] Nelson, J.L., Bernstein, P.S., Schmidt, M.C., Von Tress, M.S., Wayne Askew, E., (2003). Dietary modification and moderate antioxidant supplementation differentially affect serum carotenoids, antioxidant levels and markers of oxidative stress in older humans. *J. Nutr.* 133, 3117-3123.

[115] Blanch, A., Hernández, J.M., (2000). Red carotenoids for optimal yolk pigmentation. *Feed Mix* 8, 9-12.

[116] Nickell, D. C., Bromage, N.R., (1998). The effect of dietary lipid level on variation of flesh pigmentation in rainbow trout (*Oncorhynchus mykiss*). *Aquaculture* 161, 237-251.

[117] Alós, E., Roca, M., Iglesias, D.J., Mínguez-Mosquera, M.I., Damasceno, C.M., Thannhauser, T.W., Rose, J.K., Talón, M., Cercós, M., (2008). An evaluation of the basis and consequences of a stay-green mutation in the *navel negra* citrus mutant using transcriptomic and proteomic profiling and metabolite analysis. *Plant Physiol.* 147, 1300-1315.

[118] Aluru, M., Xu, Y., Guo, R., Wang, Z., Li, S., White, W., Wang, K., Rodermel, S., (2008). Generation of transgenic maize with enhanced provitamin A content. *J. Exp. Bot.* 59, 3551-3562..

[119] Li, F., Vallabhaneni, R., Yu, J., Rocheford, T., Wurtzel, E.T., (2008). The maize phytoene synthase gene family, overlapping roles for carotenogenesis in endosperm, photomorpho genesis, and thermal stress tolerance. *Plant Physiol.* 146, 1334-1346.

[120] Welsch, R., Wüst, F., Bär, C., Al-Babili, S., Beyer, P., (2008). A third phytoene synthase is devoted to abiotic stress-induced abscisic acid formation in rice and defines functional diversification of phytoene synthase genes. *Plant Physiol.* 147, 367-380.

[121] Busch, M., Seuter, A., Hain, R., (2002). Functional analysis of the early steps of carotenoid biosynthesis in tobacco. *Plant Physiol.* 128, 439-453.

[122] Fraser, P.D., Romer, S., Shipton, C.A., Mills, P.B., Kiano, J.W., Misawa, N., Drake, R.G., Schuch, W., Bramley, P.M., (2002). Evaluation of transgenic tomato plants expressing an additional phytoene synthase in a fruit-specific manner. *Proc. Natl. Acad. Sci. USA*. 99, 1092-1097.

[123] Zhang, J., Tao, N., Xu, Q., Zhou, W., Cao, H., Xu, J., Deng, X., (2009). Functional characterization of *Citrus PSY* gene in Hongkong kumquat (*Fortunella hindsii* Swingle). *Plant Cell Rep.* 28, 1737-1746.

[124] Burkhardt, P.K., Beyer, P., Wünn, J., Klöti, A., Armstrong, G.A., Schledz, M., Lintig, J., Potrykus, I., (1997). Transgenic rice (*Oryza sativa*) endosperm expressing daffodil (*Narcissus pseudonarcissus*) phytoene synthase accumulates phytoene, a key intermediate of provitamin A biosynthesis. *Plant J.* 11, 1071-1078.

[125] Ye, X., Al-Babili, S., Kloti, A., Zhang, J., Lucca, P., Beyer, P., (2000). Potrykus I, Engineering the provitamin A (beta-carotene) biosynthetic pathway into (carotenoid-free) rice endosperm. *Science* 287, 303-305.
[126] Rosati, C., Aquilani, R., Dharmapuri, S., Pallara, P., Marusic, C., Tavazza, R., Bouvier, F., Camara, B., Giuliano, G., (2000). Metabolic engineering of beta-carotene and lycopene content in tomato fruit. *Plant J.* 24, 413-420.
[127] Dharmapuri, S., Rosati, C., Pallara, P., Aquilania, R., Bouvierb, F., Camarab, B., Giulianoa, G., (2002). Metabolic engineering of xanthophyll content in tomato fruits. *FEBS Lett.* 519, 30-34.
[128] Diretto, G., Tavazza, R., Welsch, R., Pizzichini, D., Mourgues, F., Papacchioli, V., Beyer, P., Giuliano, G., (2006). Metabolic engineering of potato tuber carotenoids through tuber-specific silencing of lycopene epsilon cyclase. *BMC Plant Biol.* 6, 13.
[129] Takaichia, S., Mochimaru, M., (2007). Carotenoids and carotenogenesis in cyanobacteria: unique ketocarotenoids and carotenoid glycosides. *Cell. Mol. Life Sci.* 64, 2607 – 2619.
[130] Jayaraj, J., Devlin, R., Punja, Z., (2008). Metabolic engineering of novel ketocarotenoid production in carrot plants. *Transgenic Res.* 17, 489-501.
[131] Gerjets, T., Sandmann, G., (2006). Ketocarotenoid formation in transgenic potato. *J. Exp. Bot.* 57 (14), 3639-3645.
[132] Zhu, C., Naqvi, S., Breitenbach, J., Sandmann, G., Christoua, P., Capella, T., (2008). Combinatorial genetic transformation generates a library of metabolic phenotypes for the carotenoid pathway in maize. *Proc. Natl. Acad. Sci. USA*. 105, 18232-18237.

In: Citrus
Editor: Khizar Hayat
ISBN: 978-1-63117-985-3

Chapter 5

INFLUENCE OF POSTHARVEST HANDLING ON ANTIOXIDANT COMPOUNDS OF CITRUS FRUITS

Sawsen Sdiri*[*]*, Alejandra Salvador, Imen Farhat,
Pilar Navarro and Cristina Besada
Postharvest Technology Center, Instituto Valenciano de Investigaciones Agrarias, Valencia, Spain

ABSTRACT

Citrus fruits are the world's most popular and economically important fruit crop grown in tropical and subtropical climates in many countries. Citrus fruits are appreciated for their taste and aroma, and for their attractive color. In addition to their eating and refreshing quality, citrus fruits are rich in many phytochemicals, which are important for human nutrition since they possess antioxidant properties. The main part of the total antioxidant activity of citrus fruits is due to the hydrosoluble fraction of vitamin C. Apart from being an important source of vitamin C, citrus fruits are also rich in other bioactive compounds with high antioxidant capacity, such as phenolic compounds and carotenoids. The content of antioxidant compounds in citrus fruits depends on the species, cultivar, climate and other different agronomic factors. Moreover, the practices and treatments that fruits are submitted to during postharvest handling have been shown to affect the antioxidant properties of citrus fruits. As interest in the health benefits of fruits and vegetables has increased in the last few years, many recent studies have focused on improving and preserving the nutritional- and health-related quality of fresh fruits. In the present chapter, the effect of different commonly applied treatments during the postharvest handling of citrus fruits, e.g., cold storage and degreening, on antioxidant compounds are reviewed. Changes in these compounds among species and cultivar, and their evolution during maturity, are discussed.

Keywords: Citrus, vitamin C, antioxidant capacity, phenolic compounds, carotenoids, cold storage, degreening treatment, maturity stages

[*] Corresponding author address: Postharvest Technology Center, Instituto Valenciano de Investigaciones Agrarias, Carretera Moncada-Náquera km 4,5, 46113, Valencia, Spain. Email: sdiri_saw@gva.es.

INTRODUCTION

Citrus is the world's most popular and an economically important fruit crop grown in tropical and subtropical climates in a large number of countries. The worldwide production was estimated at over 100 million tons in 2009, in which 21 million tons being mandarins, clementines and satsumas [1]. World's production trends indicate that oranges constitute about 60% of the total citrus output, followed by mandarins, clementines and satsumas, which comprise about 20% of the output. The group of lemons and limes constitute 11–12%, and grapefruit and pomelos comprise roughly 5–6%. The main citrus fruit-producing countries are Brazil, China, the United States and Mexico, although the whole Mediterranean region ranks first worldwide accounting for 19% of the world citrus production. In this region, citrus fruits are produced mainly for fresh consumption [2].

Citrus fruits are attractive fruits sought by consumers overall the world for their unique taste, flavor, eating quality and health benefits. After harvest, fresh citrus fruit need to be manipulated at different stages with postharvest treatments before reaching consumers.

ANTIOXIDANT COMPOUNDS OF FRESH CITRUS FRUITS

Nowadays, consumers demand high sensory, nutritional and health-related qualities of fruit and their derivatives. Citrus fruits are recognized as being an important component of human diet that provides a range of key nutrients and many non-nutrient phytochemicals which are important for human nutrition as they possess antioxidant properties. The antioxidant and antiradical activity of citrus fruits is due mainly to the hydrosoluble fraction containing vitamin C and polyphenols, but also to the apolar fraction including carotenoids, leading to their protective effects against chronic and degenerative diseases [3-5].

Vitamin C

Citrus fruits are highlighted as an important source of vitamin C. Vitamin C is considered the most important water-soluble antioxidant that destroys oxygen-free radicals [6]. It protects compounds in extracellular and intracellular spaces in most biological systems [7]. It can directly scavenge superoxide radicals, singlet oxygens, hydrogen peroxides and hydroxyl radicals.

The vitamin C content in Citrus depends on the species and the cultivar; it has been reported that among Citrus spp., the vitamin C content in orange fruit is higher than that in mandarins [8-11]. The level of vitamin C also depends on other factors, such as ripening time, harvesting method, storage, processing, climate and other different agronomic factors [12-14].

Vitamin C is an umbrella term for ascorbic acid (AA) and dehydroascorbic acid (DHAA). AA is the dominant reduced form of Vitamin C and DHAA is the oxidized form. These are found in equilibrium in most fruits and vegetables. However, ascorbic acid is very labile and, under adverse conditions, it undergoes oxidation.

The oxidation of L-ascorbic acid, the active form of the vitamin, to DHAA does not result in loss of biological activity since DHAA is readily reconverted into L-ascorbic acid.

However, the subsequent conversion into diketogulonic acids is irreversible. Therefore, it has been suggested that vitamin C measurements in fruits and vegetables in relation to their nutritional value should include both AA and DHAA [15].

Phenolic Compounds

Citrus fruits contain phenolic compounds, especially flavonoids and phenolic acids. In recent years, more attention has been paid to the phenolic compounds of citrus fruits since many epidemiological studies have indicated that consumption of polyphenol-rich foods and beverages is associated with a reduced risk of cardiovascular diseases, stroke and certain cancer forms. It has been suggested that these compounds play an important role in the antioxidant capacity of citrus fruits [16-18]. Moreover, the presence of phenolics contributes to the sensory quality of fruit and juice through their effect on color, bitterness, astringency and flavor [19].

Among the phenolic coumpouds, flavonoids have recently aroused considerable interest because of their potential beneficial effects on human health, such as antiviral, anti-allergic, anti-inflammatory, antioxidant activities, and protection against cardiovascular diseases and certain cancer forms [5, 20-27].

Flavonoid compounds have been studied in many Citrus species, such as oranges [28, 29, 30-34], grapefruits [28-32, 34, 35] lemons [28-31, 34, 36] and limes [28-31, 34]. They are the most abundant phenolics in citrus fruits [28]. The commonest flavonoids found in Citrus spp. can be classified into different groups: flavanones, flavones, flavanols and anthocyanins (specific and unique of pigmented oranges) [21]. The highest concentrations found in Citrus spp. correspond to flavanone glycosides, followed by flavones, flavonols and fully polymethoxylated flavones [5, 28-30]. Hesperidin, narirutin, naringin, eriocitrin and neohesperidin are major flavanone glycosides [30, 31].

Polymethoxylated flavones (PMFs) are also present and exist exclusively in the Citrus genus, especially in the peels of mandarins, sweet and bitter oranges [34]. Although citrus juice contains low concentrations of PMFs, sometimes at the limit of detection, these compounds exhibit high biological activity and have been reported as having anti-inflammatory, antiviral, anti-tumor and anticarcinogenic activity [25, 37-40]. The composition of PMFs varies among *Citrus* species [28, 30, 41].

Anthocyanins, found in blood (pigmented) citrus fruits, have also been associated with potentially beneficial effects on various diseases, such as capillary fragility, diabetic retinopathy and human platelet aggregation [42]. In addition, anthocyanins are known as potent antioxidants [43, 44], and anthocyanin-rich fruit or juice has been associated with greater antioxidant capacity. Main anthocyanins include cyanidin-3-glucoside (Cy3G) and cyanidin-3-(6''-malonyl)-glucoside (Cy3MG) [45], and their level in fruits always varies among varieties. It has been reported that Cy3G has greater antioxidant activity than other more common anthocyanins [43], and that Cy3MG protects plant cells against UV-induced damage [46].

In addition to flavonoids, a major part of phenolic compounds of citrus fruits are benzoic and hydroxycinnamic acids. Previous studies have reported that hydroxycinnamic acids also possess significant antioxidant acticity and chemoprotective effects [47]. The most important phenolic acid in citrus juice is hydroxycinnamic acid and its derivatives: ferulic, ρ-coumaric, sinapic, caffeic and chlorogenic acids [48]. Hydroxycinnamic acids are a class of polyphenolic compounds that are hydroxy derivatives of cinnamic acid. Hydroxybenzoic acids, such as gallic and protocatechuic acid, are also present in low concentrations [49]. Hydroxycinnamic acid has been reported to possess significantly greater antioxidant activity than hydroxybenzoic acids [17, 50, 51].

Carotenoids

Carotenoids are important for citrus fruit quality because the orange color in peel and juice is due mainly to the presence of these pigments [52, 53]. Although the antioxidant capacity of citrus juices has been associated mainly with the hydrosoluble fraction containing polyphenols and vitamin C, the more apolar fraction, including carotenoids as well, could also contribute to the antioxidant capacity of juices.

Carotenoids exert potential action against certain cancer types, protect against age-related macular degeneration and cataracts, and prevent cardiovascular diseases [54-57]. Carotenoids also play an important indirect role in mandarin flavor by being precursors of potent aroma-active volatiles [58, 59].

Citrus fruits are a complex source of carotenoids with the largest number of carotenoids. Approximately 115 different carotenoids have been reported in citrus, including a large number of isomers [60]. Among the carotenoids present in citrus, α- and β-carotene, lycopene, β-cryptoxanthin, lutein, and zeaxanthin are major carotenoids in mandarin, with relatively high concentrations in orange fruit [61]. Some carotenoid compounds (mainly α- and β-carotene, β-cryptoxanthin) are the main precursors of provitamin A in citrus fruits [62].

Carotenoid accumulation occurs in juice sacs of citrus fruits during fruit maturation [52, 61, 63, 64]. Carotenoid content and composition in citrus fruits vary greatly among cultivars [53, 60, 61, 65].

Although the genetic factor has been shown to play an important role in citrus carotenoid composition, other factors, such as maturity stage, geographical origin, cultural practices and postharvest treatments, have been reported to affect the content and composition of carotenoids in citrus fruits [66-74].

INTERSPECIFIC AND VARIETAL INFLUENCE ON ANTIOXIDANT COMPOUNDS

The chemical variability of bioactive compounds of citrus fruits and its relationship with genetic factors has been studied by diverse authors. Based on the bioactive compounds profile (mainly phenolics and the carotenoids profile), the agrupation of different genetically closely related citrus species has been demostrated, which confirms the genotype influence on fruit composition. In general, studies have revealed more interspecific differences than intraspecific ones, although an important varietal influence has also been reported.

Differences in vitamin C content among citrus species have been widely investigated. Bermejo and Cano [75] reported that at commercial harvest stage, 'Fino' lemons showed the highest vitamin C concentration (60.51 mg/100mL juice), followed by clementine mandarins

(59.3 to 47.26 mg/100mL juice) and sweet oranges (50.22 to 44.57 mg/100mL juice), with grapefruits and pummelos displaying the lowest content. However, different results were obtained by Goulas and Manganaris [76] when comparing the ascorbic acid content of citrus fruits grown in Cyprus [orange (cv. 'Valencia'), grapefruit (cvs. 'White Marsh', 'Star Ruby', 'Rio Red') and an interspecific hybrid (*Citrus reticulata* x *Citrus sinensis*, cv. 'Mandora')]; these authors reported that Valencia fruit exhibited the highest ascorbic acid content, grapefruits gave intermediate values, while Mandora fruit had the lower content. This citrus species classification based on ascorbic acid (orange > grapefruit > mandarin) was previously reported by Xu et al. [77]. In agreement with this, Cano et al. [10] found a higher vitamin C content in sweet orange juice than in mandarins. Moreover, Al-Juhaimi and Ghafoor [78] did not observe significant differences in ascorbic acid content between mandarin and orange juice cultivated in Saudi Arabia, and they reported lower content in lemon juice. Xu et al. [77] also reported lower ascorbic acid content in lemon juice if compared to that of mandarins and orange.

Regarding phenolic compounds, it has been recently demostrated that different citrus species can be differenciated based on their phenolic compounds profile. So, Abad-García et al. [79] characterized the phenolic profile of 83 citrus juices covering sweet orange, tangerine, lemon and grapefruit species, and reported that a natural sample grouping among species, and even the citrus subclass, was observed by principal component analyses. Xu et al. [77] reported that general mandarins and oranges gave a higher content of phenolic acids as compared with grapefruits and pummelos. It must be mentioned that among phenolic compounds, anthocyanins are characteristic of blood (pigmented) citrus fruits. The main anthocyanins are cyanidin-3-glucoside (Cy3G) and cyanidin-3-(6β-malonyl)-glucoside (Cy3MG), and their level in fruit always varies among varieties [17, 45, 80].

Among phenolic compounds, special attention has been paid to flavonoid compounds because of their potential beneficial effects on human health. Data on mean flavonoids content present in the juice of different citrus species were collected in the excellent review by Gattuso et al. [81] in sweet orange, hesperidin is specially abundant (28.6mg/100mL), followed by narirutin (5.2mg/100mL) and didymin (1.89 mg/100mL); in mandarin, hesperidin (23, 24.3 mg/100 mL) is also the main component, followed by narirutin (3.92 mg/100 mL) and didymin (1.44 mg/100 mL). These findings confirm that *C. sinensis* and *C. reticulata* are closely related. It has been suggested that the sum of hesperidin and narirutin may be used to classify orange and mandarin cultivars [10], with the former possessing larger amounts [11].

The juice flavonoid composition of sour orange differs from sweet orange, but is similar to that of grapefruit and is rich in naringin (1.96 mg/100 mL), neohesperidin (0.87 mg/100 mL) and neoeriocitrin (0.77 mg/100 mL) [81]. Besides, naringenin is recognized as being a distinctive component of grapefruit juice. Lemon juice is characterized by the presence of significant amounts of hesperidin (20.5 mg/100 mL) and eriocitrin (16.7 mg/100 mL), and is also quite rich in diosmin and diosmetin 6,8-di-C-glucoside, and contains apigenin di-C-glucoside [81]. Bergamont juice is characterized by the presence of considerable amounts of poncirin (6.41 mg/100 mL) and naringin (2.23 mg/100 mL), followed closely by neohesperidin (1.60 mg/100 mL) and neoeriocitrin (1.38 mg/100 mL). Diosmetin 6,8-di-C-glucoside (3.95 mg/100 mL) and apigenin 6,8-di-C-glucoside (4.53 mg/100 mL) are present in almost equal amounts, what is related to the fact that *C. bergamia* descended from a hybrid of *C. limon* and *C. sinensis* [81]. Barreca et al. [82] reported that the main flavonoids detected in chinotto juices are neoeriocitrin (0.3 mg/100 mL), naringin (0.6 mg/100 mL) and neohesperidin (0.57 mg/100 mL).

The particular flavonoid profile of different citrus species has been corroborated by several studies. So it was that Mouly et al. [31] effectively differentiated lemon, lime, grapefruit and sweet orange by a factorial discrimination analysis of the flavanone glycoside composition in juice. Later studies confirmed that, in general, good discrimination among citrus species can be achieved by analyzing the data on their flavonoids content [28, 29, 83].

A strong impact of genotype on carotenoid composition of citrus fruits has been also reported in different studies into a wide range of varieties. Thus Fanciullino et al. [65] studied 25 genotypes that belonged to eight cultivated citrus species, and reported qualitative and quantitative differences in their carotenoids content. Mandarins, sweet orange and sour oranges were closely related, while lemons and limes were separated and came close to citron, but grapefruit and pummelos clustered together. Mandarins, oranges and clementines were the richest species in carotenoids (total content ≥ 22.48 mg/ L), followed by grapefruit, sour oranges, pummelos, but lemons, limes and citrons were poorest in pigments (total content ≤ 1.26 mg/L). Such differences in carotenoid content among citrus species (mandarin, sweet orange > grapefruit, pummelo > lemon) were later confirmed by Xu et al. [77].

Fanciullino et al. [65] reported that β-cryptoxanthin, β-carotene, cis-violaxanthin and lycopene were the major carotenoids that contributed to total content in the above-mentioned citrus species. However, some of these compounds were absent in several genotypes. Agócs et al. [84] described that considerable amounts of lutein are also found in all these species, along with β-citraurin in them all except lime. Goodner et al. [60] reported that the difference in β-cryptoxanthin concentration can be used as a discriminating factor among mandarin, orange and their hybrids since β-cryptoxanthin is detected to a lesser extent in sweet orange varieties.

In a later study, Matsumoto et al. [53] classified 39 citrus varieties based on the carotenoid profile of juice sacs. In this case, they were classified into four clusters in which carotenoid profiles were carotenoid-poor, violaxanthin-abundant, violaxanthin- and phytoene-abundant, and violaxanthin-, phytoene-, and beta-cryptoxanthin-abundant, respectively. The authors also reported that violaxanthin accumulation preceded β-cryptoxanthin accumulation in violaxanthin-, phytoene-, and β-cryptoxanthin-abundant varieties.

The presence of lycopene in citrus fruits is not a common feature. However, several mutants that have been shown to accumulate it, have aroused considerable interest in recent years since the characterization of the mutants altered in the carotenoid biosyntethic pathway is a useful experimental system to identify the molecular mechanisms regulating this process [71, 85]. Most lycopene-accumulating mutants have been identified in grapefruit (*Citrus paradisi*) and pummelo (*Citrus grandis*), but only few have been identified in orange (*Citrus sinensis*) [86-88]. In red mutants of grapefruit and pummelo, total carotenoids content has been increased up to 790 folds [89]. Besides, some mutants with a characteristic color have also been described as displaying an import accumulation of phytoene [90, 91].

After evaluating the carotenoid content of seven sweet orange cultivars, Dhuique Mayer et al. [8] reported that three of them (Sanguinelli, Pera and Shamouti) were clearly different from the rest (Salustiana, Hamlin, Maltaise and Valencia) giving the higher β-cryptoxanthin and β-carotene content. These three varieties have also been characterized by possessing the highest hespeiridin content. Major difference among cultivars have also been described in mandarins; in a study of 13 cultivars and two hybrids of clementine fruits cultivated in Italy

[92], it was observed that some cultivars were characterized by their high vitamin C content, others showed a particularly high content of polyphenols and antioxidant capacity, while others displayed a notable flavonoids content. Moreover, recently we evaluated vitamin C content, flavonoids and antioxidant capacity of nine new triploids mandarins, and reported that three were clearly differenciated from the rest, mainly because of their higher eritrocin and neoeritrocin contents and their lower narirutin and naringin contents. Interestingly, these three cultivars are closely related phylogenetically as they share the same parentals, Fortune mandarin and Ellendale tangor (data not shown).

CHANGES IN ANTIOXIDANT COMPOUNDS OF CITRUS FRUITS DURING RIPENING PROCESS

Different studies have approached changes in the main antioxidant compounds of citrus fruits during the ripening process. These research works have focused mainly on carotenoid content evolution since it is clearly responsible for fruit color. However, a relevant change in vitamin C and phenolic compounds associated with fruit maturation has also been reported.

Regarding changes in vitamin C, Nagy [93] reported that immature citrus fruits contain higher concentrations of vitamin C than ripe fruits. This pattern was later observed in Fino lemon [94] and in Navel and Valencia oranges [95]. A general decrease in vitamin C concentration as maturity advances has also been confirmed recently in *Citrus limon* (lemon), *C. reticulata* (mandarin), *C. sinensis* (sweet orange) and *C. aurantium* (bitter orange) [96], and in 20 citrus cultivars from the Mediterranean region: mandarins, hybrids, sweet oranges, grapefruits, pummelos, citrons, limes and lemons [75]. This decline in vitamin C content was particularly noteworthy for grapefruits and pummelos [75]. Despite the prevailing trend in citrus fruits being a decrease in vitamin C content as maturation progresses, some exceptions have been reported; Yoo et al. [97] described an increment in vitamin C levels in both the peel and flesh of Yuzu fruit (*Citrus junos* Sieb ex Tanaka) as maturation advances.

The research works done on changes in phenolic compounds during citrus fruit ripening have focused mainly on flavonoids and phenolic acids as they are the most abundant phenolics in citrus fruits. Similarly to the general pattern described for vitamin C, most studies have revealed a decline in the total phenolic content linked to fruit ripening. Total phenols have been reported to decline in different citrus species, such as lemon, mandarin, sweet orange, bitter orange [96] yuzu [97] or citron [98].

Similarly, flavonoids have been observed to decrease with maturation in the flesh of citron fruits: [98], grapefruit, pummelo [99, 100], chinotto [82], 'Navel' orange, clementine mandarin or satsuma mandarins [101], or 'Yuzu' [97].

Conversely, the phenolic acids trend during ripening seems to depend considerably on the species, and even on the cultivar. In a study conducted by Rapisarda et al. [102], an increment in hydroxycinnamic acids with maturation has been reported in 'Tarocco' and 'Moro' oranges. However, this pattern has not been observed in the Sanguinello, Naveline, Ovale calabrese or Valencia Late cultivars. Another trend observed in 'Ponkan' and 'Huyou' mandarins has been a sharp decrease in phenolic acids during maturation [103]. Moreover in grapefruit and orange, Peleg et al. [104] reported a distinct evolution for bound acids and free acids during the season as the former remained unchanged or rose slightly from early to late season, while the latter lowered.

During citrus fruit development, a massive accumulation of carotenoids occurs concomitantly with chlorophyll degradation. A change in the carotenoids biosynthetic pathway from β-Є-carotenoid (α-carotene and lutein) accumulation to β-β-carotenoid (β-carotene, β-cryptoxanthin, zea and violaxanthin) accumulation has been noted in the flavedo of satsuma mandarin and 'Valencia' orange with a transition of peel color from green to orange. As fruit maturation progressed, a massive accumulation of β-β-xanthophyll (β-cryptoxanthin, zea and violaxanthin) took place in both flavedo and juice sacs [61]. A substantial accumulation of β-β-xanthophyll has also been described in 'Shamouti', 'Sanguinelli' [71], 'Navelate' oranges [64] and clementine mandarin [105]. Phytoene has been reported to also be a relevant carotenoid during the ripening of certain citrus fruits. In satsuma mandarin, a massive accumulation of phytoene starts after β-β-xanthophyll increment [61]. Moreover, phytoene accumulation has also been described during the ripening of new mutants. So the characterization of the Pinalate mutant, derived from 'Navelate' orange, which produces distinctive yellow fruit instead of the typical bright orange coloring, has revealed an unusual accumulation of linear carotenoids (phytoene, phytofluene and ζ-carotene) in the flavedo of the mutant. The full-colored fruit of Pinalate contained only 10% of xanthophylls, whereas, 98% of total carotenoids in 'Navelate' were xanthophylls and apocarotenoids [90]. Another mutant, 'Cara Cara', a red-fleshed orange derived from 'Washington Navel', has shown a large accumulation of phytoene in peel and pulp. Besides, 'Cara Cara' has been characterized and identified as the only navel orange to accumulate dominant lycopene and B-carotene in flesh during ripening [106].

Therefore, while a general trend can be assumed for most antioxidant compounds during the maturation of citrus fruits, that is, a decline in vitamin C, total phenol content and flavonoids and carotenoids accumulation, we should bear in mind that certain cultivars can show a characteristic pattern during maturation.

It should also be noted that, despite the declining concentration trend of several bioactive compounds during the maturation of citrus fruits, total content per fruit tends to increase since the total volume of juice and fruit size increases as maturity advances.

EFFECT OF COLD STORAGE ON ANTIOXIDANT COMPOUNDS OF CITRUS FRUITS

Storage at low temperature is the predominant method used to preserve postharvest life and to extend marketing time of citrus fruits. Maintaining fruit at low temperature can substantially lower the biological activity of the product, slow the growth and spread of microorganisms, and reduce product moisture loss and susceptibility to get damaged from ethylene gas. Besides the use of low temperature in citrus fruit is also required in specific quarantine cold-treatments.

Changes in antioxidant activity during storage depend on varieties; for instance, antioxidant activity in 'Navelina' oranges remained relatively constant during cold storage as compared to initial values [107]. Whereas, Lafuente et al. [108] described that antioxidant activity measured by both the DPPH and ABTS methods varied in the pulp of 'Fortune' mandarins after a 32-day storage at 1.5°C. Nevertheless, Rapisarda et al. [14] reported an increase in antioxidant capacity, as measured by the DPPH assay, in blood and blond oranges after long-term cold storage at 6°C.

Citrus fruits undergo different chemical and biological changes that affect fruit quality attributes during the postharvest period [109]. Generally, the AA content of fruits and vegetables gradually diminish as storage temperature and/or duration increases [110]. Changes in vitamin C content during storage also depend on the variety.

Some studies have shown that cold storage of 'Clemenules' mandarins and 'Tarocco Messina', 'Tarocco Meli' and 'Navelina' oranges leads to a reduction in their vitamin C content; the higher the storage temperature and the longer the period, the greater the loss is [14, 107, 111]. The ascorbic acid content of 'Blood Red' sweet oranges can also be affected by storage temperature, and its level lowers after storage for 25 days at 5°C [112]. Nevertheless, a significant increase in vitamin C content in 'Cara Cara' and 'Valencia Late' oranges and in 'Fortune' mandarins after low-temperature storage has been recorded [14, 113, 114]. Palma et al. [115] did not find any changes in vitamin C content for 'Fortune' mandarins after 90 days of storage at 5°C. Cold storage at 2°C for 18 days and low-temperature transport did not promote ascorbic acid degradation of 'Ruby Red' and 'Rouge La Toma' grapefruit [116].

Changes in the phenolic compounds of citrus fruits have been the subject of many investigations. In different citrus cultivars, an increase in total phenolic contents (TPC) has been reported after long-term cold storage, which depends on the storage conditions and on the variety [14, 117]. Nevertheless, Palma et al. [115] found no differences in the TPC of 'Fortune' mandarins after a 90-days storage at 5°C.

Regarding flavanones, alterations in flavanone glycosides during cold storage (up to 12-15 days at 4°C) have been determined in segments and juice made from grapefruit, mandarin-type fruits, tangelos and oranges. A significant increase in total flavanones was observed in fruit segments after a storage period. In contrast, a diminution in total and individual flavanones was observed in juices. The concentration of three neohesperidose glycosides, mainly naringin, remained unchanged during the storage period. The increase in flavanone may be attributed to greater phenylalanine ammonia lyase (PAL) activity during low-temperature storage [117].

Generally these studies evidence an increase of some phenolic compounds under cold storage, as in the case of 'Tacle' and 'Clara' (two triploid citrus hybrids), in which flavanones and even anthocyanins and hydroxycinnamic acids increased [118]. Whereas, cold storage can, sometimes, lead to a significant reduction in the level of flavanones like in the case of a study conducted by Sdiri et al. [11] where hespiridin, narirutin, narigin and didymin decreased in 'Navelina' oranges and 'Clemenpons' mandarins and increased in 'Clemenules', 'Oronules', 'Prenules', 'Basol', 'Clemenrubi' and 'Orogros' clementines.

In a similar way, hydroxycynnamic acid levels are closely related to the variety and to storage conditions. Cold temperatures led to a rise of chlorogenic acid of 'Navelina' oranges, 'Clemenpons', 'Oronules', 'Basol', and 'Orogros' mandarins and a decrease of its levels in 'Clemenules', 'Prenules' and 'Clemenrubi' clementines after cold storage [11] and in another study caffeic acid, ferulic acid, sinapic acid and *p*-coumaric acid decreased after 104 days cold storage [14].

Anthocyanin content of blood oranges may significantly increase throughout cold storage [14, 42, 119]. For example a significant increase in anthocyanin concentration during cold storage has been seen for 'Tacle' and 'Clara', and pigment levels were 3- and 9-fold higher than those of fresh fruits after 104 days of storage [118]. Likewise in two 'Tarocco' clones, anthocyanin amounts increased from 4.89 to 23.83 mg/L (5-fold) and from 1.09 to 10.26 mg/L (9- fold) in 'T. Meli' and 'T. Messina', respectively [14]. This accumulation has been reported to be related with activation of the enzymes involved in the biosynthesis of anthocyanins by low temperature [120, 121].

Carotenoids are highly temperature-sensitive and minor variations (1°C) from the optimum temperature may affect color development. Few studies have been conducted on the relationship between storage temperature and changes in fruit color. In 'Navelina' orange fruit, a 7-week storage at 12°C showed a remarkable increase in the content of most carotenoids in fruit flavedo, but they remained the same or increased slightly at 2°C. Phytoene (initially 3 μg/g FW) and phytofluene (initially 1 μg/g FW) increased to 24 and 8-10 μg/g FW, respectively, at 12°C, and respectively remained at about 3 and 1 μg/g FW at 2°C [122]. In 'Cara Cara' navel oranges, carotenoid content in peel was maintained up to 35 days when it slightly increased [91]. In flavedo of satsuma mandarins has been also reported an increase of carotenoids during storage at 5°C [73]. Nevertheless, for 'Or' and 'Odem' mandarins, peel became paler and yellowish after only 4 weeks of storage at 2°C and 5°C [123].

Concerning juice, no significant variations were found in 'Clara' fruit juice pigments during the storage period when total carotenoids increased in 'Tacle' from the 72nd day of storage to level off until 120 days of storage [118]. In satsuma mandarins however, the level of carotenoids in pulp decreased [73]. In another study, Carmona et al. [124] reported that neither the content nor composition of carotenoid changed in the peel and pulp of citrus fruits during postharvest storage when fruit were harvested at optimum rind coloration. Nevertheless, when fruits are harvested with poor peel color, low-temperature storage of citrus fruits can limit color development [73, 125].

Effect of Postharvest Degreening Treatment on Antioxidant Compounds of Citrus Fruits

Degreening with exogenous ethylene exposure is a widely used postharvest treatment applied to accelerate the external color change of citrus fruits, mainly with those cultivars that reach internal maturity while their external peel color is still green [126].

While commercial degreening treatment is being applied, fruits are exposed to 1-5 ppm of ethylene in storage chambers. This low concentration causes a color change during the process, but does not affect fruit quality. Besides ethylene, other factors are involved in this treatment; e.g., temperature, relative humidity (RH), or oxygen and carbon dioxide in the atmosphere. The optimum temperature to cause color change depends on the cultivar and the growing area, and it varies between 18°C to 22°C for mandarins or oranges, and lies between 28°C to 30°C for lemons [127-132]. A relative humidity of about 95% is desirable to achieve satisfactory results in the color change of fruit color and to maintain quality. During degreening treatment, ventilation is required to supply the oxygen needed for ethylene to induce color changes (oxygen concentration has to be maintained above 20%) and to remove carbon dioxide from the degreening room (carbon dioxide is an ethylene antagonist and can induce off-flavors in fruit)[126].

The effect of the degreening treatment on the internal and external qualities of fruits has been extensively studied. Nevertheless the study of the effect of this post-harvest treatment on bioactive compounds has been recently done.

Regarding vitamin C, Sdiri et al. [11, 133] reported that the ascorbic acid content in 'Navelina' oranges and different clemetine cultivars ('Clemenules', 'Clemenpons', Prenules, 'Basol', 'Clemenrubí and 'Orogros') was not affected by ethylene exposure when fruit was submitted to degreening treatment under commercial conditions (2 ppm ethylene, 120 h, 21ºC). No remarkable differences were found between fruit degreened with or without ethylene. Similar results were found in 'Star Ruby' grapefruits degreened for 60 h (2ppm ethylene, 20ºC); so no differences between nondegreened and degreened fruits were encountered in the ascorbic acid levels after ethylene exposure, not even after 35 days of storage following degreening treatment [134].

An important factor to consider in the degreening process is the time required to obtain the desired fruit color, which depends principally on the cultivar and the initial fruit color which, in turn, are controlled by fruit maturity and grove conditions [135]. The effect of degreening treatment length on the vitamin C content of citrus fruits has been studied by Sdiri et al. [133], who reported that ethylene exposures of 48 h, 72 h or 120 h did not give rise to a drop in the vitamin C content of ' Clemenules' and 'Clemenpons' mandarins. Mayuoni et al. [136] detected no notable changes in vitamin C levels in Star Ruby Grapefruit and satsuma mandarins during degreening treatments which lasted from 24 h to 72 h (4ppm ethylene at 20ºC), while the slight decrease in vitamin C content observed in Navel oranges was not attributed to ethylene exposure, but to fruit storage after degreening treatment.

Regarding the effect of ethylene degreening on phenolic compounds, Sdiri et al. [11] recently studied changes in phenolic compounds (flavanones, flavones, polymethaoxy flavones, flavanols, hydroxybenzoic acids and hydroxycinnamic acids) of eight early-season commercial citrus varieties submitted to degreening treatment with or without ethylene exposure (0 ppm or 2 ppm C2H4, 120 h, 21ºC, 95% RH) which were then cold-stored under quarantine conditions (1ºC, 16 days) plus shelf life (20ºC, 7 days, 95% RH). In this study, ethylene did not affect flavanones content since the levels of these compounds in the fruits degreened with or without ethylene exposure after shelf life were the same. The only exception was found in two of all the cultivars studied ('Clemenrubi' and 'Clemenpons' clementines), which showed a higher total flavanones content than untreated fruits after shelf life study. Degreening treatment did not induce changes in any flavonone content in oranges. In clementines, although variation in the level of the individual flavone compounds depends on the cultivar, no relevant changes in total flavone content in relation to ethylene application were observed. Likewise, ethylene exposure did not affect the concentrations of flavonol, quercetin, and phenolic acids (chlorogenic and gallic acids). Similar results were found by Mayouni et al. [136] and Chaudhary et al. [134], who concluded that ethylene treatment did not significantly influence total phenolics and radical scavenging activity in 'Navel' oranges, 'Star Ruby' grapefruit and satsuma mandarins.

Studies that have addressed the effect of postharvest ethylene treatment on carotenoid accumulation have focused on the flavedo of citrus fruits since this treatment is applied usually for degreening citrus fruits [53, 69, 137]. The optimal temperature for carotenoid accumulation in the flavedo of citrus fruits falls within the 15-25ºC range. Although it is known that exogenous ethylene exposure accelerates carotenoid accumulation in flavedo, the effect of ethylene on carotenoid content in flavedo varies with temperature conditions; thus in an ethylene atmosphere, carotenoid accumulation is more dramatically enhanced than in an ethylene-free atmosphere at 20ºC [53, 69], but storage at 5ºC represses carotenoid accumulation in flavedo [73]. Moreover, several studies have reported that in flavedo, ethylene-induced carotenoids accumulation correlates with a simultaneous increase in the gene expression of carotenoid biosynthetic enzymes [69].

Despite the significant health-promoting effect that carotenoids have for humans, not many studies have addressed the effect of postharvest ethylene treatment in edible juice sacs of citrus fruits. Matsumoto et al. [73] studied carotenoid accumulation in flavedo and in juice vesicles of satsuma mandarins at different temperatures and ethylene concentrations. The results of this study suggest that carotenoids biosynthesis in citrus fruit is temperature-sensitive and that the effect of temperature on carotenoid accumulation is tissue-dependent. Thus, storage at 20ºC enhances carotenoid accumulation in flavedo and maintains carotenoid content in edible juice sacs. However storage at 5ºC and 30ºC slightly increases carotenoid content in flavedo and lowers content in edible juice sacs. However this study reveals no effect of exogeneous ethylene on carotenoid content in juice sacs of fruits stored at 20ºC and 5ºC. Similarly a recent study by Chaudhary et al. [134] have reported that degreening treatment with exogeneous ethylene has no significant effect on β-carotene and lycopene content in 'Star Ruby' grapefruit juices.

Therefore by considering these recent findings, we can conclude that degreening treatment can be used to enhance peel color of early citrus fruits with minimal effects on nutritional quality.

CONCLUSION

Citrus fruits provide a wide range of phytochemicals which are important for human nutrition with antioxidant properties. The antioxidant activity of citrus fruits is mainly due to the high content of vitamin C, polyphenols and carotenoids. The content of these bioactive compounds depends on the species, the cultivar as well as on the maturity stage.

During postharvest handling, early season citrus fruits are commonly subjected to degreening treatment with ethylene exposure in order to improve the external color. This postharvest treatment do not induce detrimental changes in antioxidant activity neither in the content of bioative compounds.

Storage at low temperature, used to preserve postharvest life and to extend marketing time of citrus fruits, can affect the content of antioxidant compounds depending on the storage conditions as well as on the species and cultivar.

REFERENCES

[1] FAO (Food and Agriculture Organization of the United Nations), (2009). Citrus Fruit, Fresh and Processed. *Annual statistics*. Available at <http://faostat.fao.org>. Accessed on 02 June, 2012.

[2] CLAM (Comité de Liaison de l'Agrumiculture Méditerranéenne), (2007). Les exportations d'agrumes du basin Méditerranéen. Statistiques, evaluations, repartitions, situation 2006-2007. pp. 121.

[3] Byers, T., Perry, G., (1992). Dietary carotenes, vitamin C, and vitamin E as protective antioxidants in human cancers. *Ann. Rev. Nutri.* 12, 139-159.

[4] Gorinstein, S., Martin-Belloso, O., Park, Y., Haruenkit, R., Lojek, A., Ciz, M., Caspi, A., Libman, A., Trakhtenberg, S., (2001). Comparison of some biochemical characteristics of different citrus fruits. *Food Chem.* 74, 309-315.

[5] Tripoli, E., La Guardia, M., Giammanco, S., Di Majo, D., Giammanco, M., (2007). Citrus flavonoids: Molecular structure, biological activity and nutritional properties: A review. *Food Chem.* 104, 466-479.

[6] Gadjeva, V., Kuchukova, D., Georgieva, R., (2005). Vitamin combinations reduce oxidative stress and improve antioxidant status in patients with iron deficiency anemia. *Comparative Clin. Pathol.* 14, 99-104.

[7] Kaur, C., Kapoor, H.C., (2001). Antioxidants in fruits and vegetables - the millennium's health. *Int. J. Food Sci. Technol.* 36, 703-725.

[8] Dhuique-Mayer, C., Caris-Veyrat, C., Ollitrault, P., Curk, F., Amiot, M.J., (2005). Varietal and interspecific influence on micronutrient contents in citrus from the Mediterranean area. *J. Agric. food Chem.* 53(6), 2140-2145.

[9] Wang, Y.C., Chuang, Y.C., Ku, Y.H., (2007). Quantitation of bioactive compounds in citrus fruits cultivated in Taiwan. *Food Chem.* 102, 1163-1171.

[10] Cano, A., Medina, A., Bermejo, A., (2008). Bioactive compounds in different citrus varieties. Discrimination among cultivars. *J. Food Comp. Anal.* 21(5), 377-381.

[11] Sdiri, S., Navarro, P., Monterde, A., Benabda, J., Salvador, A., (2012a). Effect of postharvest degreening followed by cold-quarantine treatment on vitamin C, phenolic compounds and antioxidant activity of early-season citrus fruit. *Postharvest Biol. Technol.* 65, 13-21.

[12] Lee, S.K., Kader, A.A., (2000). Preharvest and postharvest factors influencing vitamin C content of horticultural crops. *Postharvest Biol. Technol.* 20(3), 207-220.

[13] Huang, R., Xia, R., Hu, L., Lu, Y., Wang, M., (2007). Antioxidant activity and oxygen-scavenging system in orange pulp during fruit ripening and maturation. *Scientia Hort.* 113, 166-172.

[14] Rapisarda, P., Lo Bianco, M., Pannuzzo, P., Timpanaro, N., (2008a). Effect of cold storage on vitamin C, phenolics and antioxidant activity of five orange genotypes [*Citrus sinensis* (L.) Osbeck]. *Postharvest Biol. Technol.* 49, 348-354.

[15] Davey, M.W., Van Montagu, M., Inze, D., Sanmartin, M., Kanellis, A., Smirnoff, N., Benzie, I.J.J., Strain, J.J., Favell, D., Fletcher, J., (2000). Plant L-ascorbic acid: Chemistry, function, metabolism, bioavailability and effects of processing. *J. Sci. Food Agric.* 80 (7), 825-860.

[16] Wang, H., Cao, G.H., Prior, R.L., (1996). Total antioxidant capacity of fruits. *J. Agric. Food Chem.* 44, 701-705.

[17] Rapisarda, P., Tomaino, A., Lo Cascio, R., Bonina, F., De Pasquale, A., Saija, A., (1999). Antioxidant effectiveness as influenced by phenolic content of fresh orange juices. *J. Agric. Food Chem.* 47, 4718-4723.

[18] Gardner, P.T., White, T.A.C., McPhail, D.B., Duthie, G.G., (2000). The relative contributions of vitamin C, carotenoids and phenolics to the antioxidant potential of fruit juices. *Food Chem.* 68, 471-474.

[19] Sousa, W.R., da Rocha, C., Cardoso, C.L., Silva, D.H.S., Zanoni, M.V.B., (2004). Determination of the relative contribution of phenolic antioxidants in orange juice by voltammetric methods. *J. Food Comp. Anal.* 17, 619-633.

[20] Salah, N., Miller, N.J., Paganga, G., Tijburg, L., Bolwell, G.P., Rice-Evans, C., (1995). Polyphenolic flavonols as scavenger of aqueous phase radicals and as chain-breaking antioxidants. *Arch. Biochem. Biophys.* 2, 339-346.

[21] Benavente-García, O., Castillo, J., Marin, F.R., Ortuño, A., Del Río, J.A., (1997). Uses and properties of Citrus flavonoids (Reviews). *J. Agric. food Chem.* 45, 4505-4515.

[22] Kawaii, S., Tomono, Y., Katase, E., Ogawa, K., Yano, M., (1999a). Antiproliferative activity of flavonoids on several cáncer cell lines. *Biosci. Biotechnol. Biochem.* 63, 896-899.

[23] Mandalari, G., Bennett, R.N., Bisignano, G., Trombetta, D., Saija, A., Faulds, C.B., Gasson, M.J., Narbad, A., (2007). Antimicrobial activity of flavonoids extracted from bergamot (*Citrus bergamia* Risso) peel, a byproduct of the essential oil industry. *J. App. Microbiol.* 103 (6), 2056-2064.

[24] Benavente-Garcia, O., Castillo, J., (2008). Update on uses and properties of citrus flavonoids: New finding in anticancer, cardiovascular, and anti-inflammatory activity. *J. Agric. food Chem.* 56, 6185-6205.

[25] Du, Q.Z., Chen, H., (2010). The methoxyflavones in Citrus reticulata Blanco cv. Ponkan and their antiproliferative activity against cancer cells. *Food Chem.* 119, 567-572.

[26] González-Molina, E., Domímguez-Perles, R., Moreno, D.A., García-Viguera, C., (2010). Natural bioactive compounds of *Citrus limon* for food and health. *J. Pharm. Biomed. Anal.* 51, 327-345.

[27] Huang, Y.S., Ho, S.C., (2010). Polymethoxyflavones are responsible for the anti-inflammatory activity of citrus fruit peel. *Food Chem.* 119, 868-873.

[28] Nogata, Y., Sakamoto, K., Shiratsuchi, H., Ishii, T., YANO, M., Ohta, H., (2006). Flavonoid composition of fruit tissues of citrus species. *Biosci. Biotechnol. Biochem.* 70(1), 178-192.

[29] Kawaii, S., Tomono, Y., Katase, E., Ogawa, K., Yano, M., (1999b). Quantitation of flavonoid constituents in citrus fruits. *J. Agric. food Chem.* 47, 3565-3571.

[30] Peterson, J.J., Dwyer, J.T., Beecher, G.R., Bhagwat, S.A., Gebhardt, S.E., Haytowitz, D.B., Holden, J.M., (2006). Flavanones in oranges, tangerines (mandarins), tangors, and tangelos: a compilation and review of the data from the analytical literature. *J. Food Comp. Anal.* 19, S66-S73.

[31] Mouly, P. P., Arzouyan, C. R., Gaydou, E. M., Estienne, J. M., (1994). Differentiation of citrus juices by factorial discriminant analysis using liquid chromatography of flavanone glycosides. *J. Agric. Food Chem.* 42 (1), 70-79.

[32] Franke, A.A., Custer, L.J., Arakaki, C., Murphy, S.P., (2004). Vitamin C and flavonoid levels of fruits and vegetables consumed in Hawaii. *J. Food Comp. Anal.* 17, 1-35.

[33] Abeysinghe, D.C., Li, X., Sun, C.D., Zhang, W.S., Zhou, C.H., Chen, K.S., (2007). Bioactive compounds and antioxidant capacities in different edible tissues of citrus fruit of four species. *Food Chem.* 104, 1338-1344.

[34] Gattuso, G., Barreca, D., Caristi, C., Gargiulli, C., Leuzzi, U., (2007a). Distribution of flavonoids and furocoumarins in juices from cultivars of *Citrus bergamia* Risso. *J. Agric. food Chem.* 55, 9921-9927.
[35] Belajová, E., Suhaj, M., (2004). Determination of phenolic constituents in citrus juices: method of high performance liquid chromatography. *Food Chem.* 86, 339-343.
[36] Del Río, J.A., Fuster, M.D., Gómez, P., Porras, I., García-Lidón, A., Ortuño, A., (2004). *Citrus limon*: A source of flavonoids of pharmaceutical interest. *Food Chem.* 84, 457-461.
[37] Murakami, A., Nakamura, Y., Torikai, K., Tanaka, T., Koshiba, T., Koshimizu, K., Kuwahara, S., Takahashi, Y., Ogawa, K., Yano, M., Tokuda, H., Nishino, H., Mimaki, Y., Sashida, Y., Kitanaka, S., Ohigashi, H., (2000). Inhibitory effect of citrus nobiletin on phorbol ester-induced skin inflammation, oxidative stress, and tumor promotion in mice. *Cancer Res.* 60, 5059-5066.
[38] Suzuki, M., Sasaki, K., Yoshizaki, F., Fujisawa, M., Oguchi, K., Cyong, J.C., (2005). Anti-hepatitis C virus effect of citrus unshiu peel and its active ingredient nobiletin. *Am. J. Chin. Med.* 33, 87-94.
[39] Li, S., Sang, S., Pan, M.H., Lai, C.S., Lo, C.Y., Yang, C.S., Ho, C.T., (2007). Antiinflammatory property of the urinary metabolites of nobiletin in mouse. *Bioorg. Med. Chem. Letters.* 17, 5177-5181.
[40] Walle, T., (2007). Methoxylated flavones, a superior cancer chemopreventive flavonoid subclass? *Sem. Cancer Biol.* 17, 354-362.
[41] Green, C.O., Wheatley, A.O., Osagie, A.U., Morrison, E.Y.St.A., Asemota, H.E., (2007). Determination of polymethoxylated flavones in peels of selected Jamaican and Mexican citrus (*Citrus* spp.) cultivars by high-performance liquid chromatography. *Biomed. Chromatography.* 21, 48-54.
[42] Rapisarda, P., Bellomo, S.E., Intelisano, S., (2001). Storage temperature effects on blood orange fruit quality. *J. Agric. Food Chem.* 49, 3230-3235.
[43] Wang, H., Cao, G., Prior, R.L., (1997). Oxygen radical absorbing capacity of anthocyanins. *J. Agric. Food Chem.* 45, 304-309.
[44] Kähkönen, M.P., Heinonen, M., (2003). Antioxidant activity of anthocyanins and their aglycons. *J. Agric. food Chem.* 51, 628-633.
[45] Maccarone, E., Rapisarda, P., Fanella, F., Arena, E., Mondello, L., (1998). Cyanidin-3-(6-malonyl)-β-glucoside. One of the major anthocyanins in blood orange juice. *Italian J. Food Sci.* 10(4), 367-372.
[46] Takahashi, A., Takeda, K., Ohnishi, T., (1991). Light-induced anthocyanin reduces the extent of damage to DNA in UV-irradiated Centaurea cyanus cells in culture. *Plant Cell Physiol.* 32, 541-547.
[47] Natella, F., Nardini, M., Di Felice, M., Scaccini, C., (1999). Benzoic and cinnamic acid derivatives as antioxidants structure–activity relation. *J. Agric. Food Chem.* 47, 1453-1459.
[48] Kelebek, H., Selli, S., (2011). Determination of volatile, phenolic, organic acid and sugar components in Turkish cv. Dortyol (*Citrus sinensis* L. Osbeck) orange juice. *J. Sci. Food Agric.* 91, 1855-1862.
[49] Kelebek, H., Canbas, A., Selli, S., (2008). Determination of phenolic composition and antioxidant capacity of blood orange juices obtained from cvs. Moro and Sanguinello (*Citrus sinensis* (L.) Osbeck) grown in Turkey. *Food Chem.* 107, 1710-1716.

[50] Rice-Evans, C.A., Miller, N.J., Paganga, G., (1996). Structure-antioxidant activity relationships of flavonoids and phenolic acids. *Free Rad. Biol. Med.* 20, 933-956.

[51] Pulido, R., Bravo, L., Saura-Calixto, F., (2000). Antioxidant Activity of Dietary Polyphenols As Determined by a Modified Ferric Reducing/Antioxidant Power Assay. *J. Agric. Food Chem.* 48, 3396-3402.

[52] Gross, J., (1987). Pigments in fruits. In: Schweigert, B.S., (editor). *Food Science and Technology: A Series of Monographs*. Academic Press, London. pp. 87-98.

[53] Matsumoto, H., Ikoma, Y., Kato, M., Kuniga, T., Nakajima, N., Yoshida, T., (2007). Quantification of carotenoids in citrus fruit by LC-MS and comparison of patterns of seasonal changes for carotenoids among citrus varieties. *J. Agric. Food Chem.* 55 (6), 2356-2368.

[54] Narisawa, T., Fukaura, Y., Oshima, S., Inakuma, T., Yano, M., Nishino, H., (1999). Chemoprevention by the oxygenated carotenoid beta-cryptoxanthin of N-methylnitrosourea-induced colon carcinogenesis in F344 rats. *Jap. J. Cancer Res.* 90, 1061-1065.

[55] Tanaka, T., Kohno, H., Murakami, M., Shimada, R., Kagami, S., Sumida, T., Azuma, Y., Ogawa, H., (2000). Suppression of azoxymethaneinduced colon carcinogenesis in male F344 rats by mandarin juices rich in beta-cryptoxanthin and hesperidin. *Int. J. Cancer* 88, 146-150.

[56] Trumbo, P.R., Ellwood, K.C., (2006). Lutein and zeaxanthin intakes and risk of age-related macular degeneration and cataracts: An evaluation using the Food and Drug Administration's evidence-based review system for health claims. *Am. J. Clin. Nutri.* 84 (5), 971-974.

[57] Voutilainen, S., Nurmi, T., Mursu, J., Rissanen, T.H., (2006). Carotenoids and cardiovascular health. *Am. J. Clin. Nutri.* 83, 1265-1271.

[58] Winterhalter, P., Rouseff, R.L., (2002). Carotenoid-Derived aroma compounds: An introduction. *ACS Symposium Series*. 802, 1-17.

[59] Mahattanatawee, K., Rouseff, R., Valim, M.F., Naim, M., (2005). Identification and Aroma Impact of Norisoprenoids in Orange Juice. *J. Agric. Food Chem.* 53, 393-397.

[60] Goodner, K.L., Rouseff, R.L., Hofsommer, H.J., (2001). Orange, mandarin, and hybrid classification using multivariate statistics based on carotenoid profiles. *J. Agric. Food Chem.* 49 (3), 1146-1150.

[61] Kato, M., Ikoma, Y., Matsumoto, H., Sugiura, M., Hyodo, H., Yano, M., (2004). Accumulation of carotenoids and expression of carotenoid biosynthetic genes during maturation in citrus fruit. *Plant Physiol.* 134 (2), 824-837.

[62] Mares-Perlman, J.A., Millen, A.E., Ficek, T.L., Hankinson, S.E., (2002). The body of evidence to support a protective role for lutein and zeaxanthin in delaying chronic disease. *J. Nutri.* 132, 518S-524S.

[63] Ikoma, Y., Komatsu, A., Kita, M., Ogawa, K., Omura, M., Yano, M., Moriguchi, T., (2001). Expression of a phytoene synthase gene and characteristic carotenoid accumulation during citrus fruit development. *Physiol. Plant.* 111, 232-238.

[64] Rodrigo, M.J., Marcos, J.F., Zacarías, L., (2004). Biochemical and molecular analysis of carotenoid biosynthesis in flavedo of orange (*Citrus sinensis* L.) during fruit development and maturation. *J. Agric. Food Chem.* 52 (22), 6724-6731.

[65] Fanciullino, A.L., Dhuique-Mayer, C., Luro, F., Casanova, J., Morillon, R., Ollitrault, P., (2006). Carotenoid diversity in cultivated citrus is highly influenced by genetic factors. *J. Agric. Food Chem.* 54 (12), 4397-4406.

[66] Mouly, P.P., Gaydou, E.M., Lapierre, L., Corsetti, J., (1999). Differentiation of several geographical origins in single strength Valencia orange juices using quantitative comparison of carotenoid profiles. *J. Agric. Food Chem.* 47, 4038-4045.

[67] Lee, H.S., Castle, W.S., (2001). Seasonal changes of carotenoid pigments and color in Hamlin, Earlygold, and Budd Blood orange juices. *J. Agric. Food Chem.* 49, 877-882.

[68] Lester, G.E., Manthey, J.A., Buslig, B.S., (2007). Organic vs conventionally grown Rio Red whole grapefruit and juice: Comparison of production inputs, market quality, consumer acceptance, and human health-bioactive compounds. *J. Agric. Food Chem.* 55, 4474-4480.

[69] Rodrigo, M.J., Zacarías, L., (2007). Effect of postharvest ethylene treatment on carotenoid accumulation and the expression of carotenoid biosynthetic flavedo of orange (*Citrus sinensis* L. Osbeck) fruit. *Postharvest Biol. Technol.* 43, 14-22.

[70] Beltran-González, F., Perez-Lopez, A.J., Lopez-Nicolas, J.M., Carbonell-Barrachina, A.A., (2008). Effects of agricultural practices on instrumental colour, mineral content, carotenoid composition, and sensory quality of mandarin orange juice, cv. Hernandina. *J. Sci. Food Agric.* 88, 1731-1738.

[71] Fanciullino, A.L., Dhuique-Mayer, C., Froelicher, Y., Talón, M., Ollitrault, P., Morillon, R., (2008). Changes in carotenoid content and biosynthetic gene expression in juice sacs of four orange varieties (*Citrus sinensis*) differing in flesh fruit color. *J. Agric. Food Chem.* 56 (10), 3628-3638.

[72] Girennavar, B., Jayaprakasha, G.K., Mclin, S.E., Maxim, J., Yoo, K.S., Patil, B.S., (2008). Influence of electron-beam irradiation on bioactive compounds in grapefruits (*Citrus paradisi* Macf.). *J. Agric. Food Chem.* 56, 10941-10946.

[73] Matsumoto H, Ikoma Y, Kato M, Nakajima N, Hasegawa Y., (2009). Effect of Postharvest Temperature and Ethylene on Carotenoid Accumulation in the Flavedo and Juice Sacs of Satsuma Mandarin (*Citrus unshiu* Marc.) Fruit. *J. Agric. Food Chem.* 57, 4724-4732.

[74] Navarro, J.M., Perez-Perez, J.G., Romero, P., Botia, P., (2010). Analysis of the changes in quality in mandarin fruit, produced by deficit irrigation treatments. *Food Chem.* 119, 1591-1596.

[75] Bermejo, A., Cano, A., (2012). Analysis of Nutritional Constituents in Twenty Citrus Cultivars from the Mediterranean Area at Different Stages of Ripening. *Food Nutri.* 3, 639-650.

[76] Goulas, V., Manganaris, G. A., (2012). Exploring the phytochemical content and the antioxidant potential ofcitrus fruits grown in Cyprus. *Food Chem.* 131(1), 39-47.

[77] Xu, G., Ye, X., Liu, D., Ma, Y., Chen, J., (2008). Composition and distribution of phenolic acids in Ponkan (*Citrus poonenesis* Hort. ex Tanaka) and Huyou (*Citrus paradisi* Macf. Changshanhuyou) during maturity. *J. Food Comp. Anal.* 21 (5), 382-389.

[78] Al-Juhaimi, F. Y., Ghafoor, K., (2013). Bioactive compounds, antioxidant and physico-chemical properties of juice from lemon, mandarin and orange fruits cultivated in Saudi Arabia. *Pak. J. Bot.* 45 (4), 1193-1196.

[79] Abad-García, B., Berrueta, L.A., Garmón-Lobato, S., Urkaregi, A., Gallo, B., Vicente, F., (2012). Chemometric characterization of fruit juices from Spanish cultivars according to their phenolic compound contents: I. citrus fruits. *J. Agric. Food Chem.* 60 (14), 3635-3644.
[80] Proteggente, A.R., Saija, A., De Pasquale, A., Rice-Evans, C.A., (2003). The compositional characterisation and antioxidant activity of fresh juices from sicilian sweet orange (*Citrus sinensis* L. Osbeck) varieties. *Free Rad. Res.* 37 (6), 681-687.
[81] Gattuso, G., Barreca, D., Gargiulli, C., Leuzzi, U., Caristi, C., (2007b). Flavonoid composition of citrus juices. *Molecules.* 12 (8), 1641-1673.
[82] Barreca, D., Bellocco, E., Caristi, C., Leuzzi, U., Gattuso, G., (2010). Flavonoid composition and antioxidant activity of juices from chinotto (*Citrus*× *myrtifolia* Raf.) fruits at different ripening stages. *J. Agric. Food Chem.* 58 (5), 3031-3036.
[83] Sentandreu, E., Izquierdo, L., Sendra, J.M., (2007). Differentiation of juices from clementine (*Citrus clementina*), clementine-hybrids and satsuma (*Citrus unshiu*) cultivars by statistical multivariate discriminant analysis of their flavanone-7-O-glycosides and fully methoxylated flavones content as determined by liquid chromatography. *Eur. Food Res. Technol.* 224 (4), 421-429.
[84] Agócs, A., Nagy, V., Szabó, Z., Márk, L., Ohmacht, R., Deli, J., (2007). Comparative study on the carotenoid composition of the peel and the pulp of different citrus species. *Innov. Food Sci. Emerging Technol.* 8 (3), 390-394.
[85] Xu, J., Tao, N., Liu, Q., Deng, X., (2006). Presence of diverse ratios of lycopene/β-carotene in five pink or red-fleshed citrus cultivars. *Scientia Hort.* 108, 181-184.
[86] Monselise, S.P., Halevy, A.H., (1961). Detection of lycopene in pink orange fruit. *Science,* 133(3463), 1478-1478.
[87] Lee, H.S., (2001). Characterization of carotenoids in juice of red navel orange (Cara Cara). *J. Agric. Food Chem.* 49 (5), 2563-2568.
[88] Liu, Q., Xu, J., Liu, Y., Zhao, X., Deng, X., Guo, L., Gu, J., (2007). A novel bud mutation that confers abnormal patterns of lycopene accumulation in sweet orange fruit (*Citrus sinensis* L. Osbeck). *J. Exp. Bot.* 58 (15-16), 4161-4171.
[89] Xu, C.J., Fraser, P.D., Wang, W.J., Bramley, P.M., (2006). Differences in the carotenoid content of ordinary citrus and lycopene-accumulating mutants. *J. Agric. Food Chem.* 54 (15), 5474-5481.
[90] Rodrigo, M.J., Marcos, J.F., Alférez, F., Mallent M. D., Zacarías, L., (2003). Characterization of Pinalate, a novel *Citrus sinensis* mutant with a fruit-specific alteration that results in yellow pigmentation and decreased ABA content. *J. Exp. Bot.* 54 (383), 727-738.
[91] Tao, N., Hu, Z., Liu, Q., Xu, J., Cheng, Y., Guo, L., Guo, W. Deng, X,. (2007). Expression of phytoene synthase gene (Psy) is enhanced during fruit ripening of Cara Cara navel orange (*Citrus sinensis* Osbeck). *Plant Cell Rep.* 26 (6), 837-843.
[92] Milella, L., Caruso, M., Galgano, F., Favati, F., Padula, M.C., Martelli, G., (2011). Role of the cultivar in choosing Clementine fruits with a high level of health-promoting compounds. *J. Agric. Food Chem.* 59 (10), 5293-5298.
[93] Nagy, S., (1980). Vitamin C contents of citrus fruit and their products: a review. *J. Agric. Food Chem.* 28, 8-18.

[94] González-Molina, E., Moreno, D.A., García-Viguera, C., (2008). Genotype and harvest time influence the phytochemical quality of fino lemon juice (*Citrus limon* (L.) Burm. F.) for industrial use. *J. Agric. Food Chem.* 56 (5), 1669-1675.

[95] Mbogo, G.P., Mubofu, E. B., Othman, C.C., (2010). Postharvest changes in physico-chemical properties and levels of some inorganic elements in off vine ripened orange (*Citrus sinensis*) fruits cv (Navel and Valencia) of Tanzania. *African J. Biotechnol.* 9 (12), 1809-1815.

[96] Rekha, C., Poornima, G., Manasa, M., Abhipsa, V., Devi, J.P., Kumar, H. T.V., Kekuda, T.R.P., (2012). Ascorbic Acid, Total Phenol Content and Antioxidant Activity of Fresh Juices of Four Ripe and Unripe Citrus Fruits. *Chem. Sci. Transactions.* 1 (2), 303-310.

[97] Yoo, K.M., Lee, K.W., Park, J.B., Lee, H.J., Hwang, I.K., (2004). Variation in major antioxidants and total antioxidant activity of Yuzu (*Citrus junos* Sieb ex Tanaka) during maturation and between cultivars. *J. Agric. Food Chem.* 52 (19), 5907-5913.

[98] Menichini, F., Loizzo, M.R., Bonesi, M., Conforti, F., De Luca, D., Statti, G.A., de Cindio, B., Menichini, F., Tundis, R., (2011). Phytochemical profile, antioxidant, anti-inflammatory and hypoglycemic potential of hydroalcoholic extracts from *Citrus medica* L. cv Diamante flowers, leaves and fruits at two maturity stages. *Food Chem. Toxicol.* 49 (7), 1549-1555.

[99] Jourdan, P.S., McIntosh, C.A., Mansell, R.L., (1985). Naringin levels in Citrus tissues: II. Quantitative distribution of naringin in *Citrus paradisi* MacFad. *Plant Physiol.* 77 (4), 903-908.

[100] Ortuño, A., Garcia-Puig, D., Fuster, M.D., Pérez, M.L., Sabater, F., Porras, I., Garcia-Lidón, A., Del Rio, J.A., (1995). Flavanone and nootkatone levels in different varieties of grapefruit and pummelo. *J. Agric. Food Chem.* 43 (1), 1-5.

[101] Omidbaigi, R., Nasiri, M.F., (2004). Quantitative distribution of hesperidin in Citrus species, during fruit maturation and optimal harvest time. *Nat. Prod. Radiance.* 3 (1), 12-15.

[102] Rapisarda, P., Carollo, G., Fallico, B., Tomaselli, F., Maccarone, E., (1998). Hydroxycinnamic acids as markers of Italian blood orange juices. *J. Agric. Food Chem.* 46 (2), 464-470.

[103] Xu, G., Liu, D., Chen, J., Ye, X., Ma, Y., Shi, J., (2008). Juice components and antioxidant capacity of citrus varieties cultivated in China. *Food Chem.* 106(2), 545-551.

[104] Peleg, H., Naim, M., Rouseff, R.L., Zehavi, U., (1991). Distribution of bound and free phenolic acids in oranges (*Citrus sinensis*) and grapefruits (*Citrus paradisi*). *J. Sci. Food Agric.* 57 (3), 417-426.

[105] Alós, E., Cercós, M., Rodrigo, M.J., Zacarías, L., Talón, M., (2006). Regulation of color break in citrus fruits. Changes in pigment profiling and gene expression induced by gibberellins and nitrate, two ripening retardants. *J. Agric. Food Chem.* 54 (13), 4888-4895.

[106] Xu, J., Deng, X.X., (2002) Identification of main pigment in "Cara Cara" (*Citrus sinensis* L.) and evaluation of their concentration changes during fruit development and storage. *Acta Hort. Sinica.* 29, 203-208 (in Chinese).

[107] Plaza, L., Crespo, I., de Pascual-Teresa, S., de Ancos, B., Sánchez-Moreno, C., Muñoz, M., Cano, M.P., (2011). Impact of minimal processing on orange bioactive compounds during refrigerated storage. *Food Chem.* 124, 646-651.

[108] Lafuente, M.T., Ballester, A.R., Calejero, J., Gonzalez-Candelas, L., (2011). Effect of high temperature-conditioning treatments on quality, flavonoid composition and vitamin C of cold stored 'Fortune' mandarins. *Food Chem.* 128, 1080-1086.

[109] D'Aquino, S., Palma, A., Agabbio, M., Tijskens, L.M.M., Vollebregt, H.M., (2003). Response of three citrus species to different hygrometric conditions. *Acta Hort.* 604, 631-635.

[110] Adisa, V.A., (1986). The influence of molds and some storage factors on the ascorbic acid content of orange and pineapple fruits. *Food Chem.* 22, 139-146.

[111] Pérez, A.G., Luaces, P., Oliva, J., Ríos, J.J., Sanz, C., (2005). Changes in vitamin C and flavour components of mandarin juice due to curing of fruits. *Food Chem.* 91, 19-24.

[112] Rab, A., Sajid, M., Khan, N.U., Nawab, K., Arif, M., Khattak, M.K., (2012). Influence of storage temperature on fungal prevalence and quality of citrus fruits (cv. Blood Red). *Pak. J. Bot.* 44 (2), 831-836.

[113] Huang, R., Xia, R., Lu, Y., Hu, L., Xu, Y,. (2008). Effect of pre-harvest salicylic acid spray treatment on post-harvest antioxidant in the pulp and peel of 'Cara cara' navel orange (*Citrus sinensis* L. Osbeck). *J. Sci. Food Agric.* 88, 229-236.

[114] Sdiri, S., Monterde, A., Benabda, J., Rojas, C., Salvador, A., (2008). Effect of postharvest heat treatments on vitamin C content and quality of 'Fortune' mandarin (*Citrus reticulata*, Blanca). *Proceeding Int. Soc. Citric.* 11, 1351-1355.

[115] Palma, A., D´Aquino, S., Agabbio, M., Schirra, S., (2005). Changes in flavonoids, ascorbic acid, polyphenol content and antioxidant activity in cold stored 'Fortune' Mandarin. *Acta Hort.* 682, 617-622.

[116] Biolatto, A., Vazquez, D.E., Sancho, A.M., Carduza, F.J., Pensel, N.A., (2005). Effect of commercial conditioning and cold quarantine storage treatments on fruit of 'Rouge La Toma' grapefruit (*Citrus paradise* Macf.). *Postharvest Biol. Technol.* 35, 167-176.

[117] Patil, B.S., Vanamal, J., Hullman, G., (2004). Irradiation and storage influence on bioactive components and quality of early and late season 'Rio Red' grapefruit (*Citrus parasidi* Macf.). *Postharvest Biol. Technol.* 34, 53-64.

[118] Rapisarda, P., Bellomo, S., Fabroni, S., Russo, G., (2008b). Juice quality of two new mandarin-like hybrids (*Citrus clementina* Hort. ex Tan x *Citrus sinensis* L. Osbeck) containing anthocyanins. *J. Agric. Food Chem.* 56, 2074-2078.

[119] Crifò, T., Petrone, G., Lo Cicero, L., Lo Piero, A.R., (2012). Short cold storage enhances the anthocyanin contents and level of transcripts related to their biosynthesis in blood oranges. *J. Agric. Food Chem.* 60, 476-481.

[120] Lo Piero, A.R., Puglisi, I., Rapisarda, P., Petrone, G., (2005). Anthocyanins accumulation and related gene expression in red orange fruit induced by low temperature. *J. Agric. Food Chem.* 53, 9083-9088.

[121] Crifò, T., Puglisi, I., Petrone, G., Reforgiato Recupero, G., Lo Piero, A.R., (2011). Expression analysis in response to low temperature stress in blood oranges: implication of the flavonoid biosynthetic pathway. *Gene.* 476, 1-9.

[122] Carmona, L., Zacarías, L., Rodrigo, M.J., (2012). Stimulation of coloration and carotenoid biosynthesis during postharvest storage of 'Navelina' orange fruit at 12 ºC. *Postharvest Biol. Technol.* 74, 108-117.

[123] Tietel, Z., Lewinsohn, E., Fallik, E., Porat, R., (2012) Importance of storage temperatures in maintaining flavor and quality of mandarins. *Postharvest Bio. Technol.* 64(1), 175-182.

[124] Carmona, L., Zacarías, L., Rodrigo, M.J., (2007). Efecto de la temperatura de conservación en la síntesis y acumulación de carotenoids en frutos cítricos. Congreso Iberoamericano de Tecnología Postcosecha y Agroexportaciones. 453-461.

[125] Van, Wyk, A.A., Huysamer, M., Barry, G.H., (2009). Extended low-temperature shipping adversely affects rind colour of 'Palmer Navel' sweet orange [*Citrus sinensis* (L.) Osb.] due to carotenoid degradation but can partially be mitigated by optimising post-shipping holding temperature. *Postharvest Biol. Technol.* 53, 109-116.

[126] Sdiri, S.; Navarro, P., Salvador, A., (2011). Postharvest degreening treatment on citrus fruit: Effect on external and internal quality. In: D.A. Slaker, D.A., (editor). *'Nutrition and Diet Research Progress. Citrus fruits: Properties, consumption and nutrition'.* Nova Science Publishers, Inc. New York. pp 137-149.

[127] Barry, G.H., Van Wyk, A.A., (2006). Low-temperature cold shock may induce rind colour development of 'Nules Clementine' mandarin (*Citrus reticulata* Blanco) fruit. *Postharvest Biol. Technol.* 40(1), 82-88.

[128] Porat, R., Weiss, B., Cohen, L., Daus, A., Goren, R., Droby, S., (1999). Effects of ethylene and 1-methylcyclopropene on the postharvest qualities of 'Shamouti' oranges. *Postharvest Biol. Technol.* 15,155-163.

[129] Ritenour, M.A., Miller, W.M., Wardowski, W.W., (2003). Recommendations for degreening Florida fresh citrus fruits. Circular 1170. Horticultural Sciences Department, Florida Cooperative Extension Service, IFAS, University of Florida, Gainesville.

[130] Smilanick, J.L., Mansour, M.F., Sorenson, D., (2006). Pre- and Postharvest treatments to control green mold of citrus fruit during ethylene degreening. *Plant Dis.* 90, 89-96.

[131] Tugwell, B., (1999). Citrus Handling Guide. Adelaide, Australia: South Australian Research and Development Institute, ISBN 0730852458.

[132] Zhang, J.X., (2007). The potential of a new fungicide fludioxonil for stem-end rot and green mold control on Florida citrus fruit. *Postharvest Biol. Technol.* 46 (3), 262-270.

[133] Sdiri, S., Navarro, P., Salvador, A., (2012b). Antioxidant activity and vitamin C are not affected by degreening treatment of clementine mandarins. *Acta Hort.* 934 (2), 893-899.

[134] Chaudhary, P., Jayaprakasha, G.K., Porat, R., Patil, B.S., (2012). Degreening and postharvest storage influences 'Star Ruby' grapefruit (*Citrus paradisi* Macf.) bioactive compounds. *Food Chem.* 135, 1667-1675.

[135] Martínez-Jávega, J.M., Monterde, A., Navarro, P., Salvador, A., (2008). Response of new clementines to degreening treatment. *Proc. Int. Soc. Citric.* 11, 1342-1346.

[136] Mayuoni, L., Tietel, Z., Patil, B.S., Porat, R., (2011). Does ethylene degreening affect internal quality of citrus fruit? *Postharvest Biol. Technol.* 62, 50-58.

[137] Stewart, I., Wheaton, T.A., (1972). Carotenoids in citrus: Their accumulation induced by ethylene. *J. Agric. Food Chem.* 20, 448-449.

In: Citrus
Editor: Khizar Hayat

ISBN: 978-1-63117-985-3

Chapter 6

Prophylactic Propensity of Citrus Phytochemicals: Action and Mechanisms

***D. Ramful-Baboolall*[1], *V. S. Neergheen-Bhujun*[2] *and T. Bahorun*[3,*]**

[1]Department of Agricultural and Food Science, Faculty of Agriculture, University of Mauritius, Réduit, Republic of Mauritius

[2]Department of Health Sciences, Faculty of Science and ANDI Centre of Excellence for Biomedical and Biomaterials Research, University of Mauritius, Réduit, Republic of Mauritius

[3]ANDI Centre of Excellence for Biomedical and Biomaterials Research, University of Mauritius, Réduit, Republic of Mauritius

Abstract

The role played by dietary factors on health status has long been recognized but it has been only recently that epidemiological, clinical and cell-culture studies have provided a clearer insight on the chemical and physiological mechanisms of the effects of bioactive food constituents on human health. Citrus fruits are rich in phytochemicals which have been reported to contribute to optimal health and may protect against degenerative diseases such as cancer, cardiovascular diseases and diabetes. A number of mechanisms of action have been proposed for the protective effects of citrus fruits including antioxidant activity, regulation of gap-junction communication between cells, inhibition of tumor growth and nitrosation, inhibition of the enzyme topoisomerase II in cancer cells and reduction of advanced glycation end-products in diabetes models. With the background of comprehensive studies conducted on Mauritian citrus fruits, this chapter reviews some of the literature data on the modes of action of citrus phytochemicals in disease prevention and management with a focus on diabetes, cancer and neurodegenerative diseases.

* Corresponding author address: ANDI Centre of Excellence for Biomedical and Biomaterials Research, University of Mauritius, Réduit, Republic of Mauritius. Email: tbahorun@uom.ac.mu.

Keywords: Phytochemicals, citrus fruits, mechanisms of action, disease prevention, management

INTRODUCTION

Many diseases are caused by the *in vivo* action of free radicals and reactive oxygen species such as superoxide ($O_2^{\bullet-}$), hydrogen peroxide (H_2O_2), hypochlorous acid (HOCl) and the hydroxyl radicals ($OH^{\bullet}$) [1-4]. ROS-induced oxidation can result in cell membrane disintegration, membrane protein damage and DNA mutation, which can further initiate or propagate the development of diseases including cancer [5], diabetes [6], neurodegenerative diseases [7], the process of aging [8] and cardiovascular dysfunctions [8]. This kind of risk can be mitigated by suitable dietary habits including a high proportion of fruits and vegetables containing prophylactic antioxidants. Indeed, the focus of nutrition research, today, is heading towards the concept of 'Preventive Medicine'. Meta-analysis of recent epidemiologic studies indicates that the regular consumption of non-nutritive bioactive phytoconstituents, derived from plant-based diet, can reduce the risk of a number of diseases [9].

Polyphenols represent an important class of plant-derived phytochemicals which play a crucial role in health promotion and disease prevention by mechanisms related to cell differentiation, deactivation of pro-carcinogens, maintenance of DNA repair, inhibition of N-nitrosamine formation and modulation of estrogen metabolism, amongst others [10]. Dietary phytophenolics are present in a number of frequently consumed foods, especially fruits, vegetables, grains, legumes and seeds, and in beverages like teas and wines [11]. By virtue of their hydrogen and electron donating abilities and metal chelating effects [12–14], these compounds exhibit a wide range of biological properties including anti-allergenicity, anti-atherogenicity, anti-inflammatory, anti-microbial, anti-thrombotic, cardioprotective and vasodilatory actions [15–19].

Citrus fruits are an important source of such phytochemicals. They are produced in many countries around the world with geographical concentrations in certain regions and rank first in international fruit trade in terms of value, progressing from a producer-driven to a more consumer-oriented market. Oranges, grapefruits, and lemons are considered as the most consumed citrus fruits throughout the world [20]. Fresh and processed citrus fruits in the form of juices, marmalades, jams and pastes are indeed very popular. Consumption of citrus fruit or juice appears to be associated with improved blood lipid [21] and blood glucose [22] profiles, survival in the elderly [23], lower risk of cancers [24], lowering of blood pressure [25], reduced risks of stroke [26], cardiovascular and coronary heart diseases and obesity [27]. The health promoting effects of citrus fruits have been mainly related to their antioxidant vitamin C and flavonoid contents. More than sixty flavonoid compounds have so far been identified in *Citrus sp.* and a majority of them can be regrouped into flavanones, flavones and flavonols existing as glycoside or aglycone forms [3]. Citrus peels, especially, are reported to possess the highest amounts of flavonoids compared to other parts of the fruit [28]. Citrus fruits therefore represent a natural source of antioxidant prophylactics that can be judiciously exploited in the fight against ROS-mediated diseases. This chapter highlights the phytophenolic composition of citrus fruits with emphasis on their flavonoids and related antioxidative potency as well as the prophylactic potential of citrus extracts in the management of diabetes, cancer and neurodegenerative diseases.

TAXONOMY, CULTIVARS AND ANATOMY OF CITRUS FRUITS

Citrus fruits belong to the family *Rutaceae* and subfamily *Aurantioideae* [29]. They are non-climacteric hesperidium berries originating in south-eastern Asia [30]. At the origin, a small number of species existed which gave birth to a multiple number of varieties and hybrids [31]. The scientific and common names of commercially important citrus fruits and their complex array of hybrids are given in Table 1.

Table 1. Botanical names of edible *Citrus*, *Citrus* relatives and *Citrus* hybrids [32]

Botanical name				Common name
Citrus sinensis				Sweet orange
Citrus aurantium				Sour orange/Bitter orange
Citrus reticulata				Mandarin (tangerine)
Citrus paradisi				Grapefruit
Citrus grandis				Pummelo (Pamplemousses)
Citrus limon				Lemon
Citrus medica				Citron
Citrus aurantifolia				Lime
Citrus mitis				Calamondin
Poncirus trifoliata				Trifoliate orange
Fortunella margarita				Kumquat
Common hybrids				
Tangor	=	Mandarin	x	Sweet orange
Tangelo	=	Mandarin	x	Grapefruit
Lemonine	=	Lemon	x	Lime
Citrange	=	Sweet orange	x	*Poncirus*
Limequat	=	Lime	x	Kumquat
Calamansi	=	Mandarin	x	Kumquat

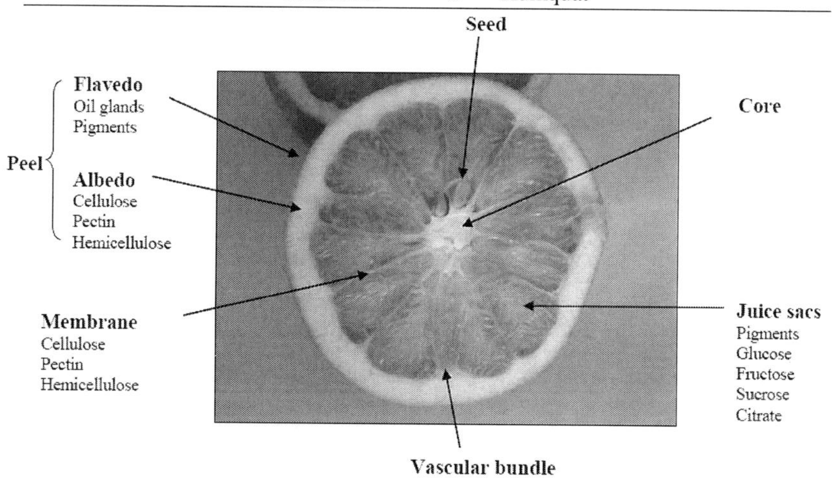

Figure 1. Equatorial cross-section of a citrus fruit.

Anatomically, citrus fruits are superior ovaries composed of 6 to 20 united carpels which form locules [33, 34]. The pericarp exterior to the locules is subdivided into the exocarp (flavedo or exterior peel), mesocarp (albedo or interior peel) and endocarp (locule or segment membrane). The juice vesicles, which are the edible portion of citrus fruit, arise from epidermal or subepidermal promordia on the surface of the endocarp and grow to fill the locular cavity [34] (Figure 1).

Flavedo

The exocarp or flavedo has a pigmentation that varies according to the species or variety and which is due to the presence of carotenoids or chlorophyll [35]. There are numerous essential oil glands in the flavedo, containing aromatic oils which can be industrially extracted and used in food flavoring, tea and aromatherapy [36].

Albedo

The mesocarp or white albedo portion of the peel consists of colourless cells which are typically eight-armed, parenchymous, highly vacuolated, and tube-like [34]. The tissue contains large air spaces, imparting a spongy nature. A network of vascular tissue branches through the albedo and extends from the main bundles that run parallel to the fruit axis to the outside of the segments at three locations per segment from where juice vesicles are attached [37]. The core of the fruit resembles the albedo and contains vascular bundles and parenchymous tissue [34].

Peel

Albedo and flavedo together make up what is called the peel or rind, and contain more bitter principles and pectin than other parts of the fruit.

Juice Vesicles

The endocarp portion of citrus fruit is the most complex, giving rise to juice sacs or vesicles [35]. Juice sac cells are highly vacuolated and the narrow cytoplasm contains lipid droplets in plastids, leucoplasts and chromoplasts [38]. Juice within the vacuole of these cells contains essentially all the titratable acids and other soluble materials such as amino acids and salts [35].

PHYTOCHEMICAL CONSTITUENTS OF CITRUS FRUITS

Citrus fruits contain hundreds of active ingredients which can affect human health in several ways. These include carbohydrates, fibre, vitamin C, potassium, folate, calcium, thiamine, niacin, vitamin B6, vitamin A (beta-carotene), phosphorous, magnesium, copper, riboflavin, pantothenic acid and a variety of phytochemicals. Phytochemicals are plant secondary metabolites having a potential for modulating human metabolism in a manner favourable for the prevention of chronic and degenerative diseases.

Polyphenols

Polyphenols encompass a wide array of naturally occurring compounds which contain one or more benzene rings, each with one or more hydroxyl group substitutions. Cinnamic acid derivatives, coumarins and flavonoids (flavanones, flavones and flavonols) are the major groups of phenolic compounds in citrus either in free form and/or as glycosides. Other groups of phenolic compounds such as hydroxycinnamates, psolarens and polymethoxylated flavones have also been detected in citrus peels [39, 40]. Phenolic acids such as caffeic, *p*-coumaric, ferulic and sinapic acids are principally located in the flavedo of citrus fruits (41, 28). The flavonoids, however, remain the most predominant phenolics in citrus fruits. Two recent studies investigated the total phenolics and flavonoids of the flavedo and pulp extracts of 21 varieties of citrus fruits grown in Mauritius. The total phenolics of the pulp extracts ranged from 406 ± 14 to 1694 ± 19 µg/g fresh weight (FW) whilst the total flavonoids varied between 133 ±6 and 965 ± 7 µg/g FW [42]. The indicative total phenols were comparable to values reported by Gorinstein et al. [43] for 3 citrus pulps which varied between 1350 and 1640 µg/g FW. These levels were lower than those of flavedo extracts of the same varieties which were between 1882 to 7667 µg/g FW [44]. Gorinstein et al. [43] also reported total polyphenols in the peels of lemons, oranges and grapefruits to be significantly higher than in the peeled fruits.

Flavonoids

Most citrus species accumulate substantial quantities of flavonoids during the development of their different organs [45, 46]. Four types of flavonoids occur in citrus species, namely the flavanones, flavones, flavonols and anthocyanins with the latter group occurring only in blood oranges [47]. Studies on the quantitative distribution of these flavonoids have shown that the flavanones predominate in all species of the genus and they occur as glycosides, in which the aglycones are linked to a sugar moiety [48]. The highest concentration of flavanones and flavanone glycosides occurs in the peel [41].

Although flavones and flavonols have been found in low concentrations in *Citrus* tissues, they have been shown to be powerful antioxidants and free radical scavengers with the highly methoxylated flavones exhibiting the highest biological activity [15].

Flavanones

In human foods, flavanones are found in tomatoes and certain aromatic plants such as mint, but they are present in high concentrations only in citrus fruits [49]. In fact they are the most important citrus flavonoids (e.g. 98% in grapefruit, 96% in limes and 90% in lemons) [50]. Flavanones are generally glycosylated by a disaccharide at position 7: either a rutinose or a neohesperidose (Figure 2) [51]. The flavanone characteristics of some common citrus fruits are presented in Table 2. Lemon peel contains two main flavanone glycosides: hesperidin and eriocitrin. Lemon, lime, mandarin and sweet orange are dominated by rutinosides (mainly hesperetin). Grapefruit and sour orange contain predominantly neohesperidosides, mainly naringenin in the former but similar amounts of naringenin, neoeriodictyol and neohesperetin in the latter. Chromatographic profiles of the intact glycosides are generally used in the identification of the botanical origin of the fruit and product such as juices, preserves and honey, and as a monitor of adulteration [52, 53].

Flavanone 7-rutinosides are usually tasteless, but flavanone 7-neohesperidosides, e.g. neohesperidin and naringin are intensely bitter and are responsible for the characteristic taste of bitter orange and grapefruit [54]. Citrus fruits and associated products are a major dietary source of flavanones, which are present both in juices and in tissues that are ingested when eating the peeled fresh fruits (albedo, segments and membranes). However, the distribution is very non-uniform, with much higher concentrations in the solid tissues compared with the juice. For example, the naringin content of grapefruit juice was reported as 295-377 mg/L, whereas the albedo, back membrane and side membranes of the fruit contained 13-16, 18-27 and 11.5-17.6 g/kg, respectively [55]. Citrus peels (albedo and flavedo) are also particularly rich, with grapefruit peel containing naringin (1-16 g/g FW), sour orange peel containing neohesperidin (0.7-31 g/kg) and sweet orange peel containing hesperidin (4.6-12.8 g/kg) [56].

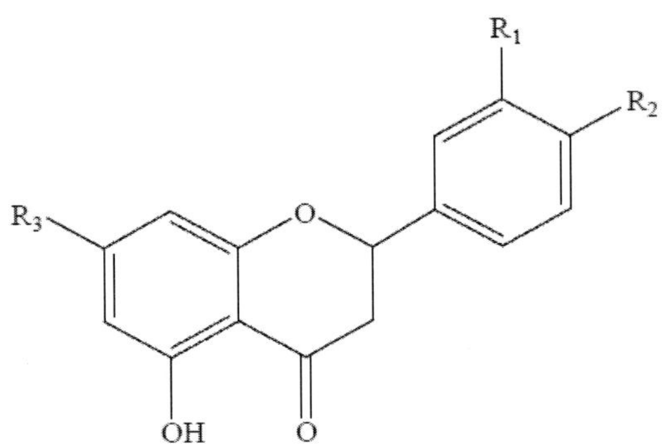

	Didymin	Hesperetin	Hesperidin	Naringenin	Naringin	Narirutin	Poncirin
R_1	H	OH	OH	H	H	H	H
R_2	OMe	OMe	OMe	OH	OH	OH	OMe
R_3	ORut[a]	OH	ORut	OH	ONeo[b]	ORut	ONeo

[a] rutinoside, [b] neohesperidoside

Figure 2. Flavanone skeleton with substitution pattern.

Table 2. Flavanone characteristics of common citrus fruits [54]

Flavanone	Sweet orange	Sour orange	Lemon	Grapefruit	Lime	Mandarin
Eriocitrin	-	-	++	-		-
Narirutin	+	-	-	++		++
Hesperidin	+++	-	+++	Trace	+++	+++
Naringin	-	+++	-	+++		-
Neohesperidin	-	++	-	Trace		-

-, absent; +, ++, +++, present in progressively greater amounts.

Flavones and Flavonols

Among the flavonoids, flavones, flavonols and their glycosides are the most common compounds [57]. They are widespread in the plant kingdom, with the exception of algae and fungi. Flavonols occur as *O*-glycosides, but flavone *O*-glycosides and *C*-glycosides are very common [58]. Common flavones and flavonols present in citrus fruits are listed in Figures 3 and 4, respectively. The formation of flavone and flavonol glycosides greatly depends on light; therefore, the highest concentrations of these compounds are found generally in leaves and outer parts of plants [58].

The skin of citrus fruits contains large quantities of polymethoxylated flavones (PMFs): tangeretin, nobiletin and sinensetin (up to 6.5 g/L of essential oil of mandarin) [49]. Polymethoxylated flavones (Figure 5) are the most hydrophobic flavonoids and they are exceptional in that they occur as the free aglycones [59, 60].

They are associated with the oil glands of the citrus peel flavedo. Composition of PMFs varies considerably among species and varieties [61, 62]. The mandarin variety Dancy has the highest total PMF content, containing approximately 5 fold the amount found in the peel of sweet orange varieties.

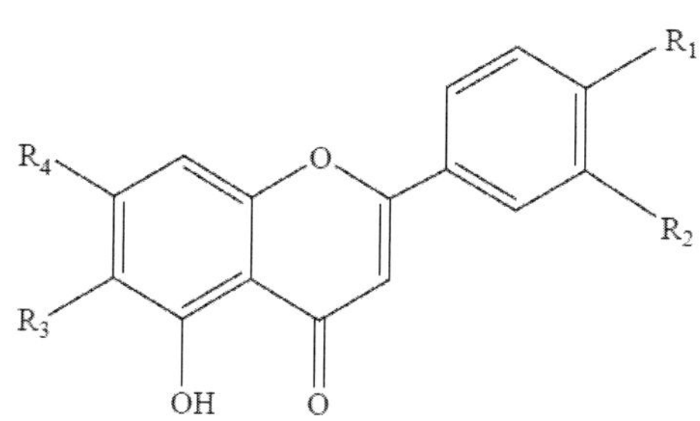

	Apigenin	Diosmin	Isorhoifolin	Luteolin	Rhoifolin
R_1	OH	OMe	OH	OH	OH
R_2	H	OH	H	OH	H
R_3	H	H	H	H	H
R_4	OH	ORut[a]	ORut	OH	ONeo[b]

[a] rutinoside, [b] neohesperidoside

Figure 3. Flavone skeleton with substitution pattern.

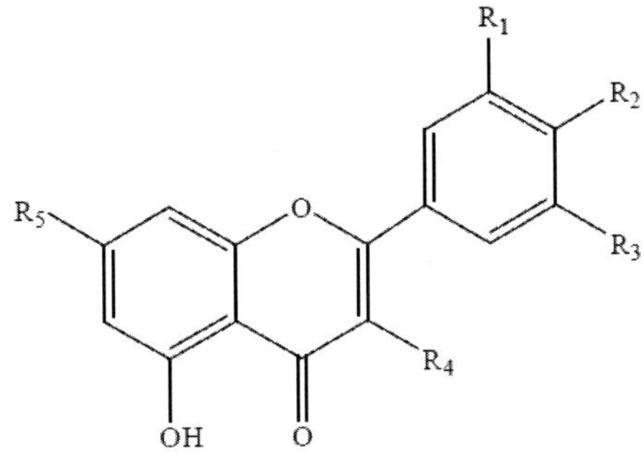

	Kaempferol	Quercetin	Rutin
R1	H	OH	OH
R2	OH	OH	OH
R3	H	H	H
R4	OH	OH	ORut[a]
R5	OH	OH	OH

[a] rutinoside

Figure 4. Flavonol skeleton with substitution pattern.

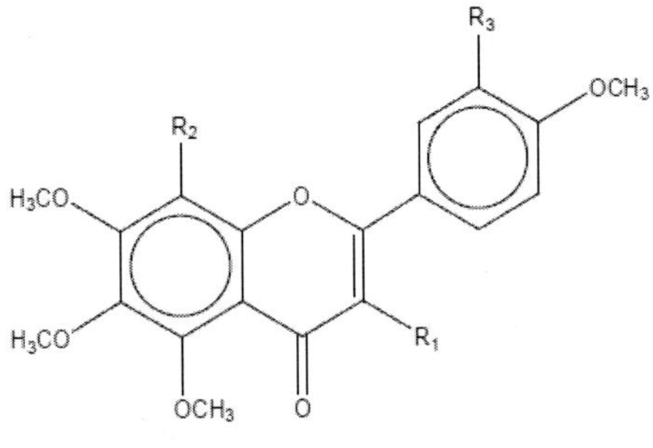

	Sinensetin	Hexamethoxyflavone	Nobiletin	Tangeretin
R1	H	OCH_3	H	H
R2	H	H	OCH_3	OCH_3
R3	OCH_3	OCH_3	OCH_3	H

Figure 5. Common polymethoxylated flavones found in citrusfruits.

In Dancy mandarins, tangeretin and nobiletin are predominant, while in sweet oranges, nobiletin, sinensetin and heptamethoxyflavone predominate [63]. Nobiletin and sinensetin have been observed in orange peel whereas tangeretin has been identified in tangerine oil. The concentration of individual polymethoxylated flavones is affected by the stage of citrus fruit development. For instance, in Tangelo Nova fruits, the highest concentration of nobiletin, sinensetin and tangeretin is observed in immature fruits [64].

ANTIOXIDANT POTENTIAL OF CITRUS PHYTOCHEMICALS

There is considerable evidence that citrus fruits may help reduce the risk, or retard the progression, of several serious diseases and disorders. The beneficial effects of the dietary citrus fruits can be attributed, not only to the vitamin C, minerals, dietary fiber, essential oils, organic acids and carotenoids, but also to their flavonoids. The biological activities of flavonoids are mainly due to their antioxidant and free radical scavenging activity and capabilities of chelating redox active metal ions [65], modulating gene expression and interacting with the cell signaling pathways [66, 67].

The free radical scavenging and antioxidant activities of phenolics are dependent upon the arrangement of functional groups about the nuclear structure. Both the number and configuration of hydroxyl groups are the main structural features influencing the antioxidant capacity of phenolics. The phenolic groups of flavonoids in fact serve as a source of a readily available "H" atoms such that the subsequent radicals produced can be delocalized over the flavonoid structure [68].Structural class, degree of hydroxylation, substitution patterns, conjugations and polymerization are generally the variants determining the chemical nature of flavonoids. Three structural groups are important for the evaluation of their antioxidant capacity [69,70]: (1) the ortho-dihydroxy (catechol) structure in the B-ring, which confers greater stability to aroxyl radicals, possibly through hydrogen bonding, and which participates in electron dislocation; (2) the 2,3-double bond, in conjugation with a 4-oxo function, responsible for electron dislocation from the B-ring; (3) the presence of both 3-(a)-and 5-(b)-hydroxyl groups (Figure 6). Obviously, flavonoid antioxidant propensity seems to be linked to a combination of these chemical and structural elements. Table 3 relates some citrus flavonoids with the functional groups involved in their antioxidant activity as shown in Figure 6.

Given that the mechanisms of action of naturally occurring antioxidants can be diverse *in vivo*, a comprehensive prediction of the antioxidant efficacy initially *in vitro* requires a multiplicity of assessing methods with various implications for molecular targets [3, 4, 71].

Table 3. Functional groups involved in the antioxidant activity of citrus flavonoids [15]

	Type of antioxidant structure (as in Figure 6)				
Flavonoid	I	II	III(a)	III(b)	Others
Naringin				✓	4'-OH
Neoeriocitrin	✓			✓	
Hesperidin				✓	3'-OH, 4'OMe
Naringenin				✓	4'-OH
Eriodictyol	✓			✓	
Hesperetin				✓	3'-OH, 4'OMe
Diosmin		✓		✓	3'-OH, 4'-Me
Apigenin		✓		✓	4'-OH
Luteolin	✓	✓		✓	
Tangeretin		✓		✓	5,6,7,8,4'-OMe
Rutin	✓	✓	✓[a]	✓	
Kaempferol		✓	✓	✓	4'-OH
Quercetin	✓	✓	✓	✓	

✓: presence of functional group as shown in Figure 6.

[a] Glycosylated in 3-OH.

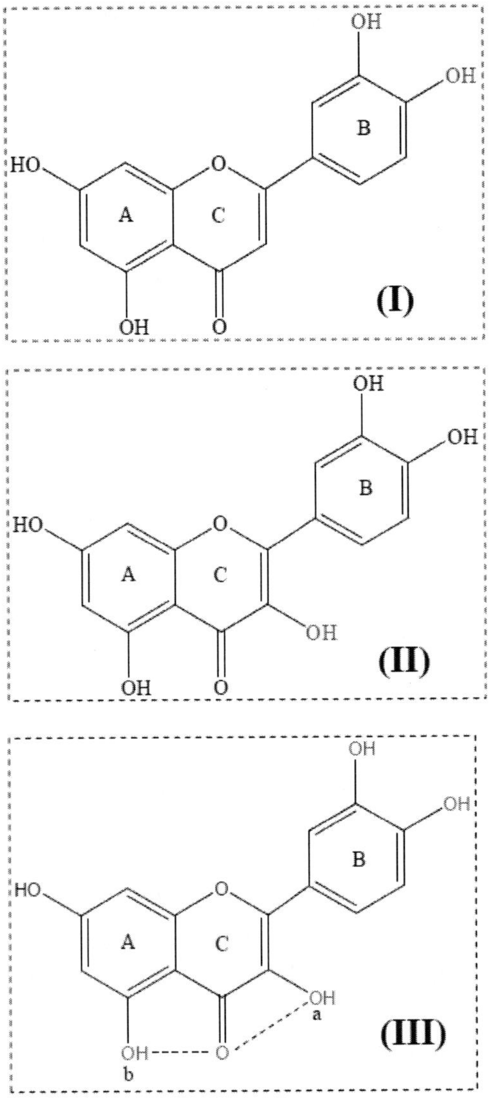

Figure 6. Functional groups of flavonoid structure with high antioxidant capacity.

It is noteworthy that synergism and concentration may also bring effects that are not observed when individual constituents are tested [72]. There is, therefore, no universal method that can measure the antioxidant capacity of all samples accurately and consistently. For instance, there have been different structural correlations observed when the antiradical propensity of several citrus flavonoids have been measured using a diversity of methods with reference to the superoxide radical [73]. In this vein, the multi antioxidant assay approach is being systematically adopted as a basis for the evaluation of plant prophylactic potential. A high number of reports highlight the antioxidant nature of citrus phenolics and flavonoids. Linoleic acid autoxidation, the liposome oxidation system, and the low-density lipoprotein (LDL) oxidation system have been used to evaluate the antioxidative activities of 6,8-di-C-β-glycosyldiosmin and 6-C-β-glycosyldiosmin and flavonoid compounds (eriocitrin, diosmin, hesperidin and narirutin) in lemon fruit with varying responses [74].

Along the same line, a comparative study between the antioxidant properties of peel (flavedo and albedo) and juice of some commercially grown citrus fruits namely, grapefruit (*Citrus paradisi*), lemon (*Citrus limon*), lime (*Citrus aurantiifolia*) and sweet orange (*Citrus sinensis*), was performed using: 2,2-diphenyl-1-picrylhydrazyl (DPPH) to assess radical scavenging capacity, β-carotene–linoleate model system in liposomes and thiobarbituric acid reactive substances (TBARS) assay to evaluate reducing power and inhibition of lipid peroxidation in brain homogenates. These assays could only collectively relate the reducing sugars, ascorbic acid, carotenoids and phenolics to the antioxidant potential [75]. Radical scavenging activities of Rio red grapefruits and sour orange fruit extracts in different *in vitro* model systems namely, 1,1-diphenyl-2-picryl hydrazyl (DPPH), phosphomolybdenum method and nitroblue tetrazolium (NBT) reduction at different concentrations, provided a clear basis for the antioxidative power of the studied extracts but again with variable superoxide radical scavenging activity [76]. In another study assessing different edible tissues of citrus fruits, namely juice sacs, segment membranes, and segments, it came out clearly that the segment membranes were high in bio-antioxidative contents [77] thereby recommending the consumption of citrus fruits with all edible tissues rather than the juice or juice sacs alone.

In Mauritius, where citrus fruits are the second most consumed fruits behind bananas, a comprehensive analysis of 21 citrus varieties by our group correlated their flavedo, albedo and pulp phenolic contents to trolox equivalent antioxidant capacity (TEAC), ferric reducing antioxidant capacity (FRAP) and hypochlorous acid (HOCl) scavenging activity. The flavone, flavanol and flavanone seemed to be the most influential antioxidative components. Nine most potent extracts in these systems were further assessed for their ability to protect DNA from damage and their iron chelating activity [42, 44]. The extracts exhibited good protecting ability in the cuphen assay and flavedo extracts generally were able to chelate metal ions effectively confirming that they were a significant source of phenolic antioxidants with potent application for the development of functional foods. There are a number of seminal reports discussing the antioxidant action mechanisms of plant phenolics [65, 78]. It is generally argued that the complex antioxidative behavior of citrus flavonoids are related to the fact that they have an antioxidant action in a hydrophilic environment, while, in a lipophilic environment, some molecules (neohesperidin, hesperetin, didymin and isosakuranetin) show a reduced antioxidant capacity, and others (naringin, narirutin, naringenin, neoeriocitrin, heridictyol) invert their behavior, becoming prooxidant [79].

It is critical to bear in mind that reported antioxidant activities are based on phenolic derivatives as present in plants using *in vitro* models. However, several studies have shown that phenolics are extensively metabolized *in vivo*, mainly during transfer across the small intestine, by colonic micro flora and in the liver, resulting in significant alteration in their redox potentials [79-81]. After undergoing phase I deglycosylation, the phenolic aglycones are converted to glucuronides, sulphates and *o*-methylated derivatives during phase II metabolism [82]. Thus, to delineate the prophylactic potential of phenolic compounds, it is essential to screen the efficacy of these phenolic derivatives as being bio available *in vivo* using cell systems, animal models and clinical trials. The physiological significance of dietary antioxidants depends on their mechanism of absorption and biotransformation, thus warranting further investigations on the bioavailability of antioxidant polyphenols.

PROPHYLACTIC POTENTIAL OF CITRUS PHYTOCHEMICALS

The prophylactic potential of citrus phytochemicals against three ROS-mediated diseases, namely diabetes, cancer and neurodegenerative diseases is discussed in the following subsections.

Diabetes

Among the various ROS-mediated pathologies, diabetes is one of the most common endocrine disorders affecting almost 6% of the world's population [83]. The incidence of diabetes is increasing, with a worldwide prevalence estimated to double by 2030, primarily because of sedentary lifestyle and obesity [84]. Diabetes mellitus (DM) is a group of metabolic diseases resulting from the defects in insulin secretion, insulin action or both and is classified into two major categories: type 1 and type 2 diabetes. Although both types of diabetes have distinct pathogenesis, hyperglycemia, and various life threatening complications are common to both. One of the consequences of hyperglycaemia is the excessive non-enzymatic glycation of proteins leading to the formation of advanced glycation end products (AGEs) which have the propensity to generate ROS. Glycation and AGE modifications lead to pathological changes contributing to diabetic complications such as cataracts, nephropathy, vasculopathy, proliferative retinopathy and atherosclerosis [85].

Several medications, including thiazolidinedione and metformin are well-known activators of anti-diabetic signaling molecules [86]. Moreover, numerous synthetic AGEs inhibitors, including aminoguanidine, improved diabetic complications in animal models and clinical trials. However, these allopathic drugs are often accompanied by a number of adverse effects [87]. It is suggested that AGEs inhibitors from natural foods/dietary biofactors may reasonably serve as valuable adjuvants. Recently, many investigators have suggested that phytochemicals exert antidiabetic effects by targeting anti-diabetic signaling molecules such as AMP-activated protein kinase (AMPK) and peroxisome proliferator-activated receptor gamma (PPAR-γ) [88-92].

Adipocyte Dysfunction: The Link Between Obesity and Diabetes

The incidence of obesity (defined as having a body mass index (BMI) of greater than 30 kg per m^2) is increasing dramatically in virtually all societies of the world, resulting in important pathological consequences such as type 2 diabetes mellitus [93]. Adipose tissue, which can average from 20–30% of total body weight in adult humans, is now recognized as an important regulator of organismal metabolism [94, 95]. It modulates metabolism by regulating systemic substrate flux and by secreting factors that modulate gene expression and metabolism in distant organs. Obesity is accompanied by important changes in adipocyte function and in systemic metabolism that have been associated with increased risk for diabetes [96, 97]. Indeed, adipocyte dysfunction in obesity has been linked to an inflammatory response in adipose tissue that is characterized by an influx of inflammatory cells. Cross talk between adipocytes and adipose tissue inflammatory cells, primarily macrophages, importantly contributes to adipocyte dysfunction. The development of the inflammatory state in adipose tissue is associated with insulin resistance in skeletal muscle.

In inflammation, proinflammatory cytokines induce the formation of large amounts of nitric oxide (NO) by inducible nitric oxide synthase (iNOS), and compounds that inhibit NO production have anti-inflammatory effects. Hämäläinen et al. [98] systematically investigated the effects of 36 naturally occurring flavonoids and related compounds belonging to eight classes (flavones, isoflavones, flavonols, flavanones, flavan-3-ols,anthocyanins, hydroxybenzoic acids, and hydroxycynnamic acids) on NO production in macrophages exposed to an inflammatory stimulus (lipopolysaccharide, LPS), and evaluated the mechanisms of action of the effective compounds. The following flavonoids present in citrus fruits namely: flavones, the flavonols (isorhamnetin, kaempferol and quercetin) and the flavanone naringenin inhibited iNOS protein and mRNA expression and also NO production in a dose-dependent manner. These active compounds inhibited the activation of nuclear factor-κB (NF-κB), which is a significant transcription factor for iNOS. Furthermore, kaempferol and quercetin also inhibited the activation of the signal transducer and activator of transcription 1 (STAT-1), another important transcription factor for iNOS [98].

One important product of adipose tissue macrophages in the obese state is a pro-inflammatory cytokine known as tumor necrosis factor-α (TNFα). TNF-α plays a pivotal role in obesity-related insulin resistance, and its expression is upregulated in the obese adipose tissue of both rodents and humans [99-101]. Additionally, several reports suggest that TNF-α indirectly promotes insulin resistance by increasing the circulating levels of free fatty acid (FFA) [102-104]. TNF-α promotes FFA secretion through adipocyte lipolysis. Although the mechanism by which TNF-α induces lipolysis has yet to be completely elucidated, studies have proposed that TNFα downregulates the expression of antilipolytic genes, such as perilipin and phosphodiesterase-3B (PDE3B) [99,105,106]. A potential molecule demonstrating anti-diabetic activity may thus downregulate the expression of this protein. Yoshida et al. [107] reported that the citrus flavonoids hesperetin and naringenin can block TNF-α-stimulated FFA secretion by inhibiting the nuclear factor-kappa B (NF-κB) and extracellular signal-related kinases (ERK) pathways in mouse adipocytes. The inhibition of the ERK pathway prevents TNF-α from downregulating the transcription of two antilipolytic genes, perilipin and phosphodiesterase 3B (PDE3B). In contrast, the inhibition of the NF-κB pathway suppresses the transcription of interleukin-6 (IL-6), which also induces FFA secretion [107].

Using a diabetes-like oxidative stress model, Ramful et al. [108] evaluated the potential protective effect of two citrus fruit extracts, namely Tangor Elendale and Tangelo Mineola, on human adipocytes. The extracts were tested on SW872 liposarcoma cells subjected or not to H_2O_2 or AGEs and apolipoprotein E (apoE) secretion was assessed in treated cells. Significant reductions in apoE secretions were observed in cells treated with albedo and pulp extracts of the citrus fruits [108]. ApoE, which is a component of lipoproteins, is known to regulate both cellular and systemic cholesterol, as well as triglyceride metabolism [109, 110]. It has been extensively studied for its potential role in the etiology of diabetes and was shown to exhibit anti-inflammatory, anti-atherogenic, and antioxidant properties [111, 112]. Recently, Tarnus et al. [110] demonstrated an increase in apoE secretion in SW872 cells subjected to stress induced by glucose or 2,2'-azobis(2-amidinopropane) dihydrochloride (AAPH), a free-radical generator. It was hypothesized that apoE may exert antioxidant effects at the adipocyte level, and its subsequent increase in expression may represent a defense response to oxidative stress [110]. The decrease in apoE secretion in cells incubated with citrus fruit extracts seems to be an adaptive response to the presence of the exogenous citrus antioxidants.

Citrus Flavonoids as Hypoglycemic Agents

A chronic hyperglycemic condition in diabetes is associated with long term damage, dysfunction, and failure of various organs, such as eyes, kidneys, nerves, heart, and blood vessels. Flavonoids, in particular citrus flavonoids, may exert antidiabetic properties by influencing glucose uptake *in vivo.* Jadhav and Puchchakayala [113] reported the acute hypoglycemic and antidiabetic activity of the flavonols quercetin and rutin in normoglycemic and streptozotocin (STZ)-nicotinamide induced diabetic rat models through blood glucose profile measurements. The proposed mechanism of action was by enhancing the peripheral utilization of glucose, either by direct stimulation of glucose uptake or via the mediation of enhanced insulin secretion, and inhibiting the glucose transporter activity from intestine [113]. The hypoglycemic effects of citrus flavanones have also been reported. Thus, naringenin is able to reduce glucose uptake and inhibit intestinal and renal Na+-glucose co-transporter (SGLT1) [114]. Both naringin and hesperidin significantly increased the glucokinase mRNA level, while naringin reduced the mRNA expression of phosphoenolpyruvate carboxykinase and glucose-6-phosphatase in the liver [115]. Recently, it was reported that a citrus extract of Dangyuja (Citrus fruit from Korea), containing high levels of flavanone glycosides, could be used to control the blood glucose level of diabetic patients by inhibiting α amylase and α glucosidase in the intestinal tract [116].

Glycation, AGEs and ROS in Diabetic Pathology

Oxidative stress and alterations in glucose metabolism are important risk factors for diabetes and its related complications. Advanced glycated end products (AGEs) and their carbonyl derivatives are believed to contribute significantly to the pathogenesis of type 2 diabetes by their interaction with specific cell membrane receptors triggering for instance the NF-κ B signalling pathway to induce the expression of pro-inflammatory mediators and elicit oxidative stress which exacerbate diabetic complications [117] (Figure 7). A great deal of efforts has been focused on the identification of useful inhibitors of protein AGEs to delay or prevent glycation so as to alleviate the phenotype of these diseases [118]. Unoki et al. [119] examined the effects of AGE on insulin sensitivity by exploring its mechanisms on the glucose uptake in adipocytes and adipocyte differentiation.

AGE was found to inhibit the differentiation of 3T3-L1 adipocyte cells as well as the glucose uptake in the absence or presence of insulin. The authors suggested that advanced glycated endproducts and receptor for advanced glycated endproducts (AGE–RAGE) interaction inhibited the glucose uptake through the over-generation of intracellular ROS, thus indicating that it is involved in the development of obesity-related insulin resistance [119]. Antioxidant compounds capable of counteracting the deleterious effects of intracellular ROS are thus promising in the diabetic state.

Flavedo extracts of the citrus fruits Tangelo Mineola and Tangor Elendale exhibited protective effects against AGEs- and H_2O_2- induced oxidative stress in human SW872 adipocytes [108]. The reduction of protein carbonyl formation at adipocyte level, as assessed by an ELISA technique, is clearly reflective of the antioxidant power of flavedo extracts of the citrus fruits. The dichloro-dihydro-fluorescein diacetate (DCFH-DA) assay also revealed the ROS scavenging properties of the two citrus fruits extracts. Indeed, intracellular ROS formation was considerably lowered in cells pretreated with citrus flavedo extracts incubated in the presence or absence of H_2O_2 [108]. It was hypothesized that the efficiency of cellular uptake and/or membrane binding combined with the radical scavenging activity likely dictated the efficacy of the citrus flavedo extracts. The physical properties of flavonoids determine their interactions with the cell membrane [120]. Hydrophobic flavonoids may become deeply embedded in membranes, where they can influence membrane fluidity and break oxidative chain reactions. More polar compounds interact with membrane surfaces via hydrogen bonding, where they are able to protect membranes from external and internal oxidative stresses. There is also some evidence that uptake *in vivo* may be related to the polarity of the compounds because the net transfer of flavonoids across the brush border of rat small intestine was found to be related to their lipophilicity, rather than their spatial conformation [121].

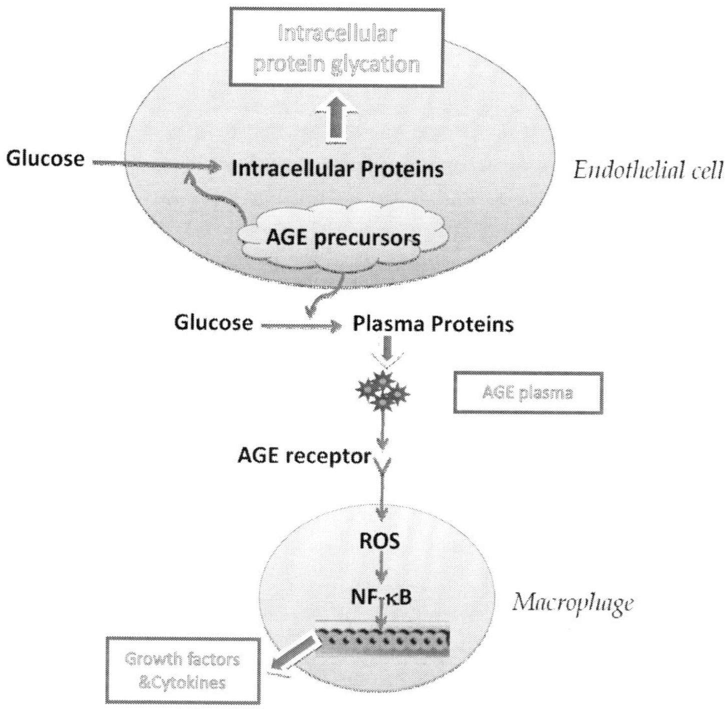

Figure 7. Damage by advanced glycation end-product (AGE) precursors at cellular level.

Citrus Fruits at the Crossroad of Cancer Chemoprevention: A Cellular and Molecular Insight

Whilst fruits have been at the crossroad of cancer chemoprevention for decades, a number of investigations are claiming citrus fruits and the bioactive flavonoids and limonoids as promising agents in this arena of research. Cancer has been described as a multifactorial disease, characterized by a number of biological capabilities acquired during the multistep development of human tumors. These hallmarks of cancer include sustaining proliferative signaling, evading growth suppressors, resisting cell death, enabling replicative immortality, inducing angiogenesis, activating invasion and metastasis; reprogramming of energy metabolism and evading immune destruction [122]. The rapidly growing armamentarium of bioactive secondary metabolites with cancer chemopreventive effects based on *in vitro*, *in vivo* and clinical studies have been categorized according to their respective effects on one or more hallmark capabilities, particularly by their effects on specific molecular targets that are involved in one way or another in enabling particular capabilities [123-124].

With over 60 types of flavonoids being identified in citrus fruits [53], this wide structural diversity may explain the potential benefits of citrus fruits against cancer through myriad mechanisms of action (Figure 8). For instance, an investigation of the structure–function relationship of citrus flavonoids in terms of their ability to alter the expression of apoptosis related proteins in the colon adenocarcinoma cells revealed that the presence of double bond between C2 and C3 and hydroxyl group at C3 and C6 are important for the proliferation inhibition and apoptosis induction ability as measured by the increased apoptosis regulator BAX or B-cell lymphoma 2 (Bax/ Bcl-2) level [125, 126]. The effect of isolated flavonoids from Korean *C. aurantium* L. peel on A549 human lung carcinoma cells showed the induction of G_2-M (a cell-cycle checkpoint) arrest by regulating proteins of cell cycle, such as cyclin B1, cdc2, cdc25c and $p21^{WAF1/CIP1}$.

The extracts were also potent activators of apoptosis via the up-regulation of the Bax pro-apoptotic protein, caspase 3 activity and cleaved poly ADP-ribose polymerase (PARP), and the down-regulation of pro-caspases (caspase-3, -6, -8 and -9) proteins. Flavonoids cause G_2-M arrest and apoptosis through the regulation cell cycle dependent and pro-apoptotic proteins [127]. Selective apoptosis has been described as an interesting approach in cancer chemoprevention and *C. aurantium* [127] and *C. grandis* [128] have shown good pro-apoptotic potential, a finding that need to be confirmed in clinical trials.

Citrus limonoids have been widely reported for their antiproliferative effects against MCF-7 breast cancer [129, 130], HT-29 colon cancer [131], panc-28 pancreatic cancer [132, 133], and SH-SY5Y neuroblastoma cells [134]. In addition, the latter induced phase II enzymes primarily glutathione S-transferase and quinone reductase, an important step in the detoxification of potential carcinogens [135-138]. Furthermore, some limonoids have the ability to induce apoptosis in rats through the suppression of anti-inflammatory proteins such as inducible nitric oxide synthase (iNOS) and cyclooxygenase (COX)-2 [139,140]. Recently an investigation of four limonoids isolated from *Citrus lemon* L. (lemon) and *Citrus aurantium* L. (sour orange) indicated that methyl nomilinate from *Citrus lemon* L. had the highest anti-proliferative potential against SW480 cells [127]. This effect correlated with the induction of G1 cell cycle arrest via reduction of cyclin-dependant kinase 4 (CDK4) levels by 31% and 53%, CDK6 levels by 34% and 46%, and cyclin D3 by 27% and 41%, in a time-dependent manner, for 24 h and 48 h, respectively. In addition, there was an upregulation of expression of CDK inhibitors such as p27Kip1, p21Waf/Cip1 and $p15^{INK4B}$ in the methyl nomilinate treated cells, compared to control cells [127].

Whilst flavonoids and limonoids have received considerable attention against cancer, studies have indicated the potential of modified citrus pectin, a complex water soluble indigestible polysaccharide obtained from the peel and pulp of citrus fruits in targeting multiple critical rate limiting steps in metastasis *in vivo* and *in vitro* [141, 142].

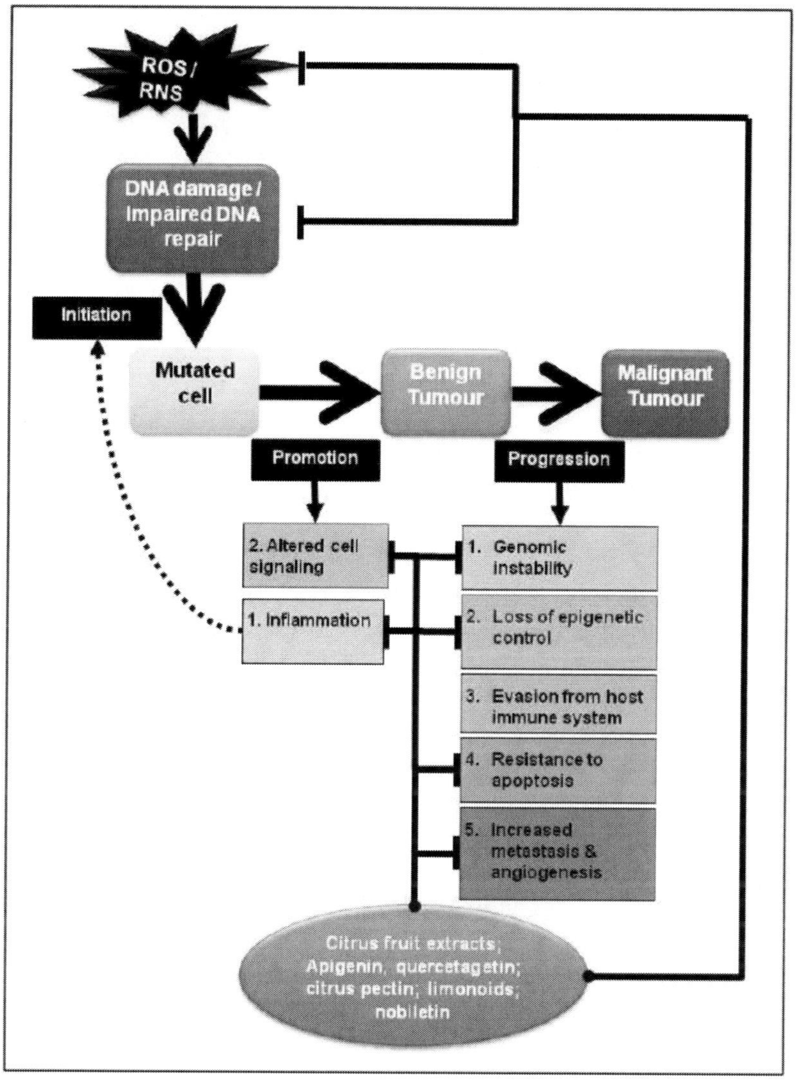

Figure 8. Schematic representation of the role of citrus fruit extracts and citrus phytochemicals on multiple cancer related biological pathways. The arrows (—|) show the inhibitory effects of citrus fruit extracts and/or the citrus flavonoids or limonoids on the different hallmarks of cancer. Data were obtained from experimental studies involving cancer cell lines and animals.

Cognition and Neurodegenerative Diseases

Neurological diseases have become a relevant problem due to an increase in ageing population. Neurodegenerative diseases (ND) affect the brain, a vital organ in the body, involved in the control of all the involuntary functions and also in memory, cognition and emotion [143].

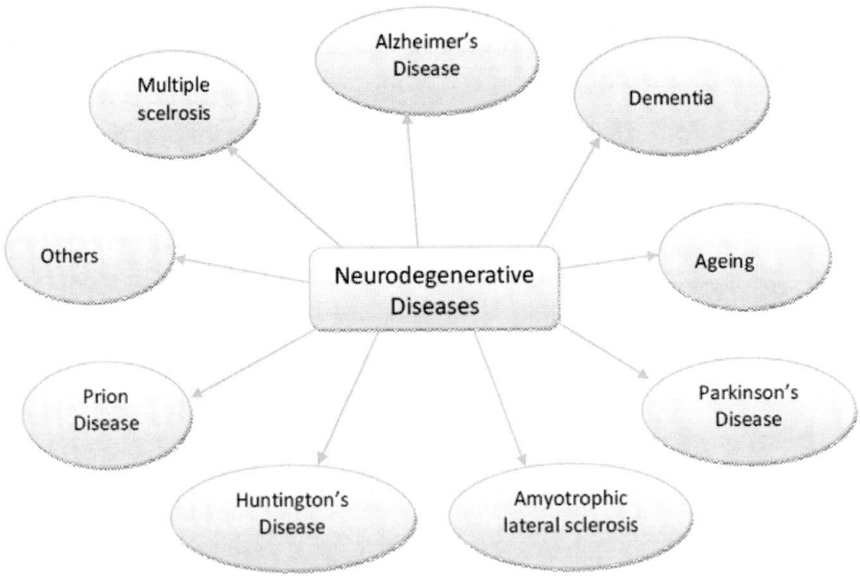

Figure 9. Common neurodegenerative diseases.

The latter leads to a deterioration, often irreversible, of the intellectual and cognitive faculties [144] usually associated with the progressive accumulation of misfolded proteins with the formation of toxic oligomers along with increasing oxidative damage and inflammation [145,146]. Common NDs are shown in Figure 9.

Ageing has been considered a major risk factor for ND. In addition, it can affect the patients' abilities of self-repair and brain functions, such as decreased memory, including recognition memory [147], short term recall [148,149], long-term memory and speed of processing [150]. As such, Alzheimer's (AD) and Parkinsons diseases (PD) seem to be on the rise and are characterized clinically by progressive memory deficits, impaired cognitive function and behavioral disorders [151] and by abnormalities in motor control respectively [152]. AD represents the most common form of dementia and ageing represented the most common risk factor for AD [153].

Different pathological hallmarks have been implicated in AD, in particular, the accumulation of amyloid-β peptide (Aβ) in the brain parenchyma which can induce apoptosis of neuronal cells [154]. Excessive Aβ accumulation, either through increased production or decreased clearance, leads to senile plaques formation. This results in a series of events which ends up with an impairment of neuronal synapses and dendrites through oxidative stress and inflammatory processes. In addition, intracellular neurofibrillary tangles (NFTs), with abnormally hyperphosphorylated tau protein (neuronal proteins of the central nervous systems) contributing to brain degeneration and disease progression, have been highlighted. Besides the activation and proliferation of brain glial cells, for example astrocytes and microglia, lead to the production of pro-inflammatory cytokines and toxins which aggravate the neurodegenerative process and oxidative damage to nuclear DNA and mitochondrial DNA have been described as potential hallmarks of the disease [155]. On the other hand PD results from dopamine deficiency in the brain and the enzyme tyrosinase appears to play a role in the production of neuromelanin and damage to neurons [156], in addition to the intraneuronal deposition of alpha synuclein proteins and irreversible loss of nigrostriatal dopaminergic neurons [146].

Oxidative stress (OS) has been involved in the pathogenesis of neurodegenerative disorders due to susceptibility of the brain to damage by ROS and as such antioxidants have been considered as interesting prophylactics since long. Besides the involvement of OS in inducing neuronal damage, it has the ability to modulate intracellular signaling which subsequently leads to neuronal death by apoptosis or necrosis [157]. The susceptibility of the brain to oxidative damage in fact, results from the high rate of oxygen consumption and glucose turnover, as well as high levels of the redox-active iron in certain regions of the brain [158], the presence of transition metals and a high content of polyunsaturated fatty acids [159].

Bioactive Phytochemicals Derived from Citrus Fruits in the Management of ND

The importance of bioactive phytochemicals in the management and treatment of ND has been greatly emphasized lately. This is because the existing treatment against ND targets mainly the symptoms and health care costs are particularly expensive due to the insidious onset of the disease, its ever-increasing levels of disability and the length of time over which the condition extends itself. Indeed, there is mounting evidence that flavonoid-rich foods can beneficially influence normal cognitive function. A combination of preclinical and epidemiological studies suggest that flavonoids might be effective at reversing neurodegenerative pathology and age-related declines in neurocognitive performance, suggestive of potential therapeutic utility, although at present a direct association between flavonoid consumption and improvement in neurological health has not been made [160].

Thus, much interest has been directed towards citrus flavonoids and the mechanisms underpinning the action of these flavonoids against ND are diverse. For instance, pretreatment with naringin and nobiletin of rat pheochromocytoma PC12 cells significantly reduced oxidative stress, via the increase of superoxide dismutase (SOD) and glutathione (GSH) activity and the decrease of malondialdehyde (MDA) levels, and apoptosis caused by H_2O_2-induced injury [161]. Hwang and Yen [162] also reported that pretreatment of PC12 cells with citrus flavanones significantly eliminated the accumulation of intracellular ROS. Hesperetin and neohesperidin reduced the level of ROS by 16–24%, while hesperidin reduced the level of ROS by 32–48% in H_2O_2-indued PC12 cells [162]. As indicated above, the brain is particularly susceptible to metal ion overload which can accentuate oxidative stress. Thus, naringin from grapefruits was reported to significantly inhibit the ferric ion-induced lipid peroxidation in mitochondrial fraction from mouse liver as well as protecting the antioxidant armoury in particular glutathione contents, glutathione peroxidase, glutathione S-transferase, superoxide dismutase and catalase activities from iron-induced depletion [163].

Naringin has been reported to mediate its neuroprotective effect in the 3-nitropropionic acid-induced neurodegeneration through its antioxidant and anti-apoptotic properties [164]. A further study confirmed the ability of naringin to upregulate the antioxidative enzymes production via activation of the nuclear factor Nrf2. Naringin-treated rats exhibited significant increase in mRNA expressions of the phase II genes NAD(P)H: quinone oxidoreductase-1 (NQO-1), heme oxygenase-1 (HO-1), glutathione S-transferase P1 (GST-P1) and gammaglutamylcysteine ligase (c-GCL), by 60.78%, 72.5%, 64.71% and 55.79% as compared with 3-NP-induced and 95.24%, 122.58%, 86.67% and 78.31% as compared with the control groups of rats [166]. In addition, inflammatory markers primarily TNF-α, COX-2 and iNOS were reduced by 23.81%, 22.76% and 34.21%, respectively when compared to 3-NP-induced rats. Thus, the authors concluded that naringin may have mitigating effects against neurodegeneration via enhancement of phase II and antioxidant gene expressions via nuclear factor erythroid 2-related factor (Nrf2) activation; thereby modulating the oxidative stress and inflammatory responses [165].

The flavanone naringenin was found to reduce lipopolysaccharide/ interferon-ɣ-(LPS/IFN-ɣ-) induced glial cell activation which causes neuronal injury. The flavonoid mediated its inhibitory actions on p38 mitogen-activated protein kinase (MAPK) phosphorylation, the prevention of the downstream activation of downstream signal transducer and activator of transcription (STAT-1) and the increased expression of iNOS [166]. Recently, Okuyama et al. [167] showed the potential of auraptene, a citrus coumarin at a dose of 25 mg/kg/day, in effectively suppressing inflammation via the inhibition of microglia activation and cyclooxygenase-2 expression by astrocytes, as well as preventing neuronal cell death in the hippocampus following ischemic insults in an ischemic mouse model.

CONCLUSION

In consideration of the fact that the prevalence of diabetes, cancer and neurodegenerative diseases seem to increase exponentially and that they share common pathological mechanisms, it can be speculated that delaying the onset of these diseases via chemoprevention by dietary biofactors like citrus fruits or citrus flavonoids can be a realistic measure. These types of dietary factors are slowly emerging as acceptable dietary lifestyle and ongoing investigations suggest high hopes for their use. They are gaining in popularity as they are harmless and participate in the natural body metabolic activities. However, scientific information is vital for the researcher, physician, policy makers and health managers with increased availability and evidence that such factors may have efficacy. This warrants further research in this field. Cellular models and animal studies have indeed provided a great deal of data on the potentiality of functional foods and their prophylactic factors but the ultimate approach remains clinical trials and this is where our efforts should concentrate.

REFERENCES

[1] Halliwell, B., (1996). Antioxidants in human health and disease. *Annu. Rev. Nutr.* 16, 33-50.

[2] Halliwell, B., Gutterridge, J.M.C., Cross, E.C., (1992). Free radicals, antioxidants, and human disease: where are we now? *J. Lab. Clin. Med.* 119, 598-620.

[3] Aruoma, O.I., (1994). Nutrition and health aspects of free radicals and antioxidants. *Food Chem. Toxicol.* 32, 671-683.

[4] Aruoma, O.I., (2003). Methodological considerations for characterizing potential antioxidant actions of bioactive components in plant foods. *Mutat. Res.* 523-524, 9-20.

[5] Huang, R.P., Golard, A., Hossain, M.Z., Huang, R., Liu, Y.G., Boynton, A.L., (2001). Hydrogen peroxide promotes transformation of rat liver non-neoplastic epithelial cells through activation of epidermal growth factor receptor. *Mol. Carcinog.* 30 (4), 209-217.

[6] Boynes, J.W., (1991). Role of oxidative stress in the development of complication in diabetes. *Diabetes.* 40, 405-411.

[7] Perry, G., Raine, K.A., Nunomura, A., Watayc, T., Sayre, L.M., Smith, M.A., (2000). How important is oxidative damage? Lessons from Alzheimer's disease. *Free Rad. Biol. Med.* 28 (5), 831-841.

[8] Hensley, K., Floyd, R.A., (2002). Reactive oxygen species and protein oxidation in aging: A look back, a look ahead. *Arch. Biochem. Biophys.* 397 (2), 377-383.

[9] Hool, L.C., (2006). Reactive oxygen species in cardiac signaling: from mitochondria to plasma membrane ion channels. *Clin. Exp. Pharmacol. Physiol.* 33 (1-2), 146-151.

[10] Shahidi, F., (2004). Functional foods: their role in health promotion and disease prevention. *J. Food Sci.* 69 (5), R146-149.

[11] Pratt, D.E., Hudson, B.J.F., (1990). Natural antioxidants not exploited commercially. In: B.J.F. HUDSON, editor. Food Antioxidants. Amsterdam: Elsevier, p 171-192.

[12] Lindsay, D.G., Astley, S.B., (2002). European research on the functional effects of dietary antioxidants – EUROFEDA. *Mol. Asp. Med.* 23, 1–38.

[13] Bajpai, M., Pande, A., Tewari, S.K., Prashad, D., (2005). Phenolic content and antioxidant activity of some food and medicinal plants. *Int. J. Food Sci. Nutr.* 4, 287–91.

[14] Valko, M., Morris, H., Cronin, M. T. D., (2005). Metals, toxicity and oxidative stress. *Curr. Med. Chem.* 12 (10), 1161–1208.

[15] Benavente-Garcia, O., Castillo, J., Marin, F.R., Ortuno, A., Del Rio, J.A., (1997). Use and properties of Citrus flavonoids. *J. Agric. Food Chem.* 45 (12), 4506-4515.

[16] Manach, C., Mazur, A., Scalbert, A., (2005). Polyphenols and prevention of cardiovascular diseases. *Curr. Opin. Lipidol.* 16, 77–84.

[17] Middleton, E., Kandaswami, C., Theoharides, T. C., (2000). The effects of plant flavonoids on mammalian cells: implications for inflammation, heart disease and cancer. *Pharmacol. Rev.* 52, 673–751.

[18] Puupponen-Pimiä, R., Nohynek, L., Meier, C., Kähkönen, M., Heinonen, M., Hopia, A., oksman-Caldentey, K.–M., (2001). Antimicrobial properties of phenolic compounds from berries. *J. Appl. Microbiol.* 90, 494–507.

[19] Samman, S., Lyons Wall, P.M., Cook, N.C., (1998). Flavonoids and coronary heart disease: Dietary perspectives. In: C.A. Rice- Evans, L. Packer, editors. *Flavonoids in health and disease.* New York: Marcel Dekker, pp. 469-482.

[20] Spreen, T.H., (2003). Projections of world production and consumption of citrus to 2010. *Fruit Process.* 13, 378-384.

[21] Kurowska, E.M., Spence, J.D., Jordan, J., Wetmore, S., Freeman, D.J., Piché, L.A., Serratore, P., (2000). HDL-cholesterol-raising effect of orange juice in subjects with hypercholesterolemia. *Am. J. Clin. Nutr.* 72 (5), 1095-1100.

[22] Gyo-Nam, K., Jung-Geun, S., Hae-Dong, J., (2009). Antioxidant and antidiabetic activity of Dangyuja (*Citrus grandis* Osbeck) extract treated with *Aspergillus saitoi. Food Chem.* 117 (1), 35-41.

[23] Fortes, C., Forastiere, F., Farchi, S., Rapiti, E., Pastori, G., Perucci, C., (2000). Diet and overall survival in a cohort of very elderly people. *Epidemiol.* 11, 440–445.

[24] Benavente-Garcia, O., Castillo, J., (2008). Update on Uses and Properties of *Citrus* Flavonoids: New Findings in Anticancer, Cardiovascular, and Anti-inflammatory Activity. J Agric. Food Chem. 56, 6185–6205.

[25] Adibelli, Z., Dilek, M., Akpolat, T., (2009). Lemon juice as an alternative therapy in hypertension in Turkey. *Int. J. Cardiol.* 135 (2), e58–59.

[26] Chen, H., Ward, M., Graubard, B., Heineman, E., Markin, R., Potischman, N., Russell, R., Weisenburger, D., Tucker, L., (2002). Dietary patterns and adenocarcinoma of the esophagus and distal stomach. *Am J. Clin. Nutr.* 75, 137–144.

[27] Gonzalez-Molina, E., Dominguez-Perles, R., Moreno, D.A., Garcia-Viguera, C., (2010). Natural bioactive compounds of citrus limon for food and health. *J. Pharm. Biomed. Anal.* 51, 327–345.

[28] Manthey, J.A., Grohman, K., (2001). Phenols in citrus peel byproducts. Concentrations of hydroxycinnamates and polymethoxylated flavones in citrus peel molasses. J. Agric. Food Chem. 49 (7), 3268-3273.

[29] Samson, J.A., (1986). Citrus. In: *Tropical Fruits*, 2nd ed. Essex: Longman group UK. Ltd. pp. 73-138.

[30] Dugo, G., Di Giacomo, A., (2002). *Citrus – The Genus Citrus*. Cornwall, U.K.: Taylor & Francis.

[31] Rouillard, G., Guého, J., (1999). *Les plantes et leur histoire à l'Ile Maurice*. Mauritius: MSM Limited.

[32] Baldwin, E. A., (1993). Citrus fruit. In: G. Seymour, J. Taylor, G. Tucker, editors. *Biochemistry of Fruit Ripening*. London: Chapman & Hall. pp. 107-137.

[33] Albrigo, L.G., Carter, R.D., (1977). Structure of citrus fruits in relation to processing. In: S. Nagy, P. E. Shaw, M. K. Veldhuis, editors. *Citrus Science and Technology*, Vol 1. Westport, CT: AVI Publishing Co. Inc.

[34] Roth, I., (1977). Species of citrus (type: hesperidium). In: *Fruits of Angiosperms*. Berlin: Gebruder Borntraeger.pp. 494-642.

[35] Cháfer, M., Ortolá, M.D., Chiralt, A., Fito, P., 2001. Orange peel products obtained by osmotic dehydration. In: P. Fito, A. Chiralt, J.M. Barat, W.E.L. Spiess, D. Behsnilian, editors. *Osmotic dehydration and vacuum impregnation*. Pennsylvania, U.S.A: Technomic Publishing Company Inc. Chapter 9.

[36] Pernise, R., Borriello, G., Ferracane, R., Borrelli, R.B., Cennamo, F., Ritieni, A., (2009). Bergamot: A source of natural antioxidants for functionalized fruit juices. *Food Chem.* 112 (3), 545-550.

[37] Koch, K.E., Lowell, C.A., Avigne, W.T., (1986). Assimilate transfer through citrus juice vescicle stalks: A nonvascular portion of the transport path. In: *Phloem Transport*. New York, NY: Alan R. Liss, Inc. pp. 247-258.

[38] Shomer, I., Ben-Gera, I., Fahn, A., (1975). Epicuticular wax on the juice sacs of citrus fruits: A possible adhesive in the fruit segments. *J. Food Sci.* 40 (5), 925-930.

[39] Kanes, K., Tisserat, B., Berhow, M., Vandercook, C., (1993). Phenolic composition of various tissues of Rutaceae species. *Phytochem*. 32 (4), 967-974.

[40] Manthay J.A., Grohmann K., (1996). Concentrations of hesperidin and other orange peel flavonoids in citrus processing by-products. J. Agric. Food Chem. 44, 811-814.

[41] Bocco, A., Cuvelier, M. E., Richard, H., Berset, C. (1998). Antioxidant activity and phenolic composition of citrus peel and seed extracts. J. Agric. Food Chem. 4, 2123–2129.

[42] Ramful, D., Tarnus, E., Aruoma, O.I., Bourdon, E., Bahorun, T. (2011). Polyphenol composition, vitamin C content and antioxidant capacity of Mauritian citrus fruit pulps. *Food Res. Int.* 44 (7), 2088-2099.

[43] Gorinstein, S., Martin-Belloso, O., Park, Y.-S., Haruenkit, R., Lojek, A., Ciz, M., Caspi, A., Libman, I., Trakhtenberg, S., (2001). Comparison of some biochemical characteristics of different citrus fruits. *Food Chem.* 74, 309–315.

[44] Ramful, D., Bahorun, T., Bourdon, E., Tarnus, E., Aruoma, O. I., (2010). Bioactive phenolics and antioxidant propensity of flavedo extracts of Mauritian citrus fruits: potential prophylactic ingredients for functional foods application. *Toxicol.* 278, 75-87.

[45] Castillo, J., Benavente-Garcia, O., Del Rio, J.A., (1992). Naringin and neohesperidin levels during development of leaves, flower, buds and fruits of *Citrus aurantium*. *Plant Physiol.* 99 (1), 67-73.

[46] Castillo, J., Benavente-Garcia, O., Del Rio, J.A., (1993). Hesperetin 7-O-glucoside and pruning in *Citrus* species (*C. aurantium* and *C. paradise*). A study of their quantitative distribution in immature fruits and as immediate precursors of neohesperidin and naringin in *Citrus aurantium*. J. Agric. Food Chem. 41 (11), 1920-1924.

[47] Horowitz, R., Gentili, B., (1977). Flavonoids constituents of Citrus. In: S. Nagy, P. E. Shaw, M. K. Veldhuis, editors. *Citrus Science and Technology*,Vol 1.Westport, CT: AVI Publishing.pp. 397-426.

[48] Lewinsohn, E., Berman, E., Mazur, Y., Gressel, J., (1989). (7) Glucosilation and (1-6) rhamnosylation of exogeneous flavanones by undifferentiated *Citrus* cell cultures. *Plant Sci.* 61, 23-8.

[49] Manach, C., Scalbert, A., Morand, C., Rémésy, C., Jiménez, L., (2004). Polyphenols: food sources and bioavailability. *Am. J. Clin. Nutr.* 79 (5), 727-747.

[50] González-Molina, E., Domínguez-Perles, R., Moreno D.A, García-Viguera, C., (2010).Natural bioactive compounds of *Citrus limon* for food and health. *J. Pharm. Biomed. Anal.* 51, 327–345.

[51] Merken, H.M., Beecher, G.R., (2000). Measurement of food flavonoids by high-performance liquid chromatography: a review. J. Agric. Food Chem. 48 (3), 577-599.

[52] Kanes, K., Tisserat, B., Berhow, M., Vandercook, C., (1993). Phenolic composition of various tissues of Rutaceae species. *Phytochem.* 32 (4), 967-974.

[53] Robards, K., Li, X., Antolovich, M., Boyd, S., (1997). Characterisation of citrus by chromatographic analysis of flavonoids. *J. Sci Food Agric.*75 (1), 87-101.

[54] Tomás-Barberán, F.A., Clifford, M.N., (2000). Flavanones, chalcones and dihydrochalcones – nature, occurrence and dietary burden. *J. Sci Food Agric.* 80 (7), 1073-1080.

[55] McIntosh, C.I., Mansell, R.L., 1997. Three-dimensional distribution of limonin, limonoate A-ring monolactone and naringin in the fruit tissues of three varities of *Citrus paradise*. J. Agric. Food Chem. 45 (8), 2876-2883.

[56] Wu, H., Calvarano, M., Giacomo, A., (1991). Some flavanones in the peel of ten citrus species and varieties in China. *Essenze E Derivati Agrumari.* 61 (2), 103-112.

[57] Bravo, L., (1998). Polyphenols: Chemistry, dietary sources, metabolism, and nutritional significance. *Nutr. Rev.* 56(11), 317-333.

[58] Herrmann, H., (1988). On the flavonol and flavone glycosides in vegetables. *Z. Lebensm. Unters. Forsch.* 186, 1-5.

[59] Mouly, P., Gaydou, E.M., Auffray, A., (1998). Simultaneous separation of flavanone glycosides and polymethoxylated flavones in citrus juices using liquid chromatography. *J. Chromatogr. A.* 800 (2), 171-179.

[60] Robards, K., Li, X., Antolovich, M., Boyd, S., (1997). Characterisation of citrus by chromatographic analysis of flavonoids. *J. Sci. Food Agric.* 75 (1), 87-101.

[61] Mizuno, M., Iinuma, M., Tanaka, T., Matoba, Y., Fujii, Y., Murata, J., Murata, H., Iwamasa, M., (1987). Chemotaxonomic studies on the genus *Citrus*. I. Distribution of flavones in the subgroup Microcarpa. *Chem. Pharm. Bull.* 35 (7), 3025-3028.

[62] Widmer, W.W., Barros, S., (1995). Flavonoids in Ambersweet orange and the impact on juice adulteration detection. In: R.J. Braddock, W.W. Widmer, C.A. Sims, editors. *Forty Sixth Annual Citrus Processors' meeting.* Gainesville, FL: University of Florida, p 21-6.

[63] Chen, J., Montanari, A.M., Widmer, W.W. (1997). Two new polymethoxylated flavones, a class of compounds with potential anticarcinogenic activity, isolated from cold pressed Dancy tangerine peel oil solids. J. Agric. Food Chem. 45 (2), 364-368.

[64] Ortuno, A., Arcas, M.C, Benavente-Garcia, O,.Del Rio, J.A., (1999). Evolution of polymethoxy flavones during development of Tangelo Nova fruits. *Food Chem.* 66, 217-220.

[65] Soobrattee, M.A., Neergheen, V.S., Luximon-Ramma, A., Aruoma, O.I., Bahorun, T., (2005). Phenolics as potential antioxidant therapeutic agents. Mechanisms and actions. *Mut. Res.* 579 (1-2), 200-213.

[66] Senthil Murugan, R., Vidya Priyadarsini, R., Ramalingam, K., Hara, Y., Karunagaran, D., Nagini, S., (2010). Intrinsic apoptosis and NF-κB signaling are potential molecular targets for chemoprevention by black tea polyphenols in HepG2 cells *in vitro* and in a rat hepatocarcinogenesis model *in vivo*. *Food Chem. Toxicol.* 48, 3281–3287.

[67] Lee, D.E., Kang, N.J., Lee, K.M., Lee, B.K., Kim, J.H., Lee K.W., Lee, H.J., (2010). Cocoa polyphenols attenuate hydrogen peroxide-induced inhibition of gap-junction intercellular communication by blocking phosphorylation of connexin 43 via the MEK/ERK signaling pathway. *J. Nutr. Biochem.* 21,680–686.

[68] Di Majo, D., Giammanco, M., La Guardia, M., Tripoli, E., Giammanco, S., Finotti, E., (2005). Flavanones in Citrus fruit: Structure antioxidant activity relationships. *Food Res. Int.* 38, 1161–1166.

[69] Bors, W., Hellers, W., Michel, C., Saran, M., (1990). Radical chemistry of flavonoids antioxidant. In: Emrit, editor. *Antioxidants in therapy and preventive medicine*,Vol 1. New York: Plenum Press.pp. 165-170.

[70] Bors, W., Hellers, W., Michel, C., Saran, M., (1990). Flavonoids as antioxidants: Determination of radical scavenging efficacies. In: Packer, L., Glazer, A.N.,(eds). *Methods in Enzymology*, Vol. 186. San Diego, CA: Academic Press.pp. 343-355.

[71] Perez-Jimenez, J., Arranz, S., Tabernero, M., Diaz- Rubio, M. E., Serrano, J., Goñi, I., Saura-Calixto, F., (2008).Updated methodology to determine antioxidant capacity in plant foods, oils and beverages: Extraction, measurement and expression of results. *Food Res. Int.* 41, 274–285.

[72] Kaur, C., Kapoor, H.C., (2001). Antioxidants in fruits and vegetables – the millennium's health. *Int. J. Food Sci. Technol.* 36 (7), 703-725.

[73] Darmon, N., Ferrandiz, V., Canal, M. T., Mitjavilla, S., (1990). Activité antiradicallaire de flavonoïdes vis-à-vis de l'anion superoxide et du radical hydroxyle. *Liaison-Groupe Polyphenols Bull.* 15, 158–162.

[74] Miyake, Y., Yamamoto, K., Morimitsu, Y., Osawa, T., (1997). Isolation of C-glucosylflavone from lemon peel and antioxidative activity of flavonoid compounds in lemon fruit. J. Agric. Food Chem. 45, 4619–4623.

[75] Guimarães, R., Barros, L., Barreira, J.C.M, Sousa, M.J., Carvalho, A.M., Ferreira, I.C.F.R., (2010). Targeting excessive free radicals with peels and juices of citrus fruits: Grapefruit, lemon, lime and orange. *Food Chem. Toxicol.* 48, 99–106.

[76] Jayaprakasha, G,K., Girennavar, B., Patil, B.S., (2008). Radical scavenging activities of Rio Red grapefruits and Sour orange fruit extracts in different in vitro model systems. *Bioresour. Technol.* 99, 4484–4494.

[77] Abeysinghe, D.C, Li, X., Sun, C.-D., Zhang, W. S., Zhou, C.H., Chen, K.S., (2007). Bioactive compounds and antioxidant capacities in different edible tissues of citrus fruit of four species. *Food Chem.* 104, 1338–1344.

[78] Tripoli, E., Guardia, M.L, Giammanco, S., Di Majo, D., Giammanco, M., (2007). Flavonoids: Molecular structure, biological activity and nutritional properties: A review. *Food Chem.* 104, 466–479.

[79] Finotti, E., Di Majo, D., (2003). Influence of solvents on the antioxidant property of flavonoids. *Die Nahrung.* 47, 186–187.

[80] Day, A.J., Williamson, G., (2003). Absorption of quercetin glycosides. In: Rice-Evans,C., Packer,L., (eds). *Flavonoids in Health and Disease.* Marcel Dekker, New York. pp. 391–412.

[81] Donovan, J.L., Waterhouse, A.L, (2003). Bioavailability of flavanol monomers. In: C. Rice-Evans, C., Packer,L., (eds). *Flavonoids in Health and Disease.* Marcel Dekker, New York. pp. 413–440.

[82] Schroeter, H., Boyd, C., Spencer, J.P.E., Williams, R.J., Cadenas, E., Rice-Evans, C., (2002). MAPK signaling in neurodegeneration: influences of flavonoids and nitric oxide. *Neurobiol. Aging.* 23, 861–680.

[83] Rudkowska, I., (2009). Functional foods for health: focus on diabetes. *Maturitas.* 62, 263-269.

[84] Wild, S., Roglic, G., Green, A., Sicree, R., King, H., (2004). Global prevalence of diabetes: estimates for the year 2000 and projections for 2030. *Diabetes Care.* 27, 1047-1053.

[85] Vinson, J., Howard, T., (1996). Inhibition of protein glycation and advanced glycation end products by ascorbic acid and other vitamins and nutrients. *Nutr. Biochem.* 7, 659-63.

[86] Souto, S.B., Souto, E.B., Braga, D.C., Medina, J.L., (2011). Prevention and current onset delay approaches of type 2 diabetes mellitus (T2DM). *Eur. J. Clin. Pharmacol.* 67, 653–661.

[87] Ho, S., Wu, S., Lin, S., Tang, Y., (2010). Comparison of anti-glycation capacities of several herbal infusions with that of green tea. *Food Chem.* 122 (3), 768-774.

[88] Choi, S.S., Cha, B.Y., Iida, K., Lee, Y.S., Yonezawa, T., Teruya, T., Nagai, T., Woo, J.T., (2011). Artepillin C, as a PPARc ligand, enhances adipocyte differentiation and glucose uptake in 3T3- L1 cells. *Biochem. Pharmacol.* 81, 925–933.

[89] Guri, A.J., Hontecillas, R., Si, H., Liu, D., Bassaganya-Riera, J., (2007). Dietary abscisic acid ameliorates glucose tolerance and obesity-related inflammation in db/db mice fed high-fat diets. *Clin. Nutr.* 26, 107–116.

[90] Ha do, T., Tuan, D.T., Thu, N.B., Nhiem, N.X., Ngoc, T.M., Yim, N., Bae, K., (2009). Palbinone and triterpenes from Moutan Cortex (Paeonia suffruticosa, Paeoniaceae) stimulate glucose uptake and glycogen synthesis via activation of AMPK in insulin-resistant human HepG2 Cells. *Bioorg. Med. Chem. Lett.* 19, 5556–5559.

[91] Hwang, J.T., Kwon, D.Y., Yoon, S.H., (2009). AMP-activated protein kinase: a potential target for the diseases prevention by natural occurring polyphenols. *New Biotechnol.* 26, 17–22.

[92] Yin, J., Zhang, H., Ye, J., (2008). Traditional Chinese medicine in treatment of metabolic syndrome. *Endocr. Metab. Immune Disorder Drug Targets.* 8, 99–111.

[93] Flier, J.S., (2004). Obesity wars: molecular progress confronts an expanding epidemic. *Cell.* 116 (2), 337–350.

[94] Scherer, P.E.,(2006). Adipose tissue: from lipid storage compartment to endocrine organ. *Diabetes.* 55 (6), 1537–1545.

[95] Fantuzzi, G., Mazzone, T., (2007). Adipose tissue and atherosclerosis: exploring the connection. Arterioscler. Thromb. Vasc. *Biol.* 27 (5), 996–1003.

[96] Bluher, M., Wilson-Fritch, L., Lezyki, J., Lausten, P.G., Corvera, S., Kahn, R., (2004). Role of insulin action and cell size on protein expression patterns in adipocytes. *J. Biol. Chem.* 279 (30), 31902–31909.

[97] Kershaw, E.E., Flier, J.S., (2004). Adipose tissue as an endocrine organ. *J. Clin. Endocrinol. Metabol.* 89 (6), 2548–2556.

[98] Hämäläinen, M., Nieminen, R., Vuorela, P., Heinonen, M., Moiiänen, E., (2007). Anti-inflammatory effects of flavonoids: genistein, kaempferol, quercetin, and daidzein inhibit STAT-1 and NF-KB activations, whereas flavone, isorhamnetin, naringenin, and pelargonidin inhibit only NF-KB activation along with their inhibitory effect on Inos expression and NO production in activated macrophages. *Mediators Inflamm.* 6, No.45673.

[99] Cawthorn, W.P., Sethi,J.K., (2008). TNF-alpha and adipocyte biology. *FEBS Lett.* 582, 117–131.

[100] Hotamisligil, G.S, Shargill, N.S., Spiegelman, B.M., (1993). Adipose expression of tumor necrosis factor-alpha: direct role in obesity-linked insulin resistance. *Science* 259, 87–91.

[101] Hotamisligil, G.S., Arner, P., Caro, J.F., Atkinson, R.L., Spiegelman, B.M., (1995). Increased adipose tissue expression of tumor necrosis factor-alpha in human obesity and insulin resistance. *J. Clin. Invest.* 95, 2409–2415.

[102] Uysal, K.T., Wiesbrock, S.M., Marino, M.W., Hotamisligil, G.S., (1997). Protection from obesity-induced insulin resistance in mice lacking TNF-alpha function. *Nature.* 389, 610–614.

[103] Miles, P.D., Romeo, O.M., Higo, K., Cohen, A., Rafaat, K., Olefsky, J.M., (1997). TNF-alpha induced insulin resistance in vivo and its prevention by troglitazone. *Diabetes.* 46, 1678–1683.

[104] Boden, G., (1997). Role of fatty acids in the pathogenesis of insulin resistance and NIDDM. *Diabetes.* 46, 3–10.

[105] Ryden, M., Arvidsson, E., Blomqvist, L., Perbeck, L., Dicker, A., Arner, P., (2004). Targets for TNF-alpha-induced lipolysis in human adipocytes. *Biochem. Biophys. Res. Commun.* 318, 168–175.

[106] Rahn Landstrom, T., Mei, J., Karlsson, M., Manganiello, V., Degerman, E., (2000). Downregulation of cyclic-nucleotide phosphodiesterase 3B in 3T3-L1 adipocytes induced by tumour necrosis factor alpha and cAMP. *Biochem. J.* 346 (Pt 2), 337–343.

[107] H., Takamura, N., Shuto, T., Ogata, K., Tokunaga J., Kawai, K., Kai, H., (2010). The citrus flavonoids hesperetin and naringenin block the lipolytic actions of TNF-a in mouse adipocytes. *Biochem. Biophys. Res. Commun.* 394, 728–732.

[108] Ramful, D., Tarnus, E., Rondeau, P., Da Silva, C. R., Bahorun, T., Bourdon, E., (2010).Citrus Fruit Extracts Reduce Advanced Glycation End Products (AGEs)- and H_2O_2-Induced Oxidative Stress in Human Adipocytes. J Agric. Food Chem. 58, 11119-11129.

[109] Mahley, R.W., (1988). Apolipoprotein E: cholesterol transport protein with expanding role in cell biology. *Science*. 240, 622-630.

[110] Tarnus, E., Wassef, H., Carmel, J.F., Rondeau, P., Roche, M., Davignon, J., Bernier, L., Bourdon, E., (2009). Apolipoprotein E limits oxidative stress-induced cell dysfunctions in human adipocytes. *FEBS Lett.* 583 (12), 2042-2048.

[111] Miyata, M., Smith, J.D., (1996). Apolipoprotein E allele-specific antioxidant activity and effects on cytotoxicity by oxidative insults and beta-amyloid peptides. *Nat. Genet.* 14, 55-61.

[112] Davignon, J., (2005). Apolipoprotein E and atherosclerosis: beyond lipid effect. *Arterioscler. Thromb. Vasc. Biol.* 25, 267-269.

[113] Jadhav, R., Puchchakayala, G., (2012). Hypoglycemic and antidiabetic activity of flavonoids: boswellic acid, ellagic acid, quercetin, rutin on streptozotocin-nicotinamide induced type 2 diabetic rats. *Int. J. Pharm. Pharm. Sci.* 4(2), 251-256.

[114] Li, J.M., Che, C.T., Lau, C.B.S., Leung, P.S., Cheng, C.H.K., (2006). Inhibition of intestinal and renal Na^+-glucose cotransporter by naringenin. *Int. J. Biochem. Cell Biol.* 38 (5-6), 985-995.

[115] Jung, U.J., Lee, M-K., Park, Y.B., Kang, M.A, Choi, M-S., (2006). Effect of citrus flavonoids on lipid metabolism and glucose-regulating enzyme mRNA levels in type-2 diabetic mice. *Int. J. Biochem. Cell Biol.*38 (7), 1134-1145.

[116] Gyo-Nam, K., Jung-Geun, S., Hae-Dong, J., (2009). Antioxidant and antidiabetic activity of Dangyuja (*Citrus grandis* Osbeck) extract treated with *Aspergillus saitoi*. *Food Chem.* 117 (1), 35-41.

[117] Stern, D.M.; Yan, S.D.; Yan, S.F.; Schmidt, A.M., (2002). Receptor for advanced glycation endproducts (RAGE) and the complications of diabetes. *Ageing Res. Rev.* 1 (1), 1-15.

[118] Pashikanti, S., De Alba, D.R., Boissonneault, G.A., Cervantes-Laurean, D., (2010). Rutin metabolites: novel inhibitors of nonoxidative advanced glycation end products. *Free Rad. Biol. Med.*48 (5), 656-663.

[119] Unoki, H., Hideaki Bujo, H., Yamagishi, S., Takeuchi, M., Imaizumi, T., Saito, Y., (2007). Advanced glycation end products attenuate cellular insulinsensitivity by increasing the generation of intracellularreactive oxygen species in adipocytes. *Diabetes Res. Clin. Pract.* 76, 236–244.

[120] Oteiza, P.I.; Erlejman, A.G.; Verstraeten, S.V.; Keen, C.L.; Fraga, C.G., (2005). Flavonoid-membrane interactions: a protective role of flavonoids at the membrane surface. *Clin. Dev. Immunol.*12 (1), 19–25.

[121] Crespy, V., Morand, C., Besson, C., Cotelle, N., Vezin, H., Demigne, C., Remesy, C., (2003). The splanchnic metabolism of flavonoids highly differed according to the nature of the compound. *Am. J. Physiol – Gastrointest. Liver Physiol.*284(6), G980–8.

[122] Hanahan, D., Weinberg, R.A., (2011). Hallmarks of Cancer: The Next Generation. *Cell.* 144, 646-674.

[123] Neergheen, V.S., Bahorun,T., Taylor,E.W., Jen, L.S., Aruoma, O.I., (2010). Targeting specific cell signaling transduction pathways by dietary and medicinal phytochemicals in cancer chemoprevention. *Toxicol.* 278(2), 229-241.

[124] Stagos, D., Amoutzias, G.D., Matakos, A., Spyroua, A., Tsatsakis, A.M., Kouretas, D., (2012). Chemoprevention of liver cancer by plant polyphenols. *Food Chem. Toxicol.* 50, 2155–2170.

[125] Chen, A.Y., Chen, Y.C., (2013). A review of the dietary flavonoid, kaempferol on human health and cancer chemoprevention. *Food Chem.* 138, 2099–2107.

[126] Murthy, K.N.C., Kim, J., Vikram, A., Patil, B.S., (2012). Differential inhibition of human colon cancer cells by structurally similar flavonoids of citrus. *Food Chem.* 132, 27–34.

[127] Kim, J., Jayaprakasha, G.K., Vikram, A., Patil, B.S., (2012). Methyl nomilinate from citrus can modulate cell cycle regulators to induce cytotoxicity in human colon cancer (SW480) cells in vitro. *Toxicol. in Vitro.* 26, 1216–1223.

[128] Lim, H.K, Moon, J.Y., Kim, H., Cho, M., Cho, S.K., (2009). Induction of apoptosis in U937 human leukaemia cells by the hexane fraction of an extract of immature *Citrus grandis* Osbeck fruits. *Food Chem.* 114, 1245–1250.

[129] Guthrie, N., Morley, K., Hasegawa, S., Manners, G.D., Vandenberg, T., (2000). Inhibition of human breast cancer cells by citrus limonoids. In: Manners, G.D, Hasegawa, S., (eds). *Citrus Limonoids.* Washington, DC: American Chemical Society, Inc. pp.164-174.

[130] Tian, Q., Miller, E.G., Hassan, A., Tang, L., Patil, B.S., (2001). Differential inhibition of human cancer cell proliferation by citrus limonoids. *Nutr. Cancer.* 40, 180-184.

[131] Jayaprakasha, G.K., Mandadi, K.K., Poulose, S.M., Jadegoud, Y., Nagana, G., Patil, B.S., (2008). Novel triterpenoid from *Citrus aurantium* L. possesses chemopreventive properties against human colon cancer cells. *Bioorg. Med. Chem.* 16, 5939-5951.

[132] Patil, J., Kim, J., Jayaprakasha, G., (2010). Berberine induces apoptosis in breast cancer cells (MCF-7) through mitochondrial-dependent pathway. *Eur. J. Pharmacol.* 645, 70–78.

[133] Patil, J.R., Murthy, K.N.C., Jayaprakasha, G.K., Chetti, M.B., Patil, B.S., (2009). Bioactive compounds from Mexican lime (*Citrus aurantifolia*) juice induce apoptosis in human pancreatic cells. *J. Agric. Food Chem.* 57, 10933–10942.

[134] Poulose, S.M, Harris, E.D., Patil, B.S., (2005). Citrus limonoids induce apoptosis in human neuroblastoma cells and have radical scavenging activity. *J. Nutr.* 135, 870-877.

[135] Kelly, C., Jewell, C., O'Brien, N.M., (2003). The effect of dietary supplementation with the citrus limonoids, limonin and nomilin on xenobiotic metabolizing enzymes in the liver and small intestine of the rat. *Nutr. Res.* 23, 681-690.

[136] Lam, L.K.T., Li, Y., Hasegawa, S., (1989) Effects of citrus limonoids on glutathione S - transferase in mice. *J. Agric. Food Chem.* 37, 878-880.

[137] Lam, L.K.T., Zhang, J., Hasegawa, S., Schut, H.A.J., (1994). Inhibition of chemically induced carcinogenesis by citrus limonoids. In: Huang, M.T., T.O., Ho, C.T., Rosen, R.T. editors. *Food Phytochemicals for Cancer Prevention I.* Washington, DC: American Chemical Society, Inc. p. 209–219.

[138] Perez, J.L., Jayaprakasha, G.K., Valdivia, V., Munoz, D., Dandekar, D.V., Ahmad, H., Patil, B.S., (2009). Limonin methoxylation influences the induction of glutathione S-transferase and quinone reductase. *J. Agric. Food Chem.* 57, 5279-5286.

[139] Tanaka, T., Maeda, M., Kohno, H., Murakami, M., Kagami, S., Miyake, M., Wada, K., (2001). Inhibition of azoxymethane-induced colon carcinogenesis in male F344 rats by the citrus limonoids obacunone and limonin. *Carcinogenesis.* 22, 193–198.

[140] Vanamala, J., Leonardi, T., Patil, B.S., Taddeo, S.S., Murphy, M.E., Pike, L.M., Chapkin, R.S., Lupton, J.R., Turner, N.D., (2006). Suppression of colon carcinogenesis by bioactive compounds in grapefruit. *Carcinogenesis.* 27, 1257–1265.

[141] Glinsky,V.V., Raz, A., (2009). Modified citrus pectin anti-metastatic properties: one bullet, multiple targets. *Carbohyd. Res.*344, 1788–1791.

[142] Nangia-Makker, P., Honjo, Y., Sarvis, R., Akahani, S., Hogan, V., Pienta, K.J., Raz, A., (2000). Galectin-3 Induces Endothelial Cell Morphogenesis and Angiogenesis. *Am. J. Pathol.*156, 899–909.

[143] Ho, Y.S., So, K.F., Chang, C.C., (2010). Anti-aging herbal medicine – How and why can they be used in aging-associated neurodegenerative diseases? *Ageing Res. Rev.* 9, 354-362.

[144] Iriti, M., Vitalini, S., Fico, G., Faoro, F., (2010). Neuroprotective herbs and foods from different traditional medicines and diets. *Molecules.* 15, 3517-3555.

[145] Rockenstein, E., Crews, L., Masliah, E., (2007). Transgenic animal models of neurodegenerative diseases and their application to treatment development. *Adv. Drug Delivery Rev.* 59, 1093-1102.

[146] Ricciarelli, R., Argellati, F., Pronzato, M.A., Domenicotti, C., (2007). Vitamin E and neurodegenerative diseases. *Mol. Asp. Med.* 28, 591-606.

[147] James, L.E., Fogler, K.A., Tauber, S.K., (2008). Recognition memory measures yield disproportionate effects of aging on learning face-name associations. *Psychol. Aging.* 23, 657-664.

[148] Gilchrist, A.L., Cowan, N., Naveh-Benjamin, M., (2008). Working memory capacity for spoken sentences decreases with adult ageing: recall of fewer but not smaller chunks in older adults. *Memory.* 16, 773-787.

[149] Gazzaley, A., Sheridan, M.A., Cooney, J.W., D'esposito, M., (2007). Age-related deficits in component processes of working memory. *Neuropsychol..* 21, 532-539.

[150] Park, D.C., Lautenschlager, G., Hedden, T., Davidson, N.S., Smith, A.D., Smith, P.P., (2002). Models of visuospacial and verbal memory across the adult life span. *Psychol. Aging.* 17, 299-320.

[151] Mattson, M.P., (2004). Pathways towards and away from Alzheimer's disease. *Nature.* 430, 631-639.

[152] Brown, R.C., Lockwood, A.H., Sonawane, B.R., (2005). Neurodegenerative Diseases: An overview of environmental risk factors. *Environ. Health Perspect.* 113, 1250-1256.

[153] Qiu, C., Kivipelto, M., Von Strauss, E., (2009). The epidemiology of Alzheimer's disease: occurrence, determinants, and strategies toward intervention. *Dialogues Clin. Neurosci.* 11, 111-128.

[154] Li, C., Ebrahimi, A., Schluesener, H., (2013). Drug pipeline in neurodegeneration based on transgenic mice models of Alzheimer's disease. *Ageing Res. Rev.* 12(1),116-140.

[155] Du, Y., Wooten, M.C., Wooten, M.W., (2009). Oxidative damage to the promoter region of SQSTM1/p62 is common to neurodegenerative disease. *Neurobiol. Dis.* 35, 302-310.

[156] Altun, M.L., Yilmaz, B.S., Orhan, I.E., Citoglu, G.S., (2013). Assessment of cholinesterase and tyrosinase inhibitory and antioxidant effects of *Hypericum perforatum* L. (St. John's wort). *Ind. Crop. Prod.* 43, 87-92.

[157] Calabrese, V., Cornelius, C., Mancuso, C., Lentile, R., Stella, Butterfield, D.A., (2010). Redox homeostasis and cellular stress response aging and neurodegeneration. *Methods Mol. Biol.* 610, 285-308.

[158] Li, J., Liu, D., Sun, L., Lu, Y,.Zhang, Z., (2012). Advanced glycation end products and neurodegenerative diseases: Mechanisms and perspective. *J. Neurol. Sci.* 317, 1-5.

[159] Reed, T.T., (2011). Lipid peroxidation and neurodegenerative disease. *Free Rad. Biol. Med.* 51, 1302-1319.

[160] Williams, R.J., Spencer, J.E., (2012). Flavonoids, cognition, and dementia: Actions, mechanisms, and potential therapeutic utility for Alzheimer disease. *Free Rad. Biol. Med.* 52, 35–45.

[161] Lu,Y.H., Su, M.Y., Huang, H.Y., Li, L., Yuan, C.G., (2006). Protective effects of the citrus flavanones to PC12 cells against cytotoxicity induced by hydrogen peroxide. *Neurosci. Lett.* 484, 6–11.

[162] Hwang, S.-L., Yen, G.-C., (2008). Neuroprotective effects of the citrus flavanones against H_2O_2-Induced cytotoxicity in PC12 Cells. *J. Agric. Food Chem.* 56 (3), 859–864.

[163] Jagetia G.C., Reddy, T.K., (2011). Alleviation of iron induced oxidative stress by the grape fruit flavanone naringin *in vitro. Chem.-Biolo. Interact.* 190, 121–128.

[164] Gopinath, K., Prakash, D., Sudhandiran, G., (2011.) Neuroprotective effect of naringin, a dietary flavonoid against 3-nitropropionic acid induced neuronal apoptosis. *Neurochem. Int.* 59, 1066–1073.

[165] Gopinath, K., Sudhandiran, G., (2012). Naringin modulates oxidative stress and inflammation in 3-nitropropionic acid-induced neurodegeneration through the activation of nuclear factor-erythroid 2-related factor-2 signalling pathway. *Neurosci.*, 227, 134–143.

[166] Vafeiadou, K., Vauzour, D., Lee, H.Y., Rodriguez-Mateos, A., Williams, R.J., Spencer, J.P.E., (2009). The citrus flavanone naringenin inhibits inflammatory signaling in glial cells and protects against neuroinflammatory injury. *Arch. Biochem. Biophys.* 484, 100–109.

[167] Okuyama, S., Minami, S., Shimada, N., Makihata, N., Nakajima, M., Furukawa, Y., (2013). Anti-inflammatory and neuroprotective effects of auraptene, a citrus coumarin, following cerebral global ischemia in mice. *Eur. J. Pharmacol.* 699, 118–123.

In: Citrus
Editor: Khizar Hayat

ISBN: 978-1-63117-985-3

Chapter 7

CITRUS MEDICA L. CV DIAMANTE: AN OVERVIEW ON THE PHYTOCHEMISTRY AND POTENTIAL HEALTH BENEFITS

Rosa Tundis**, Monica R. Loizzo, Marco Bonesi and Francesco Menichini
Department of Pharmacy, Health and Nutritional Sciences,
University of Calabria, Rende (CS), Italy

ABSTRACT

Citrus fruits, which are one of the most important commercial crops growing worldwide, have received attention for their nutritional and biological properties. The health effects of the whole fruit, as well as its juices and extracts, have been studied in relation to several diseases. Anticancer, antioxidant, antihyperlipidemic, hypoglycemic, antibacterial, anti-inflammatory and antiviral effects of *Citrus* have been reported. *Citrus* species are rich sources of ascorbic acid and other bioactive compounds such as terpenes, coumarins, carotenoids, limonoids and flavonoids. The *C. medica* was the first *Citrus* fruit to come to the notice of Europeans and was for many years the only one known. Among the better known *C. medica* cultivars are Corsican, Diamante, Etrog and Fingered Citron. *C. medica* cv Diamante is the cultivar more widely grown throughout Italy and more sought after by the industry.

This chapter aims at providing an up-to-date overview of the traditional uses, phytochemistry, and bioactivity of this *C. medica* cultivar. The relevance of *C. medica* cv Diamante is justified by the most recent findings indicating that it is a medicinal and nutritional agent useful for treating a range of human disorders.

Keywords: *Citrus*, Phytochemicals, Antioxidants, Type 2 Diabetes, Alzheimer's disease

---

* Corresponding author address: Department of Pharmacy, Health and Nutritional Sciences, University of Calabria, I-87036 Rende (CS), Italy; E-mail: rosa.tundis@unical.it.

INTRODUCTION

The *Citrus medica* was the first *Citrus* to come to the notice of Europeans and it was for many years the only one known species. This plant has an ancient origin; the more accredited provenance is from India but it probably arrived in Italy through the Hebrews who introduced its cultivation on the Calabrian coasts.

Virgil (7019 B.C.) was the first of the Latin writers to describe the *C. medica* while Theophrastus called it the Median apple and described uses similar to those given by the earlier author. Dioscorides, author of "Materia Medica" between 60 and 79 A.D., described *C. medica* as if it had become well established in the district where he lived. He referred to it as the Median and Persian apple or Cedromela, and said that the Latins named it Citria [1]. Pliny, in his "Natural History", published about 77 A.D., gave several names to the *C. medica* (Malus medica, Malus Assyria and Citrus) and described its use as a medicine, poison, antidote, perfume, and protection from moths.

In ancient times and in the Middle Ages, the *C. medica* was employed as a remedy for seasickness, pulmonary troubles, intestinal ailments and other disorders. In India, the fruit peels are a remedy for dysentery and are eaten to overcome halitosis. The candied peel is sold in China as a stomachic, stimulant, expectorant and tonic [2]. In West Tropical Africa, the *C. medica* is used as a medicine, particularly against rheumatism [3].

"Corsican", "Diamante", "Etrog" and "Fingered citron" are the better-known *C. medica* cultivars [4]. *C. medica* cv Diamante (Figure 1) is the most diffused cultivar in Italy and in particularly in Calabria where the cultivation extends along the high Thyrrenium coast from Diamante to Tortora. For this reason this area is called the "Coast of citron" (Cosenza, Italy).

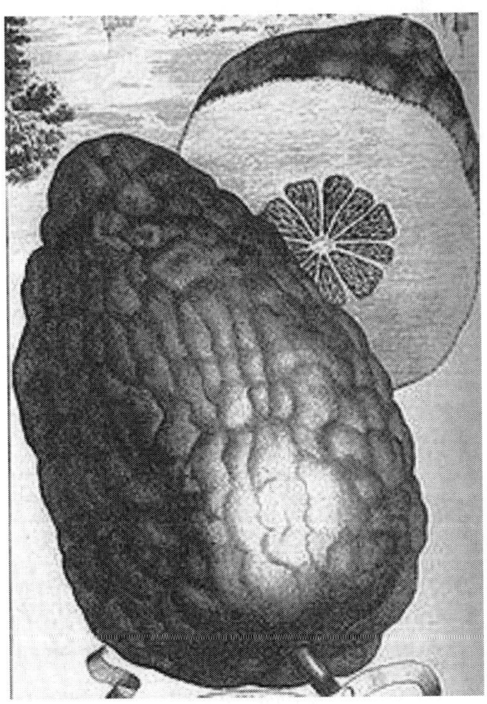

Figure 1. Ancient image of a *C. medica* cv Diamante fruit.

C. medica is a shrub or small evergreen tree, of irregular shape, with disordered growth and branching low, slow-growing, reaching 2.5-4.5 meters in height. It has a continuous flowering, with the main flowers in spring and autumn. The flowering is so distinct: flowering in spring (March-May); summer flowering (June); late flowering (September). The main and most abundant flowering is in the summer, as it provides the fruit of the best quality. The fruits are oblong, oval or ellipsoid, smooth surface, or more often wrinkled, bernocculata, often with a more or less large conical hillock to the stalk. In the full development, the fruits are very large, with a weight that can vary from 500-600 g to 1.5-2.0 kg and an average length of 20-30 cm. The fruits have a pale or greenish-yellow flesh, not very juicy, slightly sour or sweet. The peel is very rough, tough and exceptionally thick, constituting up to 70% of the fruit. Its color varies greatly depending on the maturity period, rising from deep green when the fruit is unripe, to the golden yellow of the ripe fruit [4].

CHEMICAL CONSTITUENTS

Citrus fruits are known to possess high amounts of active principles including essential oils, flavonoids, limonoids, coumarins, and carotenoids besides vitamin C, soluble fibre, minerals, vitamin B complex and related nutrients such as thiamine, riboflavin, nicotinic acid/niacin, pantothenic acid, pyridoxine, folic acid, biotin, choline, and inositol [5,6].

Some works evidenced the main phytochemical constituents of *C. medica* cv Diamante. The essential oil was obtained from the fruit peels by hydrodistillation (HD), cold-pressing (CP) and supercritical fluid extraction (SFE) [7]. A total of forty-two components were identified in the oil obtained by HD, representing 95.3% of the total oil. Thirty-six constituents were identified in the essential oil obtained by CP, representing 93.4% of the total oil. Both samples exhibited high amounts of limonene (35.4-44.5%), and γ-terpinene (24.5-26.2%). Other abundant constituents were geranial, α-pinene, and β-pinene. The high content of limonene and γ-terpinene is characteristic of this *Citrus* cultivar [8]. The essential oil obtained by HD possesses a high content of terpinen-4-ol, α-terpinene, and α-terpineol in comparison with the essential oil obtained by CP. The percentage of neral was also different in the essential oil obtained by HD and CP with percentage of 4.4% and 0.1%, respectively [7]. With SFE six compounds were identified. These data clearly indicated the selectivity of supercritical CO_2 for the extraction of the oil components. The most abundant compound was the coumarin cipropten (84.5%) indicating the capability of this extraction method at the given CO_2 density to exert a maximal solvent capability toward this highly lipophilic compound. Interestingly, the 2,3-dihydrobenzofuran and 2,3-dihydro-3,5-dihydroxy-6-methyl-4*H*-pyran-4-one were not present in the HD and CP essential oils, confirming the selectivity of the supercritical solvent at the pressure/temperature region immediately above the CO_2 supercritical point (31 °C and 73 bar) [9].

In the same year, *C. medica* cv Diamante peel essential oils were obtained from the fruits collected in two different zones characterized by different leaf nutrients and soil pedological parameters [10]. These essential oils were analyzed in order to highlight the relationships of condition of growth and *C. medica* essential oils chemical composition. The limonene was the main constituent in both zones (42.7-55.3% for zone at sea level and 40.2-55.8% for zone like hills at 300 meters above sea level), followed by γ-terpinene (18.3-24.2% for zone at sea level and 20.8-28.0% for zone like hills at 300 meters above sea level). The content of other more abundant compounds, such as thujene, α-pinene, β-pinene, β-myrcene and terpinolene, was generally higher in oils derived from plants growing at sea level. Among sesquiterpenes the main components were β-bisabolene (0.5-1.3% for zone at sea level and 0.5-1.5% for zone like hills at 300 meters above sea level), and *trans*-caryophyllene (0.2-0.5% for zone at sea level and 0.3-0.7% for zone like hills at 300 meters above sea level). The coumarins citropten and oxypeucedanin were also identified but not in all essential oils.

The composition of *C. medica* cv Diamante essential oil from three types of fruits (green citron of small size, green citron of large size and yellow citron 1 month after harvest) was previously analyzed [11]. The essential oils, extracted using three different methods, differed only in the quantitative composition. In particular, the volatile fraction of every sample of essential oil was characterized by a high content of limonene, γ-terpinene, and monoterpene aldehydes. A lower content of α-pinene, β-pinene and myrcene, sesquiterpenes, and aliphatic aldehydes was found. The essential oils were characterized by a high content of limonene followed by γ-terpinene. These data were in agreement with data reported by Verzera et al., [12] who identified limonene (51.95%) as the main component followed by γ-terpinene (27.71%). The sesquiterpene fraction was less represented; the main components were β-bisabolene (0.48%) and *trans*-α-bergamotene (0.34%). Among oxygenated compounds, carbonyl compounds showed the highest amount (4.99%), with neral and geranial as the main components [12]. Lota et al., [13] reported a high content of limonene (70.4%) and a very low abundance of γ-terpinene ($\leq$ 0.05%) for the essential oil obtained by hydrodistillation of the peel of the *C. medica* cv Diamante fruits. The peel essential oil from *C. medica* cv Diamante from Crete contained limonene as main constituent, a high content of neral and geranial, β-pinene and myrcene, and an appreciable proportion of citronellol, nerol and geraniol [14].

Nevertheless, the health benefits of *Citrus* fruit have mainly been attributed to the presence of phenolic compounds, such as flavonoids. Flavonoids are a class of naturally occurring polyphenolic compounds. Over 4000 different naturally occurring flavonoids have already been identified and the list is still growing [15]. Flavonoids are present in fruits, vegetables, nuts and plant-derived beverages such as tea and wine. Most flavonoids share a common three-ring structure of which two rings are aromatic and one ring is heterocyclic [15]. The variation in the heterocyclic ring forms the basis of the division of the flavonoids in subclasses, i.e. the flavones, isoflavones, flavonols, flavanals, flavanones, anthocyanidins and chalcones. Flavonoids inhibit lipid peroxidation (LPO), platelet aggregation and activity of enzyme systems including cyclooxygenase and lipoxygenase, and reduce the capillary permeability and fragility. Flavonoids exert these effects as antioxidants, free radical scavengers and chelators of divalent cations [16].

The content of naringenin, naringin, hesperetin, hesperidin, rutin, nobiletin, tangeretin, quercetin, diosmin, and apigenin, has been analyzed in *C. medica* cv Diamante extracts [17]. Apigenin (1) was identified in all extracts, except for mesocarp of mature fruits with values ranging from 941.0 mg/kg for flowers to 58.0 mg/kg of fresh weight for mature fruits endocarp (Figure 2). The flowers extract was characterized by the highest content of different flavonoids. Besides apigenin (1), quercetin (2) (580.8 mg/kg) and diosmin (3) (372.5 mg/kg) were also found in significant quantities. The flavone diosmin (3), abundant in the flowers extract, was detected only in the mature fruits mesocarp (18.2 mg/kg). Naringin (4) was identified only in mesocarp of immature fruits (556.0 mg/kg). Hesperidin (5), unlike of correspondent aglycone hesperetin (6), was identified in immature fruits extracts with values of 26.0 mg/kg for mesocarp and 18.4 mg/kg for endocarp [17]. Hesperedin (5) and hesperetin (6) were abundant in the flowers extract with values of 203.8 and 224.3 mg/kg. Rutin (7) was abundant in immature fruits endocarp extract (484.7 mg/kg), followed by leaves and flowers extracts with values of 264.2 and 156.5 mg/kg, respectively. The polymethoxylated flavones, nobiletin and tangeretin were not identified in any of the *C. medica* cv Diamante extracts [17]. In agreement with another study on *Citrus* fruits [18], the highest flavanones contents were found in young fruits.

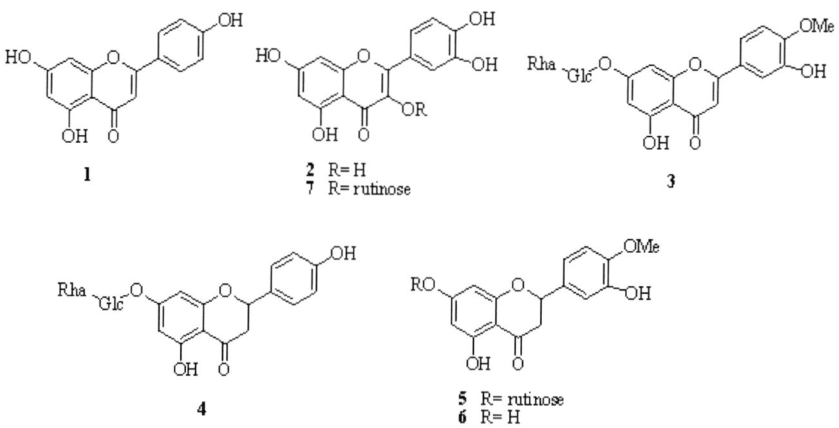

Figure 2. The chemical structures of the main *C. medica* cv Diamante flavonoids: (1), apigenin; (2), quercetin; (3), diosmin; (4), naringin; (5), hesperidin; (6), hesperetin; (7), rutin.

Antioxidant Properties

In traditional societies nutrition and health care are strongly interconnected and many plants have been consumed as food, to prepare beverage and for medicinal purposes [19]. A number of studies on the antioxidant properties of plant foods and their constituents have become very impressive [20,21].

Free radicals are reactive molecules due to the presence of one or more unpaired electron(s). They are formed in the human body either as an essential mediator in vital processes or as a byproduct [22,23]. In aerobic life forms, the reduction of oxygen comprises binding of most of the oxygen to hydrogen to give water, a process involved in the oxidative phosphorylation. However, a small part of the oxygen is only partly reduced during this redox reaction. As a result, free radicals or other reactive species, that can either oxidize other compounds or easily form radicals, will arise. These partly reduced forms of oxygen are designated as reactive oxygen species (ROS). Similarly, reactive nitrogen species (RNS) are continuously produced. ROS include singlet oxygen, superoxide, hydrogen peroxide, hydroxyl radical, ozone and hypochlorous acid, while examples of RNS are nitric oxide and peroxynitrite. Free radicals normally exist in all aerobic cells in balance with biochemical antioxidants. Oxidative stress occurs when this critical balance is disrupted because of excess of ROS, antioxidants depletion, or both. To counteract the oxidant effects and to restore redox balance, cells must reset important homeostatic parameters. When tightly regulated, ROS can act as intracellular signaling molecules [24].

ROS can determine tissue damage by reacting with nucleotides in DNA, lipids in cellular membranes, sulphydryl groups in proteins and cross-linking/fragmentation of ribonucleoproteins. In living cells, the major source of endogenous ROS is hydrogen peroxide and superoxide anion, which are generated as products of cellular metabolism such as mitochondrial respiration. Alternatively, hydrogen peroxide may be converted into water by the enzymes catalase or glutathione peroxidase [25]. The relatively unreactive superoxide anion radical is converted by superoxide dismutase (SOD) into H_2O_2, which in turn take part in the "Fenton reaction", with transition metal ion (copper or iron) as catalysts, to produce the very reactive hydroxyl radical [26].

Some works evidenced the potential antioxidant effects of *C. medica* cv Diamante. The best free radical 1,1-diphenyl-2-picrylhydrazyl (DPPH) scavenging activity was exerted by the extract obtained from the mesocarp of immature fruits (IC_{50} value of 382.0 μg/mL) followed by flowers and leaves extracts with IC_{50} values of 425.0 μg/mL and 502.0 μg/mL, respectively (Table 1). The extracts obtained from the fruits, leaves and flowers of *C. medica* cv Diamante showed the antioxidant activity in β-carotene bleaching test [17]. In particular, flowers showed the highest and interesting inhibition of linoleic acid oxidation with an IC_{50} value of 2.8 μg/mL at 30 min of incubation. These results are important if compared to the positive control propyl gallate that showed an IC_{50} value of 1.0 μg/mL. Flowers extract was characterized by apigenin and quercetin as main constituents.

Some research works reported a high correlation between phenols and flavonoids content and antioxidant activity in selected fruits [24,27,28]. Flavonoids exhibit interesting biological activities, including antiallergenic, antiviral, antiinflammatory, and vasodilating actions. However, most interest has been devoted to their antioxidant properties. Flavonoids inhibit the enzymes responsible for superoxide anion production, such as xanthine oxidase and protein kinase C [28]. Flavonoids have been also shown to inhibit cyclooxygenase, lipoxygenase, microsomal monooxygenase, glutathione *S*-transferase, mitochondrial succinoxidase, and NADH oxidase, all involved in reactive oxygen species generation [29]. A number of flavonoids efficiently chelate trace metals, which play an important role in oxygen metabolism. For exemple, free iron and copper are potential enhancers of reactive oxygen species formation [30]. In a recent study [31] quercetin was investigated in comparison with curcumin for its total antioxidant capacity (TAC), on production of ROS and nitric oxide (NO) in lipopolysaccharide (LPS)-stimulated human THP-1 acute monocytic leukemia cells. Quercetin has its TAC 3.5 fold higher than curcumin; it reduced LPS-induced ROS to near normal levels; it reduced LPS-induced NO production.

Previously, the *n*-hexane extract from the *C. medica* cv Diamante peel demonstrated anti-radical scavenging activity with an IC_{50} value of 147 μg/mL [32]. A higher level of antioxidant activity in the β-carotene-linoleic acid test system was observed with an IC_{50} value of 3 μg/mL after 30 and 60 min of incubation, indicating that their activity was not correlated with the period of incubation. The antioxidant activity may be related to the presence of monoterpenes, such as γ-terpinene, limonene, nerol, geraniol and α-terpineol that are the most abundant compounds identified in the extract [33-35].

Table 1. Radical scavenging and antioxidant activities [IC_{50} (μg/mL)] of Diamante citron extracts

Plant material	Extract	DPPH	TBA	β-Carotene bleaching test		Reference
				30 min	60 min	
Flowers	hydro-alcoholic	425.0	-	2.8	5.7	[16]
Leaves	hydro-alcoholic	502.0	-	>100	5.1	[16]
Peel	*n*-hexane	147	2472	3	3	[27]
Immature fruits						
Mesocarp	hydro-alcoholic	382.0		3.7	4.1	[16]
Endocarp	hydro-alcoholic	>1000		4.1	4.5	[16]
Mature fruits						
Mesocarp	hydro-alcoholic	>1000		36.6	45.4	[16]
Endocarp	hydro-alcoholic	>1000		3.5	7.1	[16]

PREVENTION AND MANAGEMENT OF TYPE 2 DIABETES

Diabetes mellitus (DM) is a condition in which homeostasis of carbohydrate and lipid metabolism is improperly regulated by the pancreatic hormone insulin resulting in an increased blood glucose level. The World Health Organization (WHO) submits that the number of cases for diabetes that is currently at 171 million is predicted to reach 366 million by the year 2030 [36]. The two major forms of diabetes are termed insulin-dependent diabetes mellitus (type 1 diabetes) and non-insulin-dependent diabetes mellitus (type 2 diabetes), but the WHO classification system includes evidence that diabetes mellitus is an aetiologically and clinically heterogeneous group of disorders that share hyperglycemia in common [37].

Type 2 diabetes is a heterogeneous disease resulting from a dynamic interaction between defects in insulin secretion and insulin action with increased concentrations of blood glucose, which in turn damage many of the body's systems and in particular the blood vessels. Patients with type 2 diabetes are insulin-resistant and often have a metabolic syndrome, a multifactorial intervention including aggressive treatment of arterial hypertension and dyslipidemia [38]. As most subjects are over weighted or obese, the initial treatment is optimization of the meal plan and enhancement of physical activity in order to obtain sustained weight reduction. In case of failure of life-style changes, various oral hypoglycaemic agents may be used.

The aim of antidiabetic therapy is to reach normoglycemia and to reduce insulin resistance, thereby improving metabolic control with the intention to prevent diabetic late complications. One of the therapeutic approaches for reducing post-prandial hyperglycemia in patients with type 2 diabetes is to prevent absorption of carbohydrates after foods uptake. This is done by retarding the absorption of glucose through the inhibition of the carbohydrate-hydrolyzing enzymes, α-amylase and α-glucosidase, in the digestive tract [39]. Consequently, inhibitors of these enzymes determine a reduction in the rate of glucose absorption and therefore blunting the post-prandial plasma glucose rise. These drugs also have certain adverse effects like causing hypoglycemia at higher doses, liver problems, lactic acidosis and diarrhoea [40].

For the past two decades many research articles in the field of ethno-pharmacology have focused on the anti-diabetic effects of some natural products. This increase of interest was partly due to the fact that type 2 diabetes mellitus was considered as becoming a global epidemic health problem which imposed high cost to national health services around the world [41].

The α-amylase and α-glucosidase inhibitory activity of *C. medica* cv Diamante flowers, leaves and fruits (endocarp and mesocarp) at two maturity stages were investigated [17] (Table 2). The leaves extract demonstrated an inhibitory activity against α-amylase with an IC_{50} value of 438.5 μg/mL. A comparison between results of endocarp obtained from mature fruits and immature fruits revealed that mature fruits inhibited the α-amylase with IC_{50} value 2-fold higher than that for immature fruits (IC_{50} value of 426.0 μg/mL). On the contrary the α-glucosidase was inhibited more by the immature fruits with an IC_{50} value of 472.9 μg/mL.

Correlation between phenols and flavonoids content revealed that carbohydrate-hydrolyzing enzyme inhibitory activity could not be related with these phytochemicals since flowers that are characterized by the highest content were unable to inhibit the enzymes [17].

Previously, the *n*-hexane *C. medica* cv Diamante peels extract inhibited α-amylase with an IC_{50} value of 625 μg/mL [32]. This activity was related to the content of terpenoids considering that the lipophilicity of these phytochemicals may facilitate access to the enzymatic site [42]. The *C. medica* var. Sarcodactylis essential oil demonstrated to be very beneficial to type 2 diabetes mellitus patients [43].

Table 2. Inhibitory activity of *C. medica* cv Diamante extracts against enzyme useful for maintenance of human health [IC_{50} (μg/mL)]

Plant material	Extract	α-Amylase	α-Glucosidase	AChE	BChE	Reference
Mature fruits						
Peel	Essential oil by HD	-	-	171.3	154.6	[7]
Peel	Essential oil by CP	-	-	298.8	NA	[7]
Peel	Essential oil by SFE	-	-	NA	NA	[7]
Peel	hydro-alcoholic	258.7	263.2	-	-	[16]
Peel	*n*-hexane	625	-	621	-	[27]
Mesocarp	hydro-alcoholic	707.4	633.1	-	-	[16]
Endocarp	hydro-alcoholic	426.0	574.1	-	-	[16]
Immature fruits						
Mesocarp	hydro-alcoholic	702.2	539.7	-	-	[16]
Endocarp	hydro-alcoholic	844.5	472.9	-	-	[16]
Flowers	hydro-alcoholic	>1000	>1000	-	-	[16]
Leaves	hydro-alcoholic	438.5	777.8	-	-	[16]

AChe: acetylcholinesterase; BChE: butyrylcholinesterase; HD: Hydrodistillation; CP: cold-pressing; SFE: supercritical fluid extraction; NA: no activity.

The hydroalcoholic extract of *C. medica* cv Diamante peel demonstrated to inhibit both α-amylase and α-glucosidase with IC_{50} values of 258.7 and 263.2 μg/mL, respectively. This extract was characterized by high phenols content as previously reported, and by the presence of apigenin, quercetin and hesperetin as main flavonoids [44].

Tadera et al., [45] investigated the inhibitory activity of six groups of flavonoids (flavone, flavonol, flavanone, isoflavone, flavan-3-ol, and anthocyanidin) against α-amylase and α-glucosidase. Quercetin inhibited yeast α-glucosidase with an IC_{50} value of 7 μM and porcine pancreatic α-amylase with an IC_{50} value of 0.50 mM [45]. Hesperetin (6) and apigenin (1) were less active against both enzymes showing IC_{50} values of 150 and > 200 μM, respectively, against yeast α-glucosidase, and IC_{50} values > 0.50 mM against porcine pancreatic α-amylase.

The effects of *C. medica* cv Diamante on insulin secretion were also assessed *in vitro* using the mouse insulinoma MIN6 β-cell line. This experimental model facilitates the study of agents which are thought to have direct effects on the β-cell [46]. In order to exclude non-specific release of insulin because of cytotoxicity of *C. medica* cv Diamante hydroalcoholic peel extract, cell viability was assessed by trypan blue exclusion. No cytotoxicity was detected at concentrations up to 24 mg/mL. At concentrations ranging from 1 to 24 mg/mL *C. medica* cv Diamante extract exerted direct stimulatory effects on the exocytotic release of insulin from monolayers of MIN6 cells, initiating a concentration-dependent stimulation of insulin secretion at both 2 and 20 mM glucose [44].

The maximal effects of the extract on insulin secretion were comparable to those of the known insulin secretagogues, phorbol myristate acetate (PMA) and forskolin (FSK). MIN6 cells maintained as monolayers are poorly responsive to glucose, so in subsequent experiments the cells were configured as three-dimensional pseudoislets which greatly increased their response to glucose [46,47].

The extract also enhanced glucose induced insulin secretion, although these effects were less pronounced. Thus, switching from 2 mM glucose (0-10 min) to 20 mM glucose (10 min onwards) initiated a small insulin secretory response, which was further enhanced by the inclusion of extract in the perifusion buffer (30-50 min), most noticeably at 1 mg/mL [44].

Moreover, the effects of *C. medica* cv Diamante peel extract were evaluated *in vivo* using CD-1 mice. After 30 days of treatment, blood samples were collected in order to evaluate haematological and biochemical parameters.

Data on glucose and plasma lipid concentrations (cholesterol and triglycerides) are shown in Figure 3. The oral administration (600 mg/kg) of the *C. medica* cv Diamante peel extract lowered the levels of plasma cholesterol and triglycerides [44]. Both doses (300 and 600 mg/kg) were able to reduce glucose concentration.

All other parameters, lactate dehydrogenase (LDH), glutamate-oxaloacetate transaminase (GOT), glutamate-pyruvate transaminase (GPT), creatine kinase (CK), urea, alkaline phosphatase (ALP), gamma glutamyl transferase (GGT), triglicerides, cholesterol, glucose, creatine, and prothrombin time (PT) were in the normal range and showed no significant difference [48].

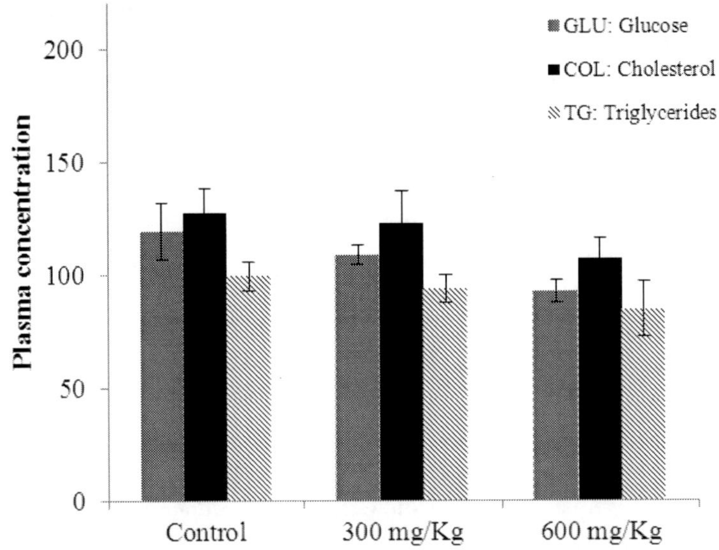

Figure 3. Plasma concentration of glucose, cholesterol and triglycerides (mg/dL) in rats treated with two experimental diets supplements (300 and 600 mg/kg) of *C. medica* cv Diamante peel extract.

ANTICHOLINESTERASE PROPERTIES

In 1907, Alois Alzheimer, a psychiatrist and neuropathologist, described the clinical and pathological findings of a 51-year-old woman with a 4 1/2 year course of progressive dementia, which subsequently became recognized as a disorder bearing his name.

Alzheimer's disease (AD) is a degenerative neurological disease that is clinically characterized by progressive cognitive dysfunction that interferes with social and occupational functioning [49]. Some relevant pathogenic events involved in AD are: a) genetic alterations, neuronal apoptosis-like processes leading to premature neuronal death and brain dysfunction; b) β-amyloid deposition in senile plaques and brain vessels, neurofibrillary tangles due to hyperphosphorilation of Tau proteins, synaptic loss; c) neurotransmitter deficits, neurotrophic alterations, neuroinmune dysfunction, neuroinflammatory processes; d) accelerated neuronal death due to excitotoxic reactions, alterations in calcium homeostasis, free radical formation and cerebrovascular dysfunction [50].

Increased levels of cholinesterase enzymes found in post-mortem brain samples of AD patients have led to the hypothesis that the cognitive decline in AD patients is related to progressive cholinergic degeneration [50]. Therefore, promising approaches for the treatment of AD are to enhance the level of cholinergic neurotransmitters in the brain by cholineresterase inhibitors [51]. Two cholinesterase enzymes, acetylcholinesterase (AChE) and butyrylcholinesterase (BChE) play an important role in decreasing choline levels in the body. During the past decade, some inhibitors of AChE and BChE have been clinically evaluated [52]. Nevertheless, all of them revealed some toxicity during prolonged use. Consequently, there is still a great demand for new drug for the treatment of AD.

The potential use of natural products has been successfully demonstrated in the field of neurodegenerative disorder treatment including AD [53,54]. Among natural sources, essential oils are attracting special attention [53-56]. The essential oil obtained by hydrodistillation from the peels of *C. medica* cv Diamante demonstrated to inhibit both AChE and BChE with IC_{50} values of 171.3 and 154.6 μg/mL, respectively [7]. A selective AChE inhibition was observed with the oil obtained by cold-pressing, while the essential oil obtained by SFE was completely inactive against both enzymes. The instituted bioactivity could be explained by the presence of some terpenes identified as major constituents [57,58].

Among them, α-pinene inhibited AChE with an IC_{50} value of 0.63 mM while β-pinene showed a 48.5% inhibition at 1 mM [51,57]. Other terpenes are also able to inhibit AChE. Particular research demonstrated the inhibition of AChE by α-terpinene (IC_{50} of 1 mM), 1,8-cineole (IC_{50} of 41 μg/mL), γ-terpinene (22.6% at 1.2 mM), *p*-cymene (39.8% at 1.2 mM), linalool (37% at 164 μg/mL), and terpineol-4-ol (24.0% at 1.2 mM) [59-63]. However, several studies demonstrated that the activity exhibited by the essential oil is probably due to the synergistic activities of several components. In fact, the monoterpenes identified in the *n*-hexane extract obtained from the peel of *C. medica* cv. Diamante peel may justify the inhibitory activity against AChE (IC_{50} value of 621 μg/mL) [32].

Conclusion

Scientific evidence strongly supports an association between a healthy diet and the prevention of chronic diseases. There is an increasing involvement of consumers in health care, resulting in lifestyle modification and incorporation of complementary and alternative medicines into their dietary routine to maintain their health and prevent disease.

In recent years, there has been increasing interest in the role of *Citrus* species in human health in particular, as antibacterial, antiviral, antioxidant, antifungal, analgesic and anti-inflammatory agents. *C. medica* cv Diamante has demonstrated antioxidant and anticholinesterase inhibitory activity. Moreover, in *in vitro* and *in vivo* studies this *Citrus* species showed interesting anti-hyperglycaemic effects. In particular, *C. medica* cv Diamante peel extract demonstrated to confer protection against induced hyperglycemia at least in part by direct stimulation of β-cells to secrete insulin. In addition, the capacity of the extract to reduce glucose, triglycerides and plasma cholesterol levels may contribute to its beneficial effects *in vivo*.

This chapter aims to highlight *C. medica* cv Diamante health properties in order to promote its use as functional food or a potential source for functional ingredients or nutraceutical products.

References

[1] Gunther, R.Y., (1959). The Greek Herbal of Dioscorides. New York: Hafner.

[2] Meena, A.K., Kandale, A., Rao, M.M., Panda, P., Reddy, G., (2011). A review on citro-pharmacognosy, phytochemistry and medical uses. *Int. Res. J. Pharm.* 2, 14-19.

[3] Arias, B.A., Ramon-Laca, L., (2005). Pharmacological properties of citrus and their ancient and medieval uses in the Mediterranean region. *J. Ethnopharmacol.* 97, 89-95.

[4] Fersini, A., Giorlando, A., Tuoto, G., (1973). Il cedro (*Citrus medica* L.). Pàtron editore: Bologna, Italy; 1973.

[5] Hamdan, D., El-Readi, M.Z., Tahrani, A., Herrmann, F., Kaufmann, D., Farrag, N., El-Shazly, A., Wink, M., (2011). Chemical composition and biological activity of *Citrus jambhiri* Lush. *Food Chem.* 127, 394-403.
[6] Cheong, M.W., Liu, S.Q., Zhou, W., Curran, P., Yu, B., (2012). Chemical composition and sensory profile of pomelo (*Citrus grandis* (L.) Osbeck) juice. *Food Chem.* 135, 2505-2513.
[7] Menichini, F., Tundis, R., Bonesi, M., de Cindio, B., Loizzo, M.R., Conforti, F., Statti, G.A., Menabeni, R., Bettini, R., Menichini, F. (2011). Chemical composition and bioactivity of *Citrus medica* L. cv Diamante essential oil obtained by hydrodistillation, cold-pressing and supercritical carbon dioxide extraction. *Nat. Prod. Res.* 25, 789-799.
[8] Poiana, M., Sicari, V., Mincione, B., (1998). A comparison between the chemical composition of the oil, solvent extract and supercritical carbon dioxide extract of *Citrus medica* L. cv. Diamante. *J. Essent. Oil Res.* 10, 145-152.
[9] Brunner, G. (1994). Gas extraction, an introduction to fundamentals of supercritical fluids and the application to separation processes. New York: Springer.
[10] Loizzo, M.R., Tundis, R., Menichini, F., Bonesi, M., Calabretta, M.L., Giuffrida, A., Intrigliolo, F., Menichini, F., (2011). Influence of nutritional status, environmental and pedological parameters on *Citrus medica* cv Diamante peel essential oil chemical composition. *Italian J. Food Sci.* 23, 146-152.
[11] Gabriele, B., Fazio, A., Dugo, P., Costa, R., Mondello L., (2009). Essential oil composition of *Citrus medica* L. cv. Diamante (Diamante citron) determined after using different extraction methods. *J. Sep. Sci.* 32, 99-108.
[12] Verzera, A., Trozzi, A., Zappala, M., Condurso, C., Cotroneo, A., (2005). Essential oil composition of *Citrus meyerii* Y. Tan. And *Citrus medica* L. cv. Diamante and their lemon hybrids. *J. Agric. Food Chem.* 53, 4890-4894.
[13] Lota, M.L., de Rocca Serra, D., Tomi, F., Bessiere, J.M., Casanova, J., (1999). Chemical composition of peel and leaf essential oils of *Citrus medica* L. and *C. limonimedica* Lush. *Flavour Fragr. J.* 14, 161-166.
[14] Vekiari, S.A., Protopapadakis, E., Gianovits-Argyriadou, N., (2004). Composition of the leaf and peel oils of *Citrus medica* L. 'Diamante' from Crete. *J. Essential Oil Res.* 16, 528-530.
[15] Harborne, J.B., Baxter, H., Moss, G.P. (1999). Phytochemical dictionary: Handbook of bioactive compounds from plants (2nd ed.). London: Taylor and Francis.
[16] Bubols, G.B., Vianna Dda, R., Medina-Remon, A., von Poser, G., Lamuela-Raventos, R.M., Eifler-Lima, V.L., Garcia, S.C. (2013). The antioxidant activity of coumarins and flavonoids. *Mini Rev. Med. Chem.* 13, 318-334.
[17] Menichini, F., Loizzo, M.R., Bonesi, M., Conforti, F., De Luca, D., Statti, G.A., de Cindio, B., Menichini, F., Tundis, R., (2011). Phytochemical profile, antioxidant, anti-inflammatory and hypoglycemic potential of hydroalcoholic extracts from *Citrus medica* L. cv Diamante flowers, leaves and fruits at two maturity stages. *Food Chem. Toxicol.* 49 1549-1555.
[18] Ortuño, A., Reynaldo, I., Fustera, M.D., Botía, J., Puiga, D.G., Sabatera, F., Lidónc, G.A., Porrasc, I., Del Río, J.A., (1997). *Citrus* cultivars with high flavonoid contents in the fruits. *Sci. Hortic.* 68, 231-236.
[19] Pieroni, A., (2000). Medicinal plants and food medicines in the folk traditions of the upper Lucca Province Italy. *J. Ethnopharmacol.* 70, 235-273.

[20] Benzie, I.F., Choi, S.W. (2014). Antioxidants in food: content, measurement, significance, action, cautions, caveats, and research needs. *Adv. Food Nutr. Res.* 71, 1-53.

[21] Gironés-Vilaplana, A., Moreno, D.A., García-Viguera, C. (2014). Phytochemistry and biological activity of Spanish *Citrus* fruits. *Food Funct.* 2014, in press.

[22] Ermakov, A.V., Konkova, M.S., Kostyuk, S.V., Izevskaya, V.L., Baranova, A., Veiko, N.N. (2013). Oxidized extracellular DNA as a stress signal in human cells. *Oxid. Med. Cell Longev.* 2013, 649747.

[23] Jomova, K, Valko, M. (2011). Advances in metal-induced oxidative stress and human disease. *Toxicology* 283, 65-87.

[24] Boots, A.W, Haenen, G.R.M.M., Bast, A., (2008). Health effects of quercetin: from antioxidant to nutraceutical. *Eur. J. Pharmacol.* 585, 325-337.

[25] Halliwell, B., (1999). Oxygen and nitrogen are pro-carcinogens. Damage to DNA by reactive oxygen, chlorine and nitrogen species: measurement, mechanism and the effects of nutrition. *Mutat. Res.* 443, 37-52.

[26] Aruoma, O.I., Halliwell, B., Dizdaroglu, M., (1989). Iron ion-dependent modification of bases in DNA by the superoxide radical-generating system hypoxanthine/xanthine oxidase. *J. Biol. Chem.* 264, 13024-13028.

[27] Velioglu, Y.S., Mazza, G., Gao, L., Oomah, B.D., (1998). Antioxidant activity and total phenolics in selected fruits, vegetables, and grain products. *J. Agric. Food Chem.* 46, 4113-4117.

[28] Terao, J., (2009). Dietary flavonoids as antioxidants. *Forum of Nutrition* 61, 87-94.

[29] Papageorgiou, N., Tousoulis, D., Katsargyris, A., Charakida, M., Androulakis, E., Siasos, G., Tentolouris, C., Stefanadis, C., (2013). Antioxidant treatment and endothelial dysfunction: is it time for flavonoids? *Recent Pat. Cardiovasc. Drug Discov.* 8, 81-92.

[30] Rubió, L., Motilva, M.J., Romero, M.P., (2013). Recent advances in biologically active compounds in herbs and spices: a review of the most effective antioxidant and anti-inflammatory active principles. *Crit. Rev. Food Sci. Nutr.* 53, 943-953.

[31] Zhang, M., Swarts, S.G., Yin, L., Liu, C., Tian, Y., Cao, Y., Swarts, M., Yang, S., Zhang, S.B., Zhang, K., Ju, S., Olek, D.J. Jr, Schwartz, L., Keng, P.C., Howell, R., Zhang, L., Okunieff, P., (2011). Antioxidant properties of quercetin. *Adv. Exp. Med. Biol.* 701, 283-289.

[32] Conforti, F., Statti, G.A., Tundis, R., Loizzo, M.R., Menichini, F., (2007). *In vitro* activities of *Citrus medica* L. cv. Diamante (Diamante citron) relevant to treatment of diabetes and Alzheimer's disease. *Phytother. Res.* 21, 427-433.

[33] Ruberto, G., Baratta, M.T., (2000). Antioxidant activity of selected essential oil components in two lipid model systems. *Food Chem.* 69, 167-174.

[34] Choi, H.S., Song, H.S., Ukeda, H., Sawamura, M., (2000). Radical scavenging activities of *Citrus* essential oils and their components: detection using 1,1-diphenyl-2-picrylhydrazyl. *J. Agric. Food Chem.* 48, 4156-4161.

[35] Grassmann, J., Elstner, E.F., Schneider, D., Weiser, D., (2001). Antioxidative effects of lemon oil and its components on copper induced oxidation of low density lipoprotein. *Arzneimittelforschung* 51, 799-805.

[36] Wild, S., Roglic, G., Green, A., Sicree, R., King, H., (2004). Global prevalence of diabetes: estimates for the year 2000 and projections for 2030. *Diabetes Care* 27, 1047-1053.
[37] World Health Organization (WHO), (2006). Definition and diagnosis of diabetes and intermediate hyperglycaemia.
[38] Molitch, M.E., (2013). Current state of type 2 diabetes management. *Am. J. Managed Care* 19(8 Suppl), s136-142.
[39] Tundis, R., Loizzo, M.R., Menichini, F., Bonesi, M., Conforti, F., De Luca, D., Menichini, F., (2012). Air-dried *Capsicum annuum* var. *acuminatum* medium and big: determination of bioactive constituents, antioxidant activity and carbohydrate-hydrolyzing enzymes inhibition. *Food Res. Inter*. 45, 170-176.
[40] Tundis, R., Loizzo, M.R., Menichini, F. (2010). Natural products as alpha-amylase and alpha-glucosidase inhibitors and their hypoglycaemic potential in the treatment of diabetes: an update. *Mini-Rev. Med. Chem*. 10, 315-331.
[41] Salimifar, M., Fatehi-Hassanabad, Z., Fatehi, M., (2013). A Review on natural products for controlling type 2 diabetes with an emphasis on their mechanisms of actions. *Curr. Diabetes Rev*. 9, 402-411.
[42] Ali, H., Houghton, P.J., Soumyanath, A., (2006). Alpha-amylase inhibitory activity of some Malaysian plants used to treat diabetes; with particular reference to *Phyllanthus amarus*. *J. Ethnopharmacol.* 107, 449-455.
[43] Peng, C.H., Ker, Y.B., Weng, C.F., Peng, C.C., Huang, C.N., Lin, L.Y., Peng, R.Y., (2009). Insulin secretagogue bioactivity of finger citron fruit (Citrus medica L. var. Sarcodactylis Hort, Rutaceae). *J. Agric. Food Chem.* 57, 8812-8819.
[44] Menichini, F., Tundis, R., Loizzo, M.R., Bonesi, M., Liu, B., Houghton, P.J., Persaud, S.J., Jones, P.M., Mastellone, V., Lombardi, P., Avallone, L., Menichini, F., (2011). *C. medica* cv Diamante peel chemical composition and influence on glucose homeostasis and metabolic parameters. *Food Chem.* 124, 1083-1089.
[45] Tadera, K., Minami, Y., Takamatsu, K., Matsuoka, T., (2006). Inhibition of alpha-glucosidase and alpha-amylase by flavonoids. *J. Nutr. Sci. Vitaminol.* 52, 149-53.
[46] Persaud, S.J., (1958). Pancreatic beta-cell line: their role in beta-cell research and diabetes therapy. In Latner, A., (editor). *Clinical Biochemistry*, (2nd ed). Philadelphia: Saunders Co. pp. 47.
[47] Hauge-Evans, A.C., Squires, P.E., Belin, V.D., Roderigo-Milne, H., Ramracheya, R.D., Persaud, S.J., et al., (2002). Role of adenine nucleotides in insulin secretion from MIN6 pseudoislets. *Mol. Cel. Endocrinol.* 191, 167-176.
[48] Bhasin, M.K., Chahal, S.M.S., (1996). A laboratory manual for human blood analysis. Kamal-raj Enterprises.
[49] Jacobsen, J.S., Reinhart, P., Pangalos, M.N., (2005). Current concepts in therapeutic strategies targeting cognitive decline and disease Modification in Alzheimer's disease. *NeuroRx.* 2, 612-626.
[50] Loizzo, M.R., Tundis, R., Menichini, F., Menichini, F., (2008). Natural products and their derivatives as cholinesterase inhibitors in the treatment of neurodegenerative disorders: an update. *Curr. Med. Chem.* 15, 1209-1228.
[51] Farfara, D., Lifshitz, V., Frenkel, D., (2008). Neuroprotective and neurotoxic properties of glial cells in the pathogenesis of Alzheimer's disease. *J. Cel. Mol. Med.* 12, 762-780.

[52] Lefevre, G., Pommier, F., Sedek, G., Allison, M., Huang, H.L., Kiese, B., Ho, Y.Y., Appel-Dingemanse, S., 2008. Pharmacokinetics and bioavailability of the novel Rivastigmine transdermal patch versus Rivastigmine oral solution in healthy elderly subjects. J. Clin. Pharmacol. 48, 246–252.

[53] Howes, M.R., Houghton, P.J., 2003. Plants used in Chinese and Indian traditional medicine for improvement of memory and cognitive function. Pharmacol. Biochem. Behav. 75, 513–527.

[54] Francotte, P., Graindorge, E., Boverie, S., de Tullio, P., Pirotte, B., (2004). New trends in the design of drugs against Alzheimer's disease. *Curr. Med. Chem.* 11, 1757-1778.

[55] Perry, N.S., Houghton, P.J., Theobald, A., Jenner, P., Perry, E.K., (2000). *In vitro* inhibition of human erythrocyte acetylcholinesterase by *Salvia lavandulaefolia* essential oil and constituent terpenes. *J. Pharm. Pharmacol.* 52, 895-902.

[56] Perry, N.S., Houghton, P.J., Jenner, P., Keith, A., Perry, E.K., (2002). *Salvia lavandulaefolia* essential oil inhibits cholinesterase *in vivo*. *Phytomedicine* 9, 48-51.

[57] Loizzo, M.R., Menichini, F., Tundis, R., Bonesi, M., Conforti, F., Nadjafi, F., Statti, G.A., Frega, N.G., Menichini, F., (2009). *In vitro* biological activity of *Salvia leriifolia* Benth essential oil relevant to the treatment of Alzheimer's disease. *J. Oleo Sci.* 58, 443-446.

[58] Loizzo, M.R., Menichini, F., Conforti, F., Tundis, R., Bonesi, M., Saab, A.M., Statti, G.A., de Cindio, B., Houghton P.J., Menichini, F., Frega, N.G., (2009). Chemical analysis, antioxidant, antiinflammatory and anticholinesterase activities of *Origanum ehrenbergii* Boiss and *Origanum syriacum* L. essential oils. *Food Chem.* 117, 174-180.

[59] Miyazawa, M., Watanabe, H., Kameoka, H., (1997). Inhibition of acetylcholinesterase activity by monoterpenoids with a *p*-menthane skeleton. *J. Agric. Food Chem.* 45, 677-679.

[60] Miyazawa, M., Watanabe, H., Umemoto, K., Kameoka, H., (1998). Inhibition of acetylcholinesterase activity by essential oils of *Mentha* species. *J. Agric. Food Chem.* 46, 3431-3434.

[61] Miyazawa, M., Yamafuji, C., (2005). Inhibition of acetylcholinesterase activity by bicyclic monoterpenoids. *J. Agric. Food Chem.* 53, 1765-1768.

[62] Miyazawa, M., Yamafuji, C., (2006). Inhibition of acetylcholinesterase activity by tea tree oil and constituent terpenoids. *Flav. Fragr. J.* 21, 198-201.

[63] Picollo, M.I., Toloza, A.C., Mougabure Cueto, G., Zygadlo, J., Zerba, E., (2008). Anticholinesterase and pediculicidal activities of monoterpenoids. *Fitoterapia* 79, 271-278.

In: Citrus
Editor: Khizar Hayat

ISBN: 978-1-63117-985-3

Chapter 8

HIGH DOSES OF SYNEPHRINE AND OCTOPAMINE ACTIVATE LIPOLYSIS IN HUMAN ADIPOCYTES, INDICATING THAT AMINES FROM *CITRUS* MIGHT INFLUENCE ADIPOSITY

Marie-Anne Carpéné*[1]*, Xavier Testar*[3] *and Christian Carpéné*[1,2]
[1]Université Paul Sabatier Toulouse III.
[2]Institut des Maladies Métaboliques et Cardiovasculaires, INSERM, Toulouse, France
[3]Departament Bioquímica i Biologia Molecular, Universitat Barcelona, Barcelona, Spain

ABSTRACT

The consumption of dietary supplements advertised as slimming agents increases with the world-wide obesity epidemics. Numerous consumers expect to loose weight consequently to the believed lipolytic and thermogenic properties of *Citrus aurantium* extracts they ingest. Indeed, amines abundant in *Citrus aurantium* (bitter orange), especially synephrine, are proposed to limit adipose tissue development. In this chapter, it will not be stated whether *Citrus* consumption is clinically relevant to treat obesity, but the results of *in vitro* tests performed on adipocytes with the amines found in *Citrus* will be analyzed after an overview of their occurrence in different *Citrus* varieties. The presence of para-synephrine, and to a lesser extent of octopamine, tyramine and methyl-tyramine in *Citrus* fruits and juices is well-recognized. Synephrine and octopamine shared a limited capacity to activate lipolysis in human fat cells, while they were more efficient in rodent fat cells. We confirmed that octopamine binds to beta$_3$-adrenergic receptors (ARs) that are weakly expressed in human adipocytes. Synephrine also acted on beta-ARs, not tyramine or methyltyramine. None of the *Citrus* amines exhibited clear activation or blockade of the alpha$_2$-ARs highly expressed in human adipocytes. The amines were unable to improve adrenaline lipolytic stimulation. At millimolar doses, they

* Corresponding author address: Dr. Christian Carpéné. INSERM U1048, I2MC, CHU Rangueil, BP 84225, 31432 Toulouse Cedex 4, France. E-mail: christian.carpene@inserm.fr.

activated glucose transport in human adipocytes. Lastly, octopamine administration in rats slightly lowered body weight gain and did not alter sensitivity to the antilipolytic and antilipogenic actions of insulin. Thus, high concentrations of synephrine and octopamine directly modify adipocyte metabolism, indicating that these amines may act on fat depots, if ingested in sufficient amounts. Further studies deserve to verify whether *Citrus* consumption (fruit juices or extracts) modifies fat accumulation.

Keywords: Obesity, Dietary amines, Tyramine, Octopamine, Synephrine, Adipocytes

INTRODUCTION

In this chapter, *Citrus* will be treated as a source of "dietary amines". To date, one of the most widely known deleterious effect of an excessive ingestion of dietary amines on human health is called the "*cheese effect*", which corresponds to a hypertensive crisis, that occurred several decades ago in depressed patients treated with irreversible inhibitors of monoamine oxidases (MAOs) [1]. Such attack occurred after consumption of tyramine-rich meals (cheeses, sausages…): once ingested, the alimentary amine tyramine was not degraded by peripheral MAOs, therefore increased sympathetic tone and provoked fatal hypertensive crisis [2]. Nowadays, this kind of serious adverse effects does not exist anymore since the use of irreversible MAO inhibitors to treat depression is limited, and the tyramine content of food items has been controlled [3].

However, as a consequence of the world-wide expansion of obesity, there is an increasing number of individuals who repeatedly ingest substantial amounts of dietary amines other than tyramine: the consumers of dietary supplements advertised as slimming drugs. Indeed, numerous companies developing weight management products or functional foods are selling a profusion of weight-lowering formulations, such as medicinal plant extracts with putative "*fat-burning*" action [4]. Some of them are claiming that *Citrus aurantium*, or more precisely synephrine or octopamine, can decrease body weight. Consequently, obese or overweight subjects, or even customers practicing fitness attracted by the putative capacity of such dietary supplements to reduce fat mass repeatedly consume these products. Such approach leads to an increased consumption of *Citrus* extracts. Synephrine and octopamine, which belong to the family of aromatic bioactive amines (Figure 1), are alkaloids univocally recognized to be abundant in *Citrus* fruits, more especially in extracts prepared from *Citrus aurantium* (bitter orange) [5]. It is essentially the non-edible parts or the unripe fruits that are very rich in these two molecules advertised as being capable to "burn fat" or to "mobilize lipids". Though it is difficult to estimate the amount of these "*Citrus* amines" consumed by the concerned costumers, such intake needs to be studied in terms of efficacy and safety.

Synephrine and octopamine are biogenic amines related to endogenous catecholamines, especially noradrenaline and adrenaline, also known as (nor)epinephrine, (Figure 1), which are neurotransmitters in the sympathetic system [6]. These amines are able to influence cardiovascular functions, but replace advantageously ephedrine that was present in ancient slimming formulations, and that has been banned in view of its serious deleterious effects [6]. However, pharmacological studies and clinical data supporting the real efficiency of synephrine and octopamine on lipid metabolism and on body weight regulation are still fragmentary [7,8]. Considering that *Citrus* fruits are widely consumed worldwide, and that many *Citrus* fruits other than bitter orange contain biogenic amines and polyamines [9], it is also important on a nutritional point of view, to better define the biological effects of their components once ingested by consumers.

Thus, this chapter will focus reader's attention on the effects of several amines found in *Citrus* on adipose tissue, although it must be kept in mind that such amines can also act on many other target tissues [10,11]. Moreover, flavonoids, phenolic compounds, carotenoids and vitamins also belong to the multiple components found in *Citrus* and in their extracts and may as well influence consumer's health or appetite by acting not only on fat cells or their precursors [12], but also on any other cell type in the organism.

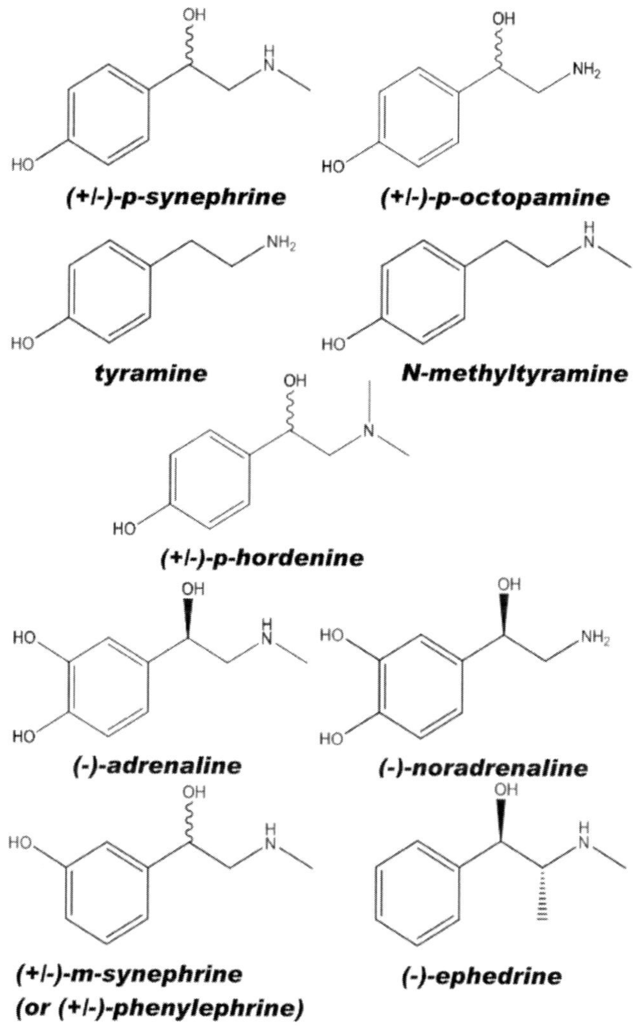

Figure 1. Structural formulae of the amines found in *Citrus* (synephrine, octopamine, tyramine, N-methyltyramine, hordenine,), and related molecules: adrenaline and noradrenaline (physiological neurotransmitters in mammals), phenylephrine (used as a vasoconstrictor drug), ephedrine (banned hypertensive amphetamine). All structures share the same phenethylamine skeleton.

In this context, we will first summarize the current pharmacology of octopamine and synephrine. Then, we will review the quantitative levels of biogenic amines present in *C.*

aurantium that have been obtained oftenly by application of various analytical methods to fruits and phytoproducts. Obviously, there is a large range of amine contents, depending on the biological source and on the laboratory technique. Thence, we will extend the survey to *Citrus* fruits other than bitter orange. Since synephrine, octopamine, tyramine and N-methyltyramine are quantitatively important alkaloids in the fruits or in their extracts, we have tested how these amines could directly regulate lipolytic activity in cells freshly isolated from abdominal subcutaneous human adipose tissues. Thereupon, the role of lipolysis in the fat store reduction will be reassessed, together with a clarification of non-shivering thermogenesis. In the following sections, we will also report verifications that were not achievable on human fat cells, and that were performed in cultured cells transfected with the human form of a membrane receptor shown to bind adrenergic substances (namely the beta3-adrenergic receptor or β_3-AR), or either in adipose tissue homogenates, and even in fat cells from rats repeatedly treated by octopamine.

Biochemistry and Pharmacology of Octopamine and Synephrine

The structural formulae of the amines found in *Citrus* are shown in Figure 1, together with several related agents belonging to the family of bioactive amines. Synephrine, together with its N-demethylated derivative, octopamine, has an asymetrical carbon atom and therefore both exist as (+)- and (-)-enantiomers. Moreover, the two amines exist as ortho-, meta- or para-forms. The nature of the major forms occurring naturally in fruits has been under debate [13-17], but at least to our knowledge, there is compelling evidence for arguing that only (-)-*p*-synephrine is found in *Citrus* species and their extracts (at least when non-adulterated with other chemical substances) [5,18,19]. It must be noted here that the presence of meta-synephrine (also known as phenylephrine, a nasal vasoconstrictor drug) reported once to be present in *Citrus* fruit juice has never been confirmed later [20]. Thus, phenylephrine is shown in Figure 1 for illustrating its similarities with *p*-synephrine, but will be not treated thereafter since not considered to naturally occur in *Citrus*.

The biogenic amine *p*-octopamine is a well-established neurotransmitter in insects or crustaceans, in which it is believed to play the role of stress hormone, as the catecholamines (adrenaline and noradrenaline) do in mammals. Different octopamine receptors (OARs) have been characterized and sequenced in invertebrates and implied in the "flight or fight" behaviour induced by octopamine [21,22]. Although these OARs do not seem to be highly expressed in mammals, other related receptors can recognize octopamine. The receptors associated to trace amines (TAARs) can bind various dietary amines (among them tyramine, phenethylamine, octopamine) and also many additional endogenous ligands [23]. Several decades ago, it remained difficult to assess whether octopamine was active directly on a precise population of receptors present in mammalian post-synaptic cells or was acting as a "false neurotransmitter" on pre-synaptic neurones, or working on both. At this time, *in vivo* and *in vitro* studies indicated that octopamine, which corresponds to the ring-dehydroxylated derivative of noradrenaline (Figure 1), interacted with mammalian adrenergic receptors of the alpha-type (α_1- and α_2-ARs) as well as synephrine, but with less affinity than noradrenaline [24]. Thereafter, the direct activation by octopamine of another adrenoreceptor type, the β_3-

AR, was reported in a single cell model: the adipocyte [25]. Thus, it was demonstrated that octopamine acted on the same target post-synaptic cells than those regulated by catecholamines. Meanwhile, it has been repeatedly observed that octopamine acts on β_3-ARs in rat, hamster and dog adipocytes [26-28]. Moreover, partial agonist properties at α_2-AR of octopamine have been confirmed in cultured mammalian cells transfected with α_2-AR-genes [29]. A β-AR activation was also proposed for synephrine, while tyramine has not been suspected to potently interact with such ARs [27].

Octopamine-induced activation of β_3-ARs resulted in a stimulation of lipolysis in white fat cells and in an activation of oxygen consumption in brown adipocytes [27]. These distinct effects have been sometimes confused and inadequately quoted in the literature. A frequent misunderstanding between lipolysis and thermogenesis deserves to be clarified:

The former action, lipolysis (also known as triglyceride breakdown) is the metabolic pathway that releases the energy stored in lipid droplets. The most important anatomical location of lipid droplets is inside the fat cells of white adipose tissue. This tissue (which is yellow in man) is widely distributed in the body. Subcutaneous and visceral white adipose depots can be distinguished; both store the excess of ingested energy under the form of triglycerides, and release such stored energy under the form of free fatty acids and glycerol that circulate in blood and can be used as substrates by skeletal and cardiac muscles, essentially during physical exercise, fasting or cold exposure. In this view, adipocyte lipolysis contributes to the *in vivo* fat mobilization, one of the catabolic steps of energy homeostasis.

The latter action, thermogenesis, is mainly observed in special adipocytes isolated from brown fat in rodents, and consists in oxidizing free fatty acids to generate heat. Such direct heat production helps the small rodents and hibernators to regulate their body temperature without need for muscle contraction or shivering, by recruiting special adipose depots mainly distributed in the trunk: the brown fat, which is much more functional in small mammals than in humans [30]. The brown fat is able to have its mitochondria under an "uncoupled state" that allows heat production rather than synthesis of highly energetic molecules, such as ATP. Therefore, during arousal of hibernators, the brown adipose tissue, once activated by catecholamines exquisitely performs both lipolysis and thermogenesis to rewarm the cold animal. The fatty acids released during lipid mobilization from white or brown adipocytes are used as fuel for non-shivering thermogenesis in brown adipocytes. The term "burning fat" should apply in this case only.

Unfortunately, "burning fat" is misused as short-cut that is attractive for customers wanting to loose weight. This is a too mere contraction of the two distinct metabolic pathways that are practically not occurring in a coordinated manner in adult humans lacking brown fat. The products of white adipose tissue lipolysis have to be oxidized in other tissues (mainly muscles) for generating more mechanical energy than heat. Such shortcoming information has prompted diverse drug industries that advertise weight-lowering products, medicinal plants or botanical extracts to propose that synephrine or octopamine could exert weight-lowering effect on human obesity by enhancing "fat burning", which is illusory or by increasing "fat mobilization", which could be true, but which does not indicate what that is the fate of the mobilized lipids? Ideally, they can be oxidized in skeletal muscle during physical exercise, while they can be re-esterified in liver or adipose tissue (lipogenesis) if energy expenditure is not increased enough. The unverified assertions "fat burning" or " "fat mobilizing" used for *Citrus* amines take advantage of the results obtained by international pharmaceutical companies during the preclinical development of synthetic β_3-adrenergic agonists generated for anti-obesity and anti-diabetes therapeutic applications. These drugs were really acting as lipolytic and thermogenic agents and clearly decreased fat mass and increased body temperature, at least in rodents and animals possessing functional brown adipose tissue [31].

After the clarification of lipolysis and thermogenesis, we have to precise that not only the lipolytic and thermogenic properties of octopamine and synephrine might be involved in their proposed slimming effects. These substitution products of ephedrine are proposed as the active principles of dietary supplements aiming at losing weight have other targets than the fat stores. Once ingested, the bioactive amines can act centrally, in the cardiovascular system and in other organs too. It is not excluded that the amines also interfere with appetite regulation. This explains why octopamine is definitively considered as a prohibited doping stimulant by the World anti-doping agency [32] while synephrine is still under examination.

In this context, it seems that preparations from *Citrus aurantium* are empirically used worldwide to treat obesity, or even less morbid overweight, since the only used argument is their richness in octopamine and more especially in synephrine (see below). However, to our knowledge, clear-cut *in vivo* demonstrations of the slimming efficacy of such pharmacological molecules are still very scarce [8]. Our objective was to make a non-exhaustive overview of the amine content in *Citrus*, then to reassess the lipolytic and lipogenic properties of the major amines found in *Citrus* fruits.

Naturally Occurring Levels of Amines in *Citrus*

As indicated above, para-synephrine has been repeatedly reported to be the main constituent of *Citrus aurantium* fruits and extracts while the other alkaloids are present in much lower concentrations [5,33-35]. Table 1 shows for bitter orange, the fruit of *Citrus aurantium*, belonging to the *Rutaceae* family, the contents of 4 amines reported by various studies. The values are given as percentage of dried material and it has been already reported that these percentages are approximately one-hundred times higher than those found in the raw material, i.e. the fresh fruit collected from the tree [33]. On a quantitative aspect, the major amine is synephrine, then octopamine and N-methyltyramine are found in similar proportions. Tyramine is less abundant and other alkaloids (e.g. hordenine) are at the limit of detection. Not only the edible parts of the fruits have been used to prepare dietary supplements claimed to promote fat mass loss [36] since the peel and the segment parts of the plant contain more alkaloids than the juice. The leaves also contain these alkaloids, though at lower concentrations. The synephrine content is negatively correlated with the maturity index of the fruit [37]. Since the content of such alkaloids is richer in unripe *Citrus aurantium* fruit than in other fruits - such as mandarins (*Citrus reticulata*) or sweet oranges (*Citrus sinensis*) - extracts from the former are frequently included in mixtures aiming at treating obesity. As bitter oranges are generally used before maturation for the preparation of extracts, Table 1 also reports the values of the standard reference material, consisting in a dried homogenate of immature bitter orange sample that is stored for standardization purposes at the National Institute of Standards and Technology [38-40]. The amine content of laboratory and commercialized extracts will not be reviewed since it essentially depends on the extraction method and on the combination or not with other botanical components or chemical agents (e.g. caffeine).

Table 1. Amine concentration in *Citrus aurantium*

Sample	Amine concentration (%) or (g/100mL of juice)				Reference
	Synephrine	N-methyltyramine	Octopamine	Tyramine	
Unripe fruit	0.045	n.d.	n.d.	n.d.	[19]
	0.252	0.027	< l.o.d.	0.005	[5]
	0.630	< l.o.d.	< l.o.d.	0.050	[45]
	0.861	0.015	0.016	0.008	[46]
	0.881 [a]	0.017 [a]	0.014 [a]	0.002 [a]	[38]
	0.884 [a]	0.018 [a]	0.013 [a]	0.003 [a]	[40]
	0.910	0.018	0.012	0.003	NIST [b]
Mature peel	0.056	n.d.	n.d.	n.d.	[19]
	0.075	< l.o.d.	0.006	< l.o.d.	[5]
Leaf	0.006	n.d.	n.d.	n.d.	[19]
Juice	0.006	n.d.	n.d.	n.d.	[20]
	0.009	n.d.	0.003	0.002	[35]

n.d.: not determined; < l.o.d.: under limit of detection; a) Standard Reference Material at National Institute of Standards and Technology, NIST #SRM3258 ; b) Mean values from NIST certificate of analysis available at: https://www-s.nist.gov/srmors/view_cert.cfm?srm=3258.

Since synephrine is an alkaloid that is similar in structure - but distinct - from ephedrine, extracts of *Citrus aurantium* have been presented as "ephedra-free" products [36] to replace banned extracts from the medicinal plants related to *Ephedra sinica*. Therefore, *Citrus aurantium* extracts have been the subject of various safety reports [8] and of analytical determinations. They have been included in numerous multi-component formulations sold as weight-loss and athletic-performance-enhancement products. Consequently, the amount of (+/-)-synephrine, the major alkaloid found in such dietary supplements and phytoproducts with supposed slimming effects varies largely, depending on different factors such as the grove, the extraction process, or the fact that the product respects what is on manufacturers' label or has been adulterated before reaching the consumer. All these aspects have been reviewed elsewhere [7,41] and will not be treated in the present chapter. The influence of the techniques used for separation/detection brings much more moderate variability, and it can be summarized that the amine levels found after High Pressure Liquid Chromatography (HPLC) or Capillary Electrophoresis (CE) analytical methods are closely similar [5,42]. Most of the studies reported in Table 1 have used HPLC to determine the amine amount in *Citrus aurantium* while only one used CE [35]. However, the latter method often appears more resolutive and sensitive, and is currently more and more used to determine amine and amino acid contents in samples for various applications in food chemistry [43].

More importantly, synephrine has been detected in other *Citrus* species, more widely consumed than the bitter orange extracts. The juice of sweet oranges (*C. sinensis*) or mandarins (*C. reticulata*) contains as much, and even more, synephrine than that of bitter oranges (*C. aurantium*): 85, 78 and 57 mg/L of fresh juice, respectively; and the juice of *C. clementina* is even richer (115 mg/L) [42]. A common feature is that the fruit is richer in alkaloids than the juice and that the percentages found in dried material are approximately fifty times more concentrated than that the levels found in fresh juice. Table 2 uses two units that are comparable (g/100 g dried material and g/100 mL juice) to report the richness in amines for fruits, leaves and juices of several *Citrus* species. Resulting comparisons show that the immature peel is richer than the mature peel, the whole fruit and the leaves.

Undoubtedly, synephrine is more abundant in the unripe fruit of *Citrus aurantium* than in any other material. Surprisingly, lemons (*Citrus limon*) contain more octopamine than synephrine in their juice [44]. Our survey also includes one study measuring the amine content not in juices from freshly squeezed fruits but from commercialized juices, with limited differences among eight tested brands [9]. Intriguingly, the mean value of synephrine content (16 mg/L, equivalent to 0.0016 g/100 mL) was roughly five fold lower in these orange juices than in those used for laboratory purposes. Fruit juices are easier to produce than the dried extracts and much more widely consumed as refreshing drinks in many societies than dietary supplements advertised for overweight or obese people and for body builders. Nonetheless, a comparison between synephrine content in orange juices and bitter orange-containing extracts can be helpful. Bitter orange juices can be more than one thousand times less concentrated in synephrine than bitter orange extracts. Moreover, orange juice contains approximately 50 times less synephrine than the whole bitter orange unripe fruit. Therefore, calculations to estimate the enrichment of synephrine intake in a subject consuming *Citrus aurantium*-based products must take into account the servings per day of other *Citrus* products (fruits, juices or marmelades). Such calculations may be inappropriate when considering that weight-lowering products often include many ingredients (like stimulants and caffeine) other than *Citrus aurantium* extracts in the finished formula.

Table 2. Amine concentrations in different *Citrus* species

Citrus species	Sample	Amine concentration (% of dry mass) or (g/100mL of juice)				Reference
		Synephrine	N-methyltyramine	Octopamine	Tyramine	
C. sinensis	fruit	0.079	n.d.	n.d.	n.d.	[19]
	leaf	0.023	n.d.	n.d.	n.d.	[19]
	juice	0.009	< l.o.d.	< l.o.d.	0.001	[44]
	brand juice*	0.002	n.d.	trace	trace	[9]
C. reticulata	fruit	0.398	n.d.	n.d.	n.d.	[42]
		0.360	n.d.	0.010	0.030	[45]
	mature peel	0.238	< l.o.d.	< l.o.d.	< l.o.d.	[18]
	immat. peel	0.623	0.005	0.006	0.005	[18]
	juice	0.008	< l.o.d.	< l.o.d.	< l.o.d.	[44]
C. unshiu	mature peel	0.307	< l.o.d.	< l.o.d.	< l.o.d.	[18]
	juice	0.010	n.d.	n.d.	n.d.	[37]
C. limon	fruit	0.041	n.d.	n.d.	n.d.	[19]
	leaf	0.010	n.d.	n.d.	n.d.	[19]
	juice	0.001	< l.o.d.	0.002	0.001	[44]
C. limonia	fruit	0.031	n.d.	n.d.	n.d.	[19]
	leaf	0.019	n.d.	n.d.	n.d.	[19]
C. deliciosa	fruit	0.118	n.d.	n.d.	n.d.	[19]
	leaf	0.054	n.d.	n.d.	n.d.	[19]
C. clementina	juice	0.012	< l.o.d.	< l.o.d.	0.002	[44]

n.d.: not determined; < l.o.d.: under limit of detection; * mean of eight marketed orange juices commercialized by different brands in Brazil, the other juice values being from freshly pressed fruits.

Of note, another dietary amine; putrescine [5,18-20,35,37,42,44-46] is present in orange juice and has not been reported in most of the studies collected in Table 1 and 2. The quantifications performed by Vieira et al., demonstrated that this polyamine was present at 33.6 mg/L in commercialized orange juices and represented the major form among the nine amines detected (total amine levels: 53.5 mg/L) [9]. Alongside putrescine, other polyamines found in *Citrus sinensis* juice are: spermine, spermidine, histamine, cadaverine; while agmatine and serotonin complete the panel [9]. Very recently, N-methylated derivatives of tryptamine have also been detected in *Citrus* [47].

To summarize, the amines present in *Citrus* are daily ingested by more numerous consumers than originally expected when considering *Citrus aurantium*-based supplements. Consuming such dietary supplements is not a prerequisite condition to consume synephrine or octopamine: drinking fruit juices is sufficient for being concerned [48].

Since there are (+)- and (-)-enantiomers of synephrine and octopamine and the both amines can exist as ortho-, meta- or para-forms, only the use of analytical enantioselective methods of separative chromatography [5] has allowed to establish that *Citrus* contains mainly the (-)-*p*-synephrine form. The occurrence of a racemization from (-) to (+)-para-form during the conditions of pH and temperature that may easily (not compulsorily) encountered during the process of *Citrus* extract preparation is widely recognized [49]. Consequently, a tremendous number of studies is needed to determine the pharmacological properties of each entity, and to determine which can be the most potent regarding a given biological effect. In the following lines, we report merely the results of the tests performed on human fat cells with mixtures of (+/-)-*p*-synephrine and of (+/-)-*p*-octopamine, irrespective of the isomer form, for the following reasons:

- Though *R*-(-)-para-synephrine is considered as the major form naturally occurring in *Citrus* [16], traces of (+)-enantiomer may occur in dietary supplements, resulting from a racemization occurring during extract production, or from an adulteration by the provider. In this context, testing the racemate gives useful overall observations since the natural form of synephrine can likely undergo racemization before being ingested by the consumer.
- Interpretations of preclinical studies performed on rodent models are often extrapolated too straight to humans, while cautions are required before doing so. Consequently, it is of poor utility and time-consuming to determine precisely the exact potency of a given amine enantiomer on a rodent cell model, especially if the latter does not possess the relevant receptor profile similar to that found in humans. Therefore, testing directly human fat cells is of great value. We took advantage that under controlled conditions, adipocytes are available for functional tests, when originating from biological wastes of plastic surgical interventions.
- For a given biological response, the potency ratio between the most active enantiomer and a racemic mixture is generally of one order of magnitude. Thus, estimations obtained with racemate can underestimate the potency of the real naturally occurring form. In fact, this could bring erroneous interpretations of limited importance when considering that ingested dietary amines do not recognize only one receptor type with a given selectivity ratio for an enantiomer relative to the other;

they also interact with a variety of transporters, carriers, or enzymes involved in the catabolism of endogenous neurotransmitters bearing an amine moiety.

We have therefore investigated various integrated functional responses of human fat cells that could be regulated by (+/-) mixtures of octopamine and synephrine not only via receptor interaction but also via interplay with other enzymes such as amine oxidases, largely expressed in adipocytes [50], including in man [51,52]. Although less concentrated in *Citrus*, tyramine and methyltyramine, were also incorporated in most of these studies.

Lipolytic Effects of Octopamine in Mouse and Human Fat Cells

We have claimed since 1999 that octopamine is a strong activator of lipolysis essentially in fat cells from rodents [27], and confirmed later that octopamine activated lipolytic pathway only partially in human adipocytes [53,54]. In all these previous studies, we found that octopamine tended to be a little more lipolytic than synephrine in rodent as in human fat cells. Though being much less concentrated than synephrine in most of the *Citrus* fruits, octopamine will be therefore presented first in the following overview of amine lipolytic capacity. In fact, we have observed that several steps of the experiments (adipose tissue digestion, adipocyte separation owing to their buoying properties, incubation duration...) could influence maximal lipolytic responses (Carpéné, unpublished observations). An update was required since small changes occurred in the adipocyte isolation protocol relative to our previous reports [25, 27]. Regarding the nature or quantity of the enzyme used for the adipose tissue digestion (collagenase *vs* liberase) we report here novel observations comparing the lipolytic activity of octopamine in mouse and human adipocytes obtained by liberase digestion of the adipose tissue (instead of collagenase for the original studies).

For these recent *in vitro* explorations of the functional responses of human adipocytes, pieces of subcutaneous adipose tissues, considered as surgical waste at the plastic surgery department of Rangueil Hospital (Toulouse, France), were obtained from a total of 24 women undergoing abdominal lipectomy. They gave their consent under the agreement of the ethic committee, and their body mass index was 25.9 ± 0.7 kg/m^2, while mean age was 30 years. It was decided to determine glycerol release into the adipocyte incubation medium since it is a production triggered by lipolytic activity that cannot be easily re-used by the fat cells themselves, while free fatty acids may be re-esterified. The maximal lipolytic response elicited by the typical β-AR-agonist isoprenaline (also named isoproterenol) was taken as 100 % reference. Table 3 shows that octopamine is a stronger lipolytic stimulator in mouse adipocytes than in human fat cells. The stimulation obtained with 0.1-1mM octopamine represented almost 90 % of the maximum of mouse fat cell capacity, while in human adipocytes, it only reached 60 % of the maximum obtained with 10 µM isoprenaline. Table 3 also shows that tyramine and dopamine were far from being as efficient as octopamine, indicating that not any biogenic amine can activate fat cell lipolysis, even when present at 1 mM concentration. Additionally, submicromolar dose of noradrenaline, which could be considered as "physiological" (100 nM), activated lipolysis up to levels that were around one-half of fat cell maximal capacity, irrespective of the species. Such observations are in agreement with our previous report indicating that maximal noradrenaline lipolytic action (1-10 μM) was hardly reaching 75 % of maximal isoprenaline while that of another dietary amine, histamine, was limited to 25 % [55]. Thus, physiological lipolytic stimulation is lower than the maximal capacity of adipocytes, which can be considered extraphysiological, recruited in extreme situations only. Such neuro-hormonal half-stimulation of triglyceride breakdown, considered as partial on a pharmacological point of view, can however denote a sustainable activation sufficient to participate to the continuous cyclic regulation of energy income/expenditure balance, therefore necessary to maintain homeostasis.

Table 3. Effect of several biogenic amines on lipolysis in human and mouse adipocytes

	Lipolytic activation (% of 10 μM isoprenaline effect)	
Species	mouse	human
Incubation condition:		
Isoprenaline 10 μM (Reference compound)	100	100
Octopamine 1 μM	22.3 ± 5.0	n.d.
Octopamine 10 μM	64.1 ±11.4	7.0 ± 4.2
Octopamine 100 μM	84.9 ± 8.7	13.8 ± 6.7
Octopamine 1 mM	88.4 ± 8.8	59.7 ± 4.8
Tyramine 1 mM	3.1 ± 0.5	18.6 ± 4.3
Dopamine 1 mM	1.2 ± 5.0	n.d.
Noradrenaline 0.1 μM	58.2 ± 8.4	58.0 ±9.2

Mean ± SEM of three mouse preparations and more than 8 human adipocyte preparations. n.d.: not done.

It was evident that half-maximal lipolysis stimulation was reached with one-hundred times lower octopamine dose in mouse than in human adipocytes (Table 3). It was also confirmed that in human fat cells, an approximately ten thousand fold higher dose of octopamine was required to reproduce noradrenaline lipolytic effect. Irrespective of the enzyme used to isolate adipocytes, the human ones were less responsive than the rodent ones, regarding octopamine activation of lipolysis. Thus, the dietary amine is definitively less potent than the endogenous catecholamine regarding lipolysis activation. As we have already observed that both octopamine and synephrine were much less lipolytic in human fat cells than in animal models [27], the results of animal experimentation remain to be cautiously extrapolated to man, even when the laboratory animal used is the mouse, intensively used in seminal research using transgenic models.

Again, a first explanation for the limitation of octopamine effect in man could be that the amine, which can be considered as an "ancestral neurotransmitter", exhibits low affinity for the human form of the β_3-AR (which does not share exact sequence identity with the murine form). Alternative justification is that human adipocytes possess a low number of $\square_3$-adrenoreceptors, not enough to trigger strong lipolytic responses, while they have sufficient β_1- and β_2-ARs to fully respond to the full β-agonist isoprenaline [56].

Octopamine, Not Tyramine, Recognizes Human β_3-ARs

The β_3-adrenergic nature of most of the octopamine effects on adipocytes have been already demonstrated by the use of pharmacological antagonists and of β_3-AR gene knock-out mice [25,27,28,53]. Similarly, the low expression of β_3-ARs in human fat cells, comparatively to rodents, has already been supported by different means [56,57]. We will only add here that there is an inter-specific difference in the number of binding sites to the radioligand (–)-3-[^{125}I]-iodocyanopindolol ([^{125}I]ICYP) that are displaceable by competition with selective β_3-AR-antagonists. Such binding site number, representative of the β_3-AR equipment, was three-fold more elevated in adipocyte membranes from rat than from man [58].

Although octopamine affinity to human β_1- or β_2-ARs have been reported to be very low [27], the hypothesis that octopamine was able to readily bind to human β_3-AR ortholog remained to be further supported. Since human adipocytes are not rich enough in β_3-ARs, we verified the octopamine capacity to compete for [^{125}I]ICYP binding in Chinese hamster ovary cells transfected with the human β_3-AR (CHO-β_3) under cell culture and binding conditions described in [27].

The competitors tested from 10 nM to 10 mM on [^{125}I]ICYP binding to CHO-β_3 cells included octopamine, adrenaline and noradrenaline (endogenous activators of adrenoreceptors), as well as tyramine (traces found in *Citrus*). For noradrenaline and adrenaline, the slope of the competition curve was particularly shallow, indicating that each amine was binding to various receptor populations with different affinity (Figure 2). Almost all the [^{125}I]ICYP binding (representing around 3500 fmol/mg protein) was inhibited by the competing amines. Octopamine behaved similarly to the endogenous catecholamines, with a trend to a lower affinity at doses of 10-100 μM. Nevertheless, it inhibited almost all the binding as did catecholamines. By contrast, tyramine was unable to displace radioligand binding, even when tested at 10 mM. Since the inhibition pattern of octopamine was close to that of the endogenous catecholamines, it can be supposed that octopamine is able to recognize β_3-ARs in human adipocytes also. However, considering that these receptors are very poorly expressed in human fat cells, and taking into account the overall low affinity of the natural amines for these β_3-ARs, relative to other AR-subtypes, it is conceivable that the stimulation of only so few receptors in human fat cells was far from triggering a response as elevated than that promoted by the physiological stimulators (nor)adrenaline, or by the pharmacological agent isoprenaline, which activated the more numerous β_1- and β_2-ARs.

Our observation of a substantial binding of octopamine to β_3-ARs in a transfected cell system is in agreement with the loss of octopamine lipolytic effect found in mouse adipocytes from mice with genetic invalidation of the β_3-AR gene [28]. Tyramine clearly showed that a molecule without any affinity for β_3-ARs is largely less active on human fat cell lipolysis [54]. This reinforced the idea that activation of the third subtype of β-adrenoreceptors was necessary and sufficient to observe a weak lipolytic action of octopamine.

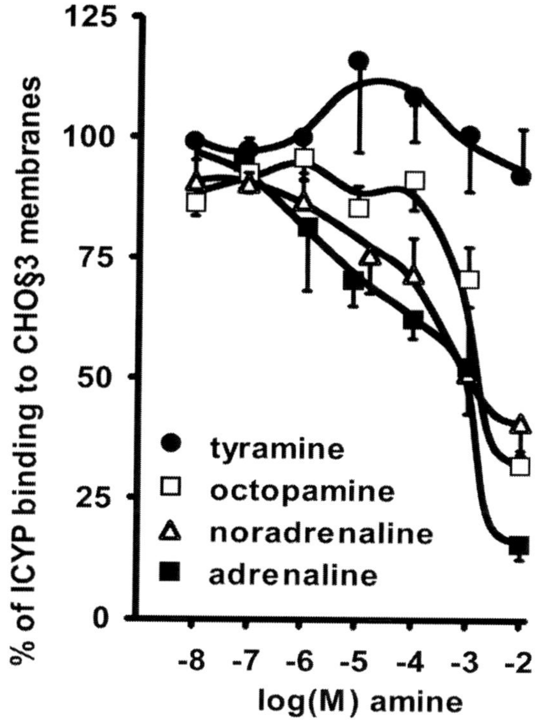

Figure 2. Displacement of [^{125}I]-Iodocyanopindolol binding to membranes of Chinese hamster ovary cells transfected with human β_3-ARs. The indicated concentrations of the following amines: tyramine (closed circles), (±) octopamine (open squares), (-)noradrenaline (triangles) and (-)adrenaline (closed squares) were incubated for 60 min with thawed membranes (approx. 75 µg protein/mL) from CHO-cells transfected with the gene for human β_3-AR and 3 nM of [^{125}I]ICYP. Values are expressed as percentage of the [^{125}I]ICYP binding found when incubated alone with membranes. Mean ± SEM of 3 experiments.

SYNEPHRINE, TYRAMINE AND N-METHYLTYRAMINE EFFECTS ON HUMAN ADIPOCYTE LIPOLYSIS

Complementary determinations were performed on another group of ten female donors, the mean BMI of which was 25.2, and the mean age was 41 years.

Lipolysis Activation

Figure 3 shows the glycerol release by human adipocytes in response to various amines. Again, positive control is the maximal stimulation of lipolysis by response to the β-AR-agonist of reference, isoprenaline, which reached 6- to 7-fold increase over basal values. Under these conditions, basal lipolysis was 0.12 ± 0.01, while maximal stimulation was 0.82 ± 0.08 µmoles of glycerol released per 100 mg of cell lipids during 90 min, in response to isoprenaline 10 µM (equivalent to 2.47 µg/mL) (n = 5). The maximal stimulation obtained with the higher dose tested of each amine, given between parentheses as percent of isoprenaline-dependent activation, allowed to establish the following relative rank order: isoprenaline (100)>> synephrine (34) > tyramine (25) ≥ methyltyramine (20). The high dose of 1000 μg/mL was necessary for tyramine and methyl-tyramine to reach their maximal effect, while 100 μg/mL was sufficient for synephrine. Although all amines can be qualified as exhibiting partial lipolytic activity with poor potency, synephrine was more potent than tyramine or its methylated derivative. In view of its large amount found in *Citrus* extracts and of its action on adipocytes, synephrine appears therefore as the active principle candidate of the lipid-mobilizing effects of *Citrus* extracts. Again, the incapacity of the biogenic amines to reach the maximal lipolytic efficiency of isoprenaline may be due to several mechanisms. Besides the above-mentioned scarcity of β_3-ARs in human fat cells, other reasons for incomplete lipolytic activation may be: 1) partial agonism at the receptors (beta-adrenergic or others) stimulated by the amines, or 2) simultaneous action at different types of receptors or proteins: activating *vs* limiting triglyceride breakdown. Whatever the mechanism(s) involved, the resulting partial activation may have an *in vivo* interest: avoiding overstimulation and desensitization. Another well-known example of an agent that cannot totally reproduce *in vitro* the isoprenaline lipolytic activation is adrenaline. This neurohormone stimulates all the β-AR subtypes and also the α_2-ARs. The resulting effect is a balance between activation of lipolytic and antilipolytic pathways, respectively [28,31]. The search of a putative antilipolytic component of the amines found in *Citrus* was therefore performed on a pre-stimulated state of lipolysis, i.e. in the presence of isobutyl-methyl-xanthine (IBMX), since the pharmacological blockade of amine-induced lipolysis by β-adrenergic antagonists has been already achieved [27].

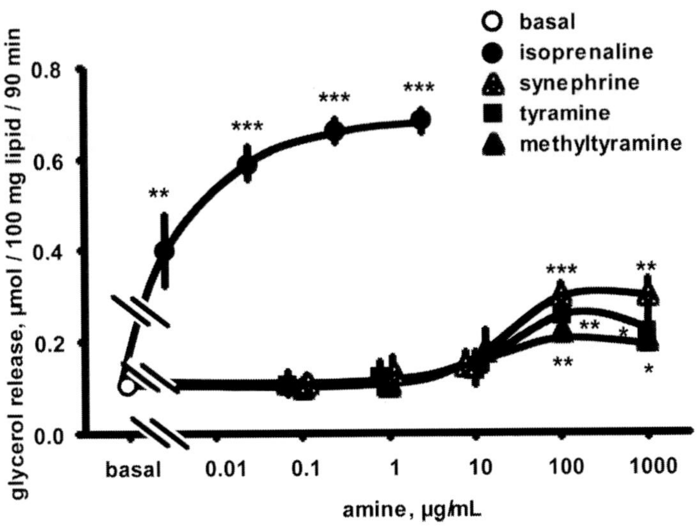

Figure 3. Lipolytic responses of human adipose cells to biogenic amines. Adipocytes freshly isolated from subcutaneous abdominal fat were incubated for 90 min with (-) isoprenaline hydrochloride (black circles) or the indicated amines:(±) synephrine hydrochloride (open triangles), tyramine hydrochloride (closed squares), and N-methyltyramine hydrochloride (closed triangles). X-axis corresponds to the increasing doses of tested agents, and is expressed as μg/mL. Lipolysis (Y-axis) is expressed as μmoles of glycerol released/100 mg cell lipid/90 min. The amount of cell lipid was 18 ± 1 mg/vial. Mean ± SEM of five different human adipocyte preparations. Different from basal glycerol release without any addition (open circle) at: * $p< 0.05$; ** $p< 0.01$; *** $p< 0.001$.

Lipolysis Inhibition

IBMX elicited a sub-maximal activation of lipolysis, since at 1mM it stimulated up to 87 ± 4 % of the maximal response to isoprenaline (n = 10). The activation by this agent not interfering with adrenergic receptors represented a 6.4 ± 0.6 fold increase over basal. Tyramine and methyl-tyramine exerted a tendency to limit IBMX activation, which represented around 36 % and 43 % inhibition of lipolysis at 1000 μg/mL (not shown). Synephrine did not hamper at all the effect of IBMX. On the contrary, it exhibited a tendency to increase by 26 % the lipolytic response (not shown). Thus, amines found in *Citrus* were devoid of clear-cut antilipolytic properties. Under the same experimental conditions, widely recognized α_2-AR agonists were able to deeply depress IBMX-induced lipolysis. It was the case for the selective α_2-AR-agonist brimonidine (bromo-imidazolin-ylaminoquinoxaline, or UK 14304), which inhibited at 1 μM by more than 90 % the IBMX action (Figure 4).

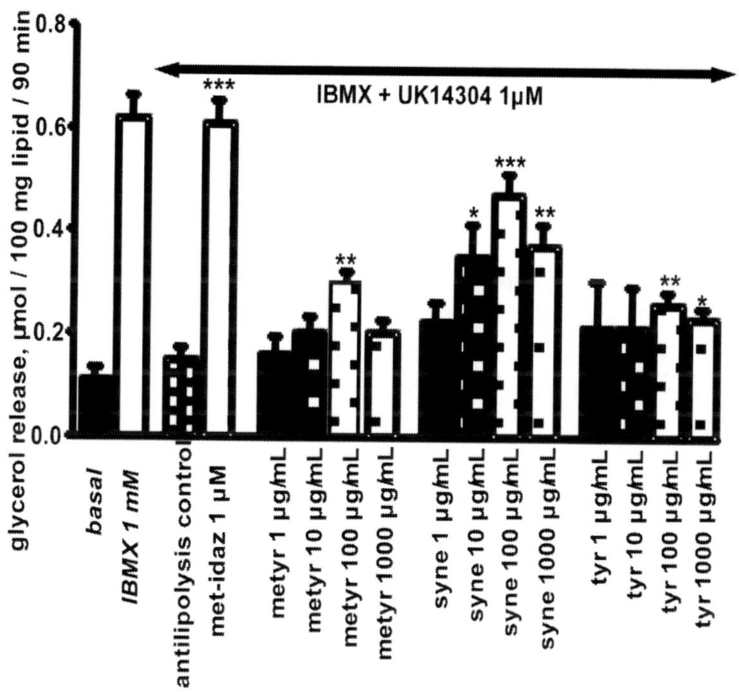

Figure 4. Modulation of brimonidine inhibition of IBMX-induced lipolysis by *Citrus* amines. Stimulation of basal lipolysis (dark column) by 1 mM IBMX (white column) was inhibited by 1 μM of the α_2-AR-agonist brimonidine (UK 14304, shaded column). Such control antilipolysis was more or less reversed by the addition of the followed agents at the indicated concentrations: methoxy-idazoxan (an α_2-AR-antagonist, met-idaz), methyl-tyramine (metyr), synephrine (syne) or tyramine (tyr). Mean ± SEM of five cases. Different from control antilipolysis (IBMX + UK 14304) at: * $p < 0.05$, ** $p < 0.01$, *** $p < 0.001$.

This suggested that the tested amines were unable to strongly activate α_2-ARs. However, a possible interaction of amines with α_2-AR that may be of α_2-adrenergic-antagonist nature could not be excluded, especially when considering that synephrine has been suspected to act as an α_2-AR antagonist in a study performed on transfected cell system [59].

As commented above, lipolysis returned to almost basal level when incubated with IBMX and brimonidine for 90 min. This antilipolytic effect has already been demonstrated to be the consequence of the α_2-AR activation by brimonidine [31] and constituted a control condition that allowed us to test the capacity of molecules to inhibit α_2-ARs. Accordingly, such antilipolysis control was completely prevented by the α_2-AR-antagonist of reference: methoxy-idazoxan (Figure 4). It was verified in complementary experiments that methoxy-idazoxan at 1 µM was unable to modify basal (0.11 ± 0.01 *vs* 0.12 ± 0.01 µmol/100 mg lipid/90 min) or IBMX-stimulated lipolysis (0.84 ± 0.08 *vs* 0.83 ± 0.08 µmol/100 mg lipid/90 min). In these conditions, tyramine and methyl-tyramine were unable to reverse the antilipolytic effect of brimonidine, except partially at the dose of 100 µg/mL. Thus, they did not behave as classical α_2-AR-antagonists. The incapacity of methyl-tyramine (and of tyramine, to a lesser extent) to further inhibit α_2-adrenergic antilipolysis when tested at a higher dose was possibly related to a weak partial agonist action, detectable at high dose only, and responsible for the above-mentioned weak inhibition of IBMX-induced lipolysis.

On the opposite, synephrine induced a recovery of the lipolysis hampered by the α_2-AR-agonist, suggesting an antagonism at α_2-ARs. However, it is important to keep in mind that the latter amine is: 1) slightly lipolytic on its own; 2) exhibiting a trend to improve the lipolytic response to IBMX even in the absence of brimonidine (see above). It is therefore likely that the partial reversion of the antilipolytic effect of brimonidine by synephrine was not the consequence of a direct α_2-AR blockade, but was rather resulting from the β-AR-mediated lipolytic properties of the amine.

Our observations showing that increasing doses of amines could not totally prevent the brimonidine antilipolytic effect do not allow to consider the amines found in *Citrus* as potential α_2-AR-antagonists. The fact that they did not reinforce the brimodinine-induced antilipolysis confirmed that the tested amines do not behave as full α_2-AR-agonists. A mild effect favouring lipolysis was particularly clear in the case of synephrine, and more likely due to partial β-adrenergic activation of lipolysis rather than resulting from an interference with α_2-ARs. In spite of having been previously reported to interact with α-ARs [24], synephrine did not exhibit clearly an α_2-adrenergic component: not as antilipolytic as the α_2-agonist brimonidine, and not blocking the action of the latter as well as methoxy-idazoxan, an α_2-antagonist of reference (Figure 4).

Endogenous catecholamines and atrial natriuretic peptides, known to increase during physical exercise, promote lipid mobilization in man, and since exercise if often practised during weight loss programmes, it was of interest to test the influence of *Citrus* amines on adipocytes under conditions that mimic physical activity. It was therefore decided to test the influence of the amines on adrenaline-induced lipolysis.

INFLUENCE OF *CITRUS* AMINES ON ADRENALINE-INDUCED LIPOLYSIS

Adrenaline (dose-dependently) stimulated human adipocyte lipolysis (Figure 5). However, the dose-response curve did not clearly exhibit a plateau since lipolysis was still increasing between 10 and 100 µM of adrenaline. In addition, the highest adrenaline activation (at 10 μM) was far from reaching the maximal response obtained with 10 μM isoprenaline (0.68 ± 0.03 μmoles of glycerol released per 100mg lipids in 90 min, n = 5, not shown). A clear-cut potentiation of the lipolytic activity of epinephrine was obtained in the presence of 10 μM methoxy-idazoxan (α_2-AR antagonist that was inactive on basal or isoprenaline-induced lipolysis, not shown). Indeed, it is the blockade of the α_2-adrenergic antilipolytic component of adrenaline that allowed the catecholamine to be more lipolytic. Thus, in the presence of an α_2-AR antagonist, adrenaline approached at 100 μM the maximal stimulation obtained with isoprenaline (Figure 5).

None of the tested amines was able to clearly potentiate adrenaline action (Figure 5). Thus, octopamine, synephrine, tyramine and its methylated metabolite were devoid of α_2-adrenergic blocking properties, and their β-adrenergic component was not strong enough to improve adrenaline-induced lipolysis, at least when added at 100 μM (octopamine) or at 50 μM (other amines). Only a trend to potentiate the threshold doses (0.01 and 0.1 μM) and the highest dose (100 μM) of adrenaline was detected with octopamine 100 μM. Thus, it was tested whether a larger dose of octopamine (1 mM) was able to further enhance a stronger stimulation induced by 10 μM adrenaline.

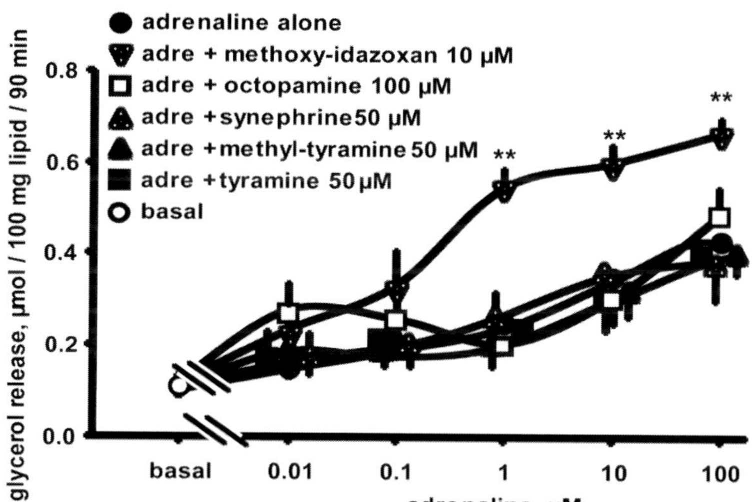

Figure 5. Lipolytic dose-response to adrenaline: influence of *Citrus* amines and of α_2-adrenergic blockade. Human adipocytes were incubated for 90 min without (basal, open circles) or with increasing concentrations of (-) adrenaline alone (adre, black circles) or in combination with the indicated concentrations of: methoxy-idazoxan (α_2-AR antagonist, inverted triangles), (±) octopamine (open squares), (±) synephrine (open triangles), tyramine (closed squares), and N-methyltyramine (closed triangles). Mean ± SEM of five different human adipocyte preparations. Different from corresponding adrenaline alone at: ** $p < 0.01$.

However, the glycerol release was equivalent to 0.55 ± 0.08, 0.35 ± 0.09, and 0.50 ± 0.04 μmoles of glycerol released per 100mg lipids in 90 min, for octopamine, adrenaline, and adrenaline + octopamine, respectively (n = 8, non significant difference: NS). Then, the influence of octopamine was tested on isoprenaline-induced lipolysis. Again, there was not evident addition of the lipolytic effects since glycerol release was equivalent to 0.25 ± 0.07, 0.72 ± 0.09, and 0.67 ± 0.13 μmoles/100 mg lipids/90 min, for octopamine 100 μM, isoprenaline 0.1 μM, and their combination, respectively (n = 8, NS). Thus, octopamine was unable to improve lipolytic activation by a pure β-AR agonist, while it was able to moderately improve the action of adrenaline that acts via both β- and α_2-ARs. Our proposed explanation for all these observations performed in human adipocytes is that octopamine activates β_3-ARs and can bring at 100 μM only additional 10 % of maximal lipolytic response (as shown in Table 3) to any other lipolytic agent, while it is also a weak partial agonist at α_2-ARs, hampering faintly adrenaline from activating the antilipolytic α_2-ARs (Figure 5). Such weak interaction of octopamine with α_2-ARs has been directly demonstrated by fluorescence resonance energy transfer analysis [29].

Together, our data demonstrate that the tested amines were practically unable to facilitate *in vitro* the lipolytic response to adrenaline. It may be deduced that among the amines found in *Citrus*, synephrine, tyramine and methyl-tyramine do not offer the potential to boost the adrenergic activation of lipolysis in man. Such lack of potentiation observed under controlled experimental conditions dramatically contrasts with the "fat burning" or "extreme lipomobilizing action" properties attributed to *Citrus* extracts, irrespective of the fact that they may be adulterated by other chemicals or naturally occurring lipolytic components (e.g. caffeine). Such disappointing lack of triggering action on lipid hydrolysis in man, even in a pre-stimulated situation, could be due to a complex profile of *Citrus* amines at different adrenergic and non-adrenergic receptors, varying from "partial agonist" to "inactive agent". This dramatically contrasts with the case of rodent adipocytes, in which the above-mentioned amines [27] and *Citrus* extracts [60] promoted substantial triglyceride breakdown.

In fact, when one considers that adrenaline itself is a mixed alpha1-alpha2, beta1, beta2, and beta3 adrenergic agonist and a substrate of the amine oxidases expressed in fat cells, it is not intriguing to observe that it exhibits a peculiar multi-component pattern of lipolysis activation, with shallow dose-response and limited maximal activation. This is resulting from the so-called α_2-AR / β-AR balance [31]. Definitively, it can be concluded that neither octopamine nor synephrine activate β-ARs or α-ARs as efficiently as the endogenous catecholamines. This agrees with the poor vascular effects observed with repeated administration of (non-adulterated) *Citrus aurantium* extracts [61].

THE ADVANTAGES AND LIMITS OF *IN VITRO* STUDIES OF *CITRUS* AMINE EFFECTS

The main advantage of our observations performed on human adipocytes is that they are highly relevant for the actions expected to occur after *Citru*s consumption. However, the fate of the biogenic amines once ingested has to be taken into account: there is no clear idea of how/how much ingested molecules reach the adipocyte environment. More data about the crossing of gut, blood and brain barriers are required for a better understanding. Additionally, once present in the adipose tissue, are the amines solely binding to membrane receptors or are they internalized and metabolized inside fat cells? It is likely that amines from *Citrus* undergo amine oxidation via the amine oxidases that are highly expressed in human fat cells, at the cell surface (semicarbazide-sensitive amine oxidase) [52] or at the mitochondrial level (monoamine oxidase) [51]. Since various dietary amines are oxidized and activate glucose uptake in adipocytes [52], we tested whether amines from *Citrus* were endowed with similar properties.

Table 4. Effect of several amines on glucose uptake in human adipocytes

	Transport activation (% of 100 nM insulin effect)	
Incubation condition	Mean ± SEM	number of cases
Insulin 100 nM (reference)	100	15
Benzylamine 100 μM	29.3 ± 6.2	15
Benzylamine 1 mM	26.2 ±6.3	15
Octopamine 100 μM	23.4 ± 7.4	9
Octopamine 1 mM	28.2 ± 6.7	15
Synephrine 100 μM	14.4 ± 7.3	6
Synephrine 1 mM	19.0 ± 6.2	6

The indicated amines were incubated 45 min at 37 °C with human adipocyte preparations before performing a glucose transport assay as described by [52].

The reference substrate of semicarbazide-sensitive amine oxidase (SSAO), namely benzylamine, partially stimulated glucose uptake into human adipocytes when incubated at 100 μM for 45 min. Increasing benzylamine dose did not increase partial activation since at 0.1 or 1 mM the amine reproduced a quarter of the maximal effect of insulin on glucose transport (Table 4). At 0.1 and 1 mM, octopamine stimulated hexose transport similarly, while synephrine reproduced less than 20 % of insulin effect. Glucose transport is the first step of triglyceride assembly and it could be supposed that the amines activating such step may facilitate lipogenesis. Consequently, it is of utmost importance to further delineate the action of synephrine and other *Citrus* components not only on the lipolysis but also on the lipogenic pathway. Our observations indicate that supplementation with *Citrus* components, expected to mobilize fat, could be suspected to help glucose handling at the expense of facilitating lipid storage in fat cells, an action rather opposite to their claimed slimming properties. However, synephrine and octopamine might exhibit even more limited glucose uptake activation than lipolysis activation relative to the adipocyte maximal capacities.

Finally, the somewhat modest lipolytic properties of synephrine and octopamine we observed were limited to *in vitro* conditions. More pharamacokinetics and bioavailability data are necessary to bring more relevant observations [8]. Moreover, other *Citrus* components may be able to promote fat depletion by increasing lipid mobilization in another independent manner and this deserves to be further studied *in vivo*, in rodent models during chronic treatments, or ideally, in humans during nutritional assays.

The fact that the tested amines did not alter the lipolytic effect of adrenaline while they were mimicking part of its lipolytic action, and the observation that they also partially mimic insulin activation of glucose utilization prompted to ask how these amines interact with insulin. In other words, it was of interest to determine whether synephrine or octopamine was facilitating or hampering insulin actions. Verifying whether *Citrus* components facilitate or counteract the effect of insulin in fat cells requires a myriad of pharmacological experiments. To date, we only investigated their effects of the regulation of glucose transport and lipolysis by the pancreatic hormone. The next section will illustrate how repeated octopamine administration alters or not the adipocyte insulin sensitivity

Influence of Octopamine Prolonged Treatment on Insulin Responsiveness in Rat Adipocytes

Octopamine prolonged treatment was performed in rats and a special attention was paid to detect a putative alteration in the adipocyte responsiveness to insulin. To emphasize *in vivo* actions of octopamine on the regulation of fat deposition/accumulation, we treated male obese Zucker rats by octopamine during four weeks. To this aim, two groups of five rats each of equivalent age and body mass were constituted (6-7 weeks; 220 g), individually housed with *ad libitum* access to food and water. The treated rats received daily i.p. octopamine hydrochloride injections (15 mg/kg bw) while the control rats received daily injection of vehicle (NaCl 0.9 %). The total of the food consumed during the 28 days of treatment showed that octopamine administration exerted a somewhat anorectic effect since there was a limitation of food intake in the treated group (Figure 6A).

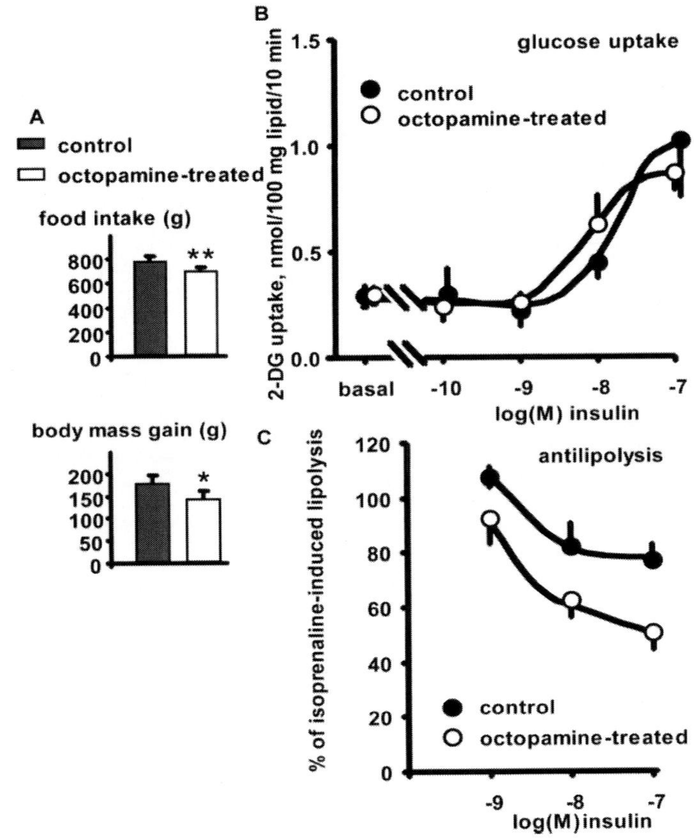

Figure 6. Influence of octopamine treatment on food intake and body weight gain in obese rats, and on insulin lipogenic and antilipolytic effects in adipocytes. A: cumulated food intake and body mass gain during the 4-week treatment period in the indicated experimental groups: control (closed symbols) and octopamine-treated (15 mg/kg bw/d, open symbols). B: 2-deoxy-glucose (2-DG) uptake was determined in the absence (basal) or in the presence of increasing doses of insulin. C: Data are given as percentage of the lipolysis stimulated by isoprenaline (set at 100 %) with return to basal lipolysis set at 0 %. Mean ± SEM of five determinations per group. Different from corresponding control at: * $p < 0.05$; ** $p < 0.01$.

Concomitantly, the body mass gain was limited in the group receiving octopamine (Figure 6A), suggesting that a prolonged treatment may exert a slimming effect as advertised in numerous websites dedicated to beneficial effects of octopamine-containing dietary supplements.

Glucose uptake stimulation and lipolysis inhibition were determined in response to 1-100 nM of the pancreatic hormone. Neither the basal nor the insulin-stimulated hexose transport was altered after octopamine treatment (Figure 6B). Thus, prolonged octopamine administration did not modify the intensity and sensitivity of glucose uptake in fat cells, the first step of *de novo* lipogenesis, exquisitely regulated by insulin. Similarly, the dose-dependent antilipolytic effect of insulin was similar in control and octopamine-treated rats (Figure 6C). Octopamine treatment exhibited a trend to improve the antilipolytic response to insulin. Taken together, these observations allow to state that octopamine supplementation did not alter insulin sensitivity and cannot be considered as diabetogenic.

CROSSING OBSERVATIONS FROM PROLONGED *IN VIVO* AND ACUTE *IN VITRO* TREATMENTS

Though most of our investigations were performed *in vitro* on isolated fat cells, the fact that the octopamine *in vivo* treatment induced a moderate slimming effect in obese rats suggests that its use for anti-obesity treatment may be relevant in man, once many complementary verifications will be performed. Several criticisms and numerous concerns must be raised before establishing a so optimistic extrapolation to man. First of all, to reach the level of octopamine administration tested in our model (estimating that all the injected amine approached targets under intact form), it was estimated that a daily ingestion of approx 7 g of *Citrus aurantium* extracts was needed per animal. Taking into account that the routine food consumption of such obese rat is 25 g/d, this requires a diet supplementation bringing at least 28 % of the diet under the form of *Citrus* extracts. Thus, even when considering the most concentrated of the extracts, it appears that an active dose of dietary octopamine cannot be brought easily under this form. Such concern can be solved by considering that synephrine is the main active principle of *Citrus* extracts. Synephrine shares most of the effects of octopamine, and is about one hundred folds more concentrated in *Citrus* fruits, it can be proposed that only 70 mg of extract (i.e. a diet supplemented with only 0.3 % synephrine) will bring a sufficient amount of amine per rat to reproduce the beneficial influence of octopamine. While such supplementation has not been reported so far, it is important to note that treatment during 10 days with 5.6 mg of *Citrus aurantium* extracts/kg of body weight was insufficient to induce a significant loss of fat mass in rats fed a high-calorie diet [62]. As the extracts were expected to contain 6 % synephrine, it can be concluded that the daily ingestion of synephrine at 0.33 mg/kg bw was insufficient to mobilize fat in diet-induced obese rats [62]. Similarly, a single oral gavage of fasting rat with the same *Citrus* dosage was also unable to reduce food intake for the consecutive 24 hours.

Larger daily doses of *Citrus* extracts, up to 4000 mg/kg bw, did not reduce body weight gain even after 28 days of daily oral gavage in rodents [63, 64]. More intriguingly, these two last studies, which compared the administration of synephrine under the form of the pure agent or under the form of *Citrus* extracts (containing 6 - 8 % synephrine) revealed several differences between the amine and the botanical extract. The former study of Arbo et al., showing that oral gavage with *Citrus aurantium* extracts (400-4000 mg/kg) did not reduce body weight gain in male mice, reported that the equivalent doses of synephrine supposed to be ingested by such treatments (30-300 mg/kg/d) were almost totally blocking body growth, (while both increased circulating glutathione) [63].

The study of Hansen et al., [64], reported a lack of effect on body weight with synephrine at 10 or 50 mg/kg/d, irrespective of its form of oral administration (pure or *Citrus* extract) in female rats. However, the cardiovascular disturbances generated by bitter orange extracts were more important than those found with the equivalent amounts of synephrine, indicating that other components of the botanical extracts may be responsible of the deleterious cardiac effects [64].

Notably, the combination of *Citrus aurantium* extracts at low doses with *Rhodolia rosea* (5.6 + 20 mg/kg) exhibited slimming and anorexic effects [62]. Similarly, larger doses of *Citrus aurantium* limited body weight gain only when administered in combination with caffeine at 25 mg/kg [64], suggesting that the potential anti-obesity effects of *Citrus aurantium* take advantage of being enhanced by other phytochemicals. Thus, combinatory therapy may be an approach that will reveal the usefulness of the *Citrus aurantium*, or the amines it contains in combating metabolic diseases

CONCLUSION

The amines found in *Citrus* can directly stimulate adipocyte functions when incubated at doses ranging between 1 μM and 1 mM. Synephrine and octopamine appear to activate the lipolytic β-adrenergic pathway and not to activate the antilipolytic α_2-ARs. Being the most abundant in *Citrus* fruits, (the peel being more enriched than the juice), and able to stimulate lipolysis in adipocytes, synephrine is the most likely candidate for being the major active principle of bitter orange extracts. However, there are at least two concerns preventing these *in vitro* observations to constitute relevant probes of an anti-obesity action of synephrine though already claimed by providers and manufacturers of body weight lowering products. The first concern is that both synephrine and octopamine are definitively less active in human than in rodent adipocytes. The second concern is that bioavailability/pharmacokinetics data of these amines are scarce and the required amount to be ingested in order to reproduce the direct effects of adipocytes appears poorly defined. According to a manufacturer of bitter orange extracts advertised for weight loss, the ingestion of 100-120 mg synephrine per day would be sufficient to induce slimming effects. If one considers that several fresh orange juices contain up to 80-100 mg synephrine/L (also applies for mandarin), the daily consumption of one litre would be sufficient to mimic the effects of the extracts, while no epidemiological survey has revealed such remarkable action. If one considers that 100 μg/mL synephrine is necessary to acutely produce a significant increase of lipolysis in isolated human adipocytes, then it can be considered that the recommended amount (100 mg) of synephrine ingested (via pills containing *Citrus aurantium* extracts or via litres of orange juice) has to be accumulated and concentrated in the equivalent of one litre only in the extracellular milieu surrounding fat depots to be as concentrated as in our *in vitro* experiments and this is hardly conceivable. Whatsoever, experimental diets enriched in *Citrus* extracts given to rodent models have not been demonstrated to exert clear body weight lowering effects, while oral synephrine limits mouse growth at doses between 30 and 300 mg/kg [63, 64]. Regarding man, the first clinical studies performed with *Citrus aurantium* extracts are far from demonstrating an impressive effect on body weight gain [8,61].

We reveal that chronic treatment with octopamine did not alter insulin sensitivity and it could be supposed that the same is valid for synephrine. As it has already been established that octopamine treatment decreases the hyper-insulinemia of obese rats [65], the *Citrus* amines cannot therefore been suspected to worsen prediabetic or diabetic states often found in obese or overweight subjects. On the opposite, taking into account their previously reported positive effect on glucose uptake [28] and re-demonstrated here in human fat cells, octopamine and synephrine warrant to be further tested as agents favouring insulin action on glucose handling.

Synephrine and octopamine are less lipolytic in human than in rat adipocytes, and they are less lipolytic than the endogenous (nor)adrenaline. It has been claimed that the ingestion of a multi-drug mixture, which contains synephrine as one of the active principles, is followed by an increase in circulating glycerol; but such observation does not constitute a probe of the relevant *in vivo* lipolytic action of this amine [66], which deserves to be established more clearly. The thermogenic effects of octopamine and synephrine have been demonstrated in rodent brown fat cells only [27] and the paucity of brown adipose tissue in man does not support a participation of non-shivering thermogenesis for their putative slimming action in man.

Moreover it appears likely that, once ingested, the amines act on various other targets than adipocytes. Thus, the claimed lipid mobilizing action of synephrine and octopamine will be not only a direct consequence of adipocyte lipolysis activation but should also result from other modes of actions (mainly central) of these catecholamine derivatives, suspected to exert anorexic and cardiovascular effects [62,67], while their actions on hepatic metabolism are less known [11], though consistent with an enhanced catabolism. Recent review of the safety of such *Citrus* extracts tested in clinical studies has also led to a novel aspect: components other than synephrine may be involved in adverse cardiovascular effects [8]. In adipocytes, the actions of components from *Citrus* extracts other than the biogenic amines can also be envisaged, and demonstrating whether the anti-adipogenic actions of flavonoids from *Citrus* extracts, observed in cultured mouse preadipocytes [12] may occur in man, is an issue that must be resolved. Finally, the abundance of putrescine in *Citrus* fruits [9] has been underestimated and it must be verified to which extent this polyamine also acts directly on adipocytes.

ACKNOWLEDGMENTS

The authors acknowledge the co-workers of AdipOlab team directed by Philippe Valet and the staff of plastic surgery of Rangueil Hospital for their invaluable help in facilitating access to surgical wastes (Univ. Toulouse, CHU & INSERM U1048, France). This work was partly supported by “Communauté de Travail des Pyrénées”. 2-Methoxy-idazoxan (RX 821002) and bromoxidine (UK 14304) were generous gifts from late Dr. H. Paris (INSERM,

Toulouse), CHOhuβ3 membranes were kindly provided by L. Emorine and S. Krief (CNRS, Toulouse).

REFERENCES

[1] Finberg, J.P., Youdim, M.B., (1988). Potentiation of tyramine pressor responses in conscious rats by reversible inhibitors of monoamine oxidase. *J. Neural Transm. Suppl.* 26, 11-16.

[2] Sandler, M., Glover, V., Ashford, A., Esmail, A. (1980). The inhibition of tyramine oxidation and the tyramine hypertensive response ("cheese effect") may be independent phenomena. *J. Neural Transm.* 48, 241-247.

[3] McCabe-Sellers, B.J., Staggs, C.G., Bogle, M.L., (2006). Tyramine in foods and monoamine oxidase inhibitor drugs: A crossroad where medicine, nutrition, pharmacy, and food industry converge. *J. Food Composition Anal.* 19, S58-S65.

[4] Astell, K.J., Mathai, M.L., Su, X.Q., (2013). A review on botanical species and chemical compounds with appetite suppressing properties for body weight control. *Plant Foods Hum. Nutr.* 68, 213-221.

[5] Pellati, F., Benvenuti, S., (2007). Chromatographic and electrophoretic methods for the analysis of phenethylamine alkaloids in *Citrus aurantium*. *J. Chromatogr. A.* 1161, 71-88.

[6] Broadley, K.J., (2010). The vascular effects of trace amines and amphetamines. *Pharmacol. Ther.* 125, 363-375.

[7] Haaz, S., Fontaine, K.R., Cutter, G., Limdi, N., Perumean-Chaney, S., Allison, D.B., (2006). Citrus aurantium and synephrine alkaloids in the treatment of overweight and obesity: an update. *Obes. Rev.* 7, 79-88.

[8] Stohs, S.J., Preuss, H.G., Shara, M., (2012). A review of the human clinical studies involving Citrus aurantium (bitter orange) extract and its primary protoalkaloid p-synephrine. *Int. J. Med. Sci.* 9, 527-538.

[9] Vieira, S.M., Theodoro, K.H., Gloria, M.B.A., (2007). Profile and levels of bioactive amines in orange juice and orange soft drink. *Food Chemistry.* 100, 895-903.

[10] Broadley, K.J., Akhtar Anwar, M., Herbert, A.A., Fehler, M., Jones, E. M., Davies, W. E., Kidd, E.J., Ford, W. R., (2009). Effects of dietary amines on the gut and its vasculature. *Br. J. Nutr.* 101, 1645-1652.

[11] Peixoto, J.S., Comar, J.F., Moreira, C.T., Soares, A.A., de Oliveira, A.L., Bracht, A., Peralta, R.M., (2012). Effects of Citrus aurantium (bitter orange) fruit extracts and p-synephrine on metabolic fluxes in the rat liver. *Molecules.* 17, 5854-5869.

[12] Kim, G.S., Park, H.J., Woo, J.H., Kim, M.K., Koh, P.O., Min, W., Ko, Y.G., Kim, C.H., Won, C.K., Cho, J.H., (2012). Citrus aurantium flavonoids inhibit adipogenesis through the Akt signaling pathway in 3T3-L1 cells. *BMC Complement Altern. Med.* 12, 31.

[13] Pellati, F., Benvenuti, S., Melegari, M., (2005). Enantioselective LC analysis of synephrine in natural products on a protein-based chiral stationary phase. *J. Pharmaceut. Biomed. Anal.* 37, 839-849.

[14] Allison, D.B., Cutter, G., Poehlman, E.T., Moore, D.R., Barnes, S., (2005). Exactly which synephrine alkaloids does Citrus aurantium (bitter orange) contain? *Int. J. Obes. (Lond).* 29, 443-446.

[15] Rossato, L.G., Costa, V.M., Limberger, R.P., Bastos, M.d.L., Remião, F., (2011). Synephrine: from trace concentrations to massive consumption in weight-loss. *Food Chem. Toxicol.* 49, 8-16.

[16] Stohs, S.J., (2011). Synephrine: from trace concentrations to massive consumption in weight-loss (comment). *Food Chem. Toxicol.* 49, 1472-1473.

[17] Rossato, L.G., (2011). Synephrine: From trace concentrations to massive consumption in weight-loss (reply). *Food Chem. Toxicol.* 49, 1474–1475.

[18] Pellati, F., Benvenuti, S., (2007). Fast high-performance liquid chromatography analysis of phenethylamine alkaloids in Citrus natural products on a pentafluorophenylpropyl stationary phase. *J. Chromatogr. A.* 1165, 58-66.

[19] Arbo, M.D., Larentis, E.R., Linck, V.M., Aboy, A.L., Pimentel, A.L., Henriques, A.T., Dallegrave, E., Garcia, S.C., Leal, M.B., Limberger, R.P., (2008). Concentrations of p-synephrine in fruits and leaves of Citrus species (*Rutaceae*) and the acute toxicity testing of Citrus aurantium extract and p-synephrine. *Food Chem. Toxicol.* 46, 2770-2775.

[20] Penzak, S.R., Jann, M.W., Cold, J.A., Hon, Y.Y., Desai, H.D., Gurley, B.J., (2001). Seville (sour) orange juice: synephrine content and cardiovascular effects in normotensive adults. *J. Clin. Pharmacol.* 41, 1059-1063.

[21] Stevenson, P.A., Hofmann, H.A., Schoch, K., Schildberger, K., (2000). The fight and flight responses of crickets depleted of biogenic amines. *J. Neurobiol.* 43, 107-120.

[22] Stevenson, P.A., Rillich, J., (2012). The decision to fight or flee - insights into underlying mechanism in crickets. *Front Neurosci.* 6, 118.

[23] Zucchi, R., Chiellini, G., Scanlan, T.S., Grandy, D.K., (2006). Trace amine-associated receptors and their ligands. *Br. J. Pharmacol.* 149, 967-978.

[24] Brown, C.M., McGrath, J.C., Midgley, J.M., Muir, A.G., O'Brien, J.W., Thonoor, C.M., Williams, C.M., Wilson, V.G., (1988). Activities of octopamine and synephrine stereoisomers on alpha-adrenoceptors. *Br. J. Pharmacol.* 93, 417-429.

[25] Galitzky, J., Carpéné, C., Lafontan, M., Berlan, M., (1993). Stimulation spécifique des récepteurs β3-adrénergiques du tissu adipeux par l'octopamine. *C. R. Acad. Sci.(Paris).* 316, 519-523.

[26] Yen, S.T., Li, M.H., Hsu, C.T., Lee, T.L., Cheng, J.T., (1998). Stimulatory effect of octopamine on β3-adrenoceptors to lower the uptake of [14C]-deoxy-D-glucose into rat adipocytes *in vitro. J. Autonomic Pharmacol.* 18, 13-19.

[27] Carpéné, C., Galitzky, J., Fontana, E., Atgié, C., Lafontan, M., Berlan, M., (1999). Selective activation of beta$_3$-adrenoceptors by octopamine: comparative studies in mammalian fat cells. *Naunyn-Schmiedeberg's Arch. Pharmacol.* 359, 310-321.

[28] Visentin, V., Morin, N., Fontana, E., Prévot, D., Boucher, J., Castan, I., Valet, P., Grujic, D., Carpéné, C., (2001). Dual action of octopamine on glucose transport into adipocytes: inhibition via b$_3$-adrenoceptor activation and stimulation via oxidation by amine oxidases. *J. Pharmacol. Exp. Ther.* 299, 96-104.

[29] Zürn, A., Zabel, U., Vilardaga, J.P., Schindelin, H., Lohse, M.J., Hoffmann, C., (2009). Fluorescence resonance energy transfer analysis of alpha 2a-adrenergic receptor

activation reveals distinct agonist-specific conformational changes. *Mol. Pharmacol.* 75, 534-541.

[30] Nedergaard, J., Bengtsson, T., Cannon, B., (2007). Unexpected evidence for active brown adipose tissue in adult humans. *Am. J. Physiol. Endocrinol. Metab.* 293, E444-452.

[31] Carpéné, C., Bousquet-Mélou, A., Galitzky, J., Berlan, M., Lafontan, M., (1998). Lypolytic effects of beta$_1$-,beta$_2$-, and beta$_3$-adrenergic agonists in white adipose tissue of mammals. *Annals N. Y. Sci.* 839, 186-189.

[32] WADA (2013). World anti-doping agency prohibited list. Available at <http://www.wada-ama.org/en/world-anti-doping-program/sports-and-anti-doping-organizations/international-standards/prohibited-list/>. Accessed on January, 2014.

[33] Pellati, F., Benvenuti, S., Melegari, M., Firenzuoli, M., (2002). Determination of adrenergic agonists from extracts and herbal products of *Citrus aurantium* L. var. *amara* by LC. *J. Pharm. Biomed. Anal.* 29, 1113-1119.

[34] Percy, D.W., Adcock, J.L., Conlan, X.A., Barnett, N.W., Gange, M.E., Noonan, L.K., Henderson, L.C., Francis, P.S., (2010). Determination of Citrus aurantium protoalkaloids using HPLC with acidic potassium permanganate chemiluminescence detection. *Talanta*. 80, 2191-2195.

[35] Mercolini, L., Mandrioli, R., Trerè, T., Bugamelli, F., Ferranti, A., Raggi, M.A., (2010). Fast CE analysis of adrenergic amines in different parts of Citrus aurantium fruit and dietary supplements. *J. Sep. Sci.* 33, 2520-2527.

[36] Stohs, S.J., Shara, M. (2007). A review of the safety and efficacy of Citrus aurantium in weight management. *In:* Bagchi D., Preuss H.G., editors. *Obesity: epidemiology, pathophysiology, and prevention. Boca Raton (FL), CRC Press*. 371–382.

[37] Dragull, K., Breksa, A.P.I., Cain, B., (2008). Synephrine content of juice from Satsuma mandarins (*Citrus unshiu Marcovitch*). *J. Agric. Food Chem.* 56, 8874-8878.

[38] Putzbach, K., Rimmer, C.A., Sharpless, K.E., Sander, L.C., (2007). Determination of Bitter Orange alkaloids in dietary supplements standard reference materials by liquid chromatography with ultraviolet absorbance and fluorescence detection. *J. Chromatogr. A.* 1156, 304-311.

[39] Putzbach, K., Rimmer, C.A., Sharpless, K.E., Wise, S.A., Sander, L.C., (2007). Determination of bitter orange alkaloids in dietary supplement standard reference materials by liquid chromatography with atmospheric-pressure ionization mass spectrometry. *Anal. Bioanal. Chem.* 389, 197-205.

[40] Nelson, B.C., Putzbach, K., Sharpless, K.E., Sander, L.C., (2007). Mass spectrometric determination of the predominant adrenergic protoalkaloids in bitter orange (*Citrus aurantium*). *J. Agric. Food Chem.* 55, 9769-9775.

[41] Stohs, S.J., Preuss, H.G., Shara, M., (2011). The safety of Citrus aurantium (Bitter Orange) and its primary protoalkaloid p-synephrine. *Phytother. Res.* 25, 1421-1428.

[42] Chen, G., Zhang, L., Zhao, J., Ye, J., (2002). Determination of hesperidin and synephrine in pericarpium Citri reticulatae by capillary electrophoresis with electrochemical detection. *Anal. Bioanal. Chem.* 373, 169-173.

[43] Poinsot, V., Carpéné, M.A., Bouajila, J., Gavard, P., Feurer, B., Couderc, F., (2012). Recent advances in amino acid analysis by capillary electrophoresis. *Electrophoresis*. 33, 14-35.

[44] Uckoo, R.M., Jayaprakasha, G.K., Nelson, S.D., Patil, B.S., (2011). Rapid simultaneous determination of amines and organic acids in citrus using high-performance liquid chromatography. *Talanta*. 83, 948-954.

[45] Tang, F., Tao, L., Luo, X., Ding, L., Guo, M., Nie, L., Yao, S., (2006). Determination of octopamine, synephrine and tyramine in Citrus herbs by ionic liquid improved 'green' chromatography. *J. Chromatogr. A*. 1125, 182-188.

[46] Roman, M.C., Betz, J.M., Hildreth, J., (2007). Determination of synephrine in bitter orange raw materials, extracts, and dietary supplements by liquid chromatography with ultraviolet detection: single-laboratory validation. *J. AOAC Int.* 90, 68-81.

[47] Servillo, L., Giovane, A., Balestrieri, M.L., Casale, R., Cautela, D., Castaldo, D., (2013). Citrus genus plants contain N-methylated tryptamine derivatives and their 5-hydroxylated forms. *J. Agric. Food Chem.* 61, 5156-5162.

[48] Stohs, S.J., (2013). Problems with Citrus aurantium Information in "A Review on Botanical Species and Chemical Compounds with Appetite Suppressing Properties for Body Weight Control". *Plant Foods Hum. Nutr.* 68, 329-331.

[49] Pellati, F., Cannazza, G., Benvenuti, S., (2010). Study on the racemization of synephrine by off-column chiral high-performance liquid chromatography. *J. Chromatogr. A*. 1217, 3503-3510.

[50] Tong, J.H., D'Iorio, A., Kandaswami, C., (1979). On the characteristics of mitochondrial monoamine oxidase in pancreas and adipose tissues from genetically obese mice. *Can. J. Biochem.* 57, 197-200.

[51] Pizzinat, N., Marti, L., Remaury, A., Leger, F., Langin, D., Lafontan, M., Carpéné, C., Parini, A., (1999). High expression of monoamine oxidases in human white adipose tissue: evidence for their involvement in noradrenaline clearance. *Biochem. Pharmacol.* 58, 1735-1742.

[52] Morin, N., Lizcano, J.M., Fontana, E., Marti, L., Smih, F., Rouet, P., Prévot, D., Zorzano, A., Unzeta, M., Carpéné, C., (2001). Semicarbazide-sensitive amine oxidase substrates stimulate glucose transport and inhibit lipolysis in human adipocytes. *J. Pharmacol. Exp. Ther.* 297, 563-572.

[53] Fontana, E., Morin, N., Prévot, D., Carpéné, C., (2000). Effects of octopamine on lipolysis, glucose transport and amine oxidation in mammalian fat cells. *Comp. Biochem. Physiol. C: Comp. Pharmacol.* 125, 33-44.

[54] Mercader, J., Wanecq, E., Chen, J., Carpéné, C., (2011). Isopropylnorsynephrine is a stronger lipolytic agent in human adipocytes than synephrine and other amines present in *Citrus aurantium*. *J. Physiol. Biochem.* 67, 443-452.

[55] Carpéné, C., Morin, N., Fontana, E., Visentin, V., Prévot, D., Marti, L., Lafontan, M., (2001). Histamine weakly stimulate lipolysis and is poorly oxidized by amine oxidases in human subcutaneous fat cells. *Inflamm. Res.* 50, S140-S141.

[56] Carpéné, C., Castan, I., Collon, P., Galitzky, J., Moratinos, J., Lafontan, M., (1994). Adrenergic lipolysis in guinea pig is not a β_3-adrenergic response : comparison with human adipocytes. *Am. J. Physiol.* 266, R905-R913.

[57] Thomas, R.F., Liggett, S.B., (1993). Lack of β_3-adrenergic receptor mRNA expression in adipose and other metabolic tissues in the adult human. *Mol. Pharmacol.* 43, 343-348.

[58] Carpéné, C., Iffiú-Soltész, Z., (2011). Monoaminergic systems and anti-obesity drug discovery: chronic administration of sympathicomimetic amines, re-uptake inhibitors, or amine oxidase inhibitors? *In : Anti-Obesity Drug Discovery and Development (Atta-ur-Rahman & Iqbal Choudhary M. Editors) Bentham Sciences Publishers*. 1, 114-130.

[59] Ma, G., Bavadekar, S.A., Schaneberg, B.T., Khan, I.A., Feller, D.R., (2010). Effects of synephrine and beta-phenethylamine on human alpha-adrenoceptor subtypes. *Planta Med.* 76, 981-986.

[60] Tsujita, T., Takaku, T., (2007). Lipolysis induced by segment wall extract from Satsuma mandarin orange (*Citrus unshiu* Mark). *J. Nutr. Sci. Vitaminol. (Tokyo).* 53, 547-551.

[61] Kaats, G.R., Miller, H., Preuss, H.G., Stohs, S.J., (2013). A 60day double-blind, placebo-controlled safety study involving *Citrus aurantium* (bitter orange) extract. *Food Chem. Toxicol.* 55, 358-362.

[62] Verpeut, J.L., Walters, A.L., Bello, N.T., (2013). *Citrus aurantium* and *Rhodiola rosea* in combination reduce visceral white adipose tissue and increase hypothalamic norepinephrine in a rat model of diet-induced obesity. *Nutr. Res.* 33, 503-512.

[63] Arbo, M.D., Schmitt, G.C., Limberger, M.F., Charão, M.F., Moro, A.M., Ribeiro, G.L., Dallegrave, E., Garcia, S.C., Leal, M.B., Limberger, R.P., (2009). Subchronic toxicity of *Citrus aurantium* L. (*Rutaceae*) extract and *p*-synephrine in mice. *Regul. Toxicol. Pharmacol.* 54, 114-117.

[64] Hansen, D.K., George, N.I., White, G.E., Pellicore, L.S., Abdel-Rahman, A., Fabricant, D., Administration, F.A.D., (2012). Physiological effects following administration of *Citrus aurantium* for 28 days in rats. *Toxicol. Appl. Pharmacol.* 261, 236-247.

[65] Bour, S., Visentin, V., Prévot, D., Carpéné, C., (2003). Moderate weight-lowering effect of octopamine treatment in obese Zucker rats. *J. Physiol. Biochem.* 59, 175-182.

[66] Bloomer, R.J., Fisher-Wellman, K.H., Hammond, K.G., Schilling, B.K., Weber, A.A., Cole, B.J., (2009). Dietary supplement increases plasma norepinephrine, lipolysis, and metabolic rate in resistance trained men. *J. Int. Soc. Sports Nutr.* 6, 4-13.

[67] Inchiosa, M.A., (2011). Experience (mostly negative) with the use of sympathomimetic agents for weight loss. *J. Obes.* 2011, 764584.

In: Citrus
Editor: Khizar Hayat

ISBN: 978-1-63117-985-3

Chapter 9

FEATURES OF THE INSECTICIDAL ACTION OF *CITRUS SINENSIS* ESSENTIAL OIL AGAINST *MUSCA DOMESTICA*

***Yanina E. Rossi*[1]*, María L. González*[1]*, María C. Carpinella*[1]*, Diego G. Andrione*[1] *and Sara M. Palacios*[1,*]**

[1]Laboratorio de Química Fina y Productos Naturales,
Universidad Católica de Córdoba, Córdoba, Argentina

ABSTRACT

The insecticidal action of *Citrus sinensis* essential oil (EO) (LC_{50} = 3.9 mg/dm^3) against the house fly *Musca domestica* is reviewed with special emphasis on the process of detoxification and on the actual intoxication of the insect once it is fumigated with the EO. The first metabolic pathway of terpenes is the oxidation by P450, followed by a neurotoxic effect with characteristic features that make flies sensitive to these compounds. The same response was observed for the most abundant terpene of the *C. sinensis* EO, the (4*R*)(+)-limonene (LC_{50} = 6.2 mg/dm^3). By comparing the activity of the EO with (4*R*)(+)-limonene, we propose an explanation of the enhanced activity of the first with respect to the compound. The toxicity of *C. sinensis* EO showed a second order response with the temperature, with a maximum at 26°C. The neurotoxic effect of *C. sinensis* and (4*R*)(+)-limonene was assayed on the enzyme acetylcholinesterase (AChE) activity and the biogenic amines levels were determined. (4*R*)(+)-Limonene showed a low activity against AChE, with an inhibitory percentage of 22.6% at 0.61 M (equivalent to 84 mg/mL).

The levels of tyrosine, dopamine, tyramine and octopamine in *M. domestica* head after fumigation with the EO or (4*R*)(+)-limonene were analyzed by HPLC and compared with the corresponding levels of untreated flies. Fumigation with *C. sinensis* EO or (4*R*)(+)-limonene increased 8 times the levels of dopamine but they did not affect the concentration of octopamine compared with control flies. The level of tyrosine, the precursor molecule of dopamine, was enhanced 3.3 and 3.6 times when flies were

---

* Phone: +54 0351 4938060. Fax: +54 0351 4938061. E-mail: sarapalacios@ucc.edu.ar.

submitted to both fumigants, respectively, indicating that terpenes affect the chemistry of the neurological system.

Keywords: *Citrus sinensis*, (4*R*)(+)-limonene, *Musa domestica*, Insecticidal action

INTRODUCTION

Many aromatic plants and their essential oils (EO) are used as flavoring agents in a wide range of food, in cosmetic, perfume and confectionary industries [1]. *Citrus* essential oils also possess insecticidal activity against various pests such as flies [2-4], mosquitoes [5-7], stored grain insects [8, 9] and cockroaches [10]. This activity has also been reported for *Citrus sinensis* EO [4, 10].

The house fly, *Musca domestica* L. (Diptera) is an important hygienic pest of humans and dairy animals with the potential to act as a mechanical vector of more than one hundred intestinal pathogens for humans and animals [11], thus leading to economic losses in healthcare and agronomic livestock [12]. Moreover, the current method of housefly control with chemical insecticides has led to the development of resistance [13], apart from the risk associated with the use of these chemicals, which require search for alternative insecticides such as essential oils. These natural compounds show low toxicity to warm-blooded mammals [14], present high volatility and have a relatively low cost [15].

EOs are lipophilic in nature and interfere with the basic metabolic, biochemical, physiological and behavioral functions of insects [16]. Little is known about the physiological actions of essential oils and their constituents on insects [17-22], but treatments with these cause symptoms that suggest a neurotoxic mode of action [17, 18, 23, 24]. Furthermore, García et al. indicated that although insecticidal modes of action are mainly related to their effect on the acetylcholinesterase (AChE) and octopaminergic system, some effects on the hormone and pheromone system and on cytochrome P450 monooxygenase has also been reported [25].

Palacios et al. [4] have studied the fumigant toxicity of *C. sinensis* EO against the fly *M. domestica* in a 30 min exposure period at 26°C, requiring doses of 3.9 mg/dm^3 (equivalent to 4.6 μL/L) to induce 50% mortality in *M. domestica* adults. (4*R*)(+)-Limonene, the most abundant terpene of this EO, has shown less toxicity (LC_{50} of 6.2 mg/dm^3). This chapter discusses the effects of absorption, metabolism and neurological action of *C. sinensis* EO and (4*R*)(+)-limonene in *M. domestica.*

ABSORPTION AND METABOLISM OF *C. SINENSIS* ESSENTIAL OIL

Determination of the Terpenes Absorbed by House Flies

In a study in which *M. domestica* adults were fumigated with *C. sinensis* EO, considerable mortality (100%) was observed at relatively low doses of 8 mg/dm^3 [26]. The EO was composed by (4*R*)(+)-limonene (95%) followed by β-pinene (2.2%), β-myrcene (0.5%), linalool (0.8%), α-pinene (0.7%), γ-terpineol (0.3 %) and α-terpineol (0.2%) [26].

The *M. domestica* adults that died after treatment with *C. sinensis* EO (8 mg/dm^3) were transferred to a GC-vial and sealed. The head space composition was determined using an SPME fiber in order to detect both the terpenes absorbed by the flies and any compound formed as a result of the insect metabolism. The chromatographic analysis detected five terpenes, three EO components, (4*R*)(+)-limonene, α-pinene, β-pinene and two new compounds identified as carveol and carvone. Considering the sum of the relative amounts of the three terpenes [(4*R*)(+)-limonene, α-pinene and β-pinene] in *C. sinenesis* EO as 100%, resulting in 97%, 0.7% and 2.2%, respectively (Table 1), the dead flies showed the three terpenes plus carveol and carvone in a relative proportion of 50%, 6.2%, 12.5%, 6.3% and 25%, respectively (Table 1). The authors demonstrated that (4*R*)(+)-limonene was metabolized to carveol and carvone by *M. domestica* recovering 46.2%, 15.3% and 38.5%, respectively (Table 1 and Figure 1).

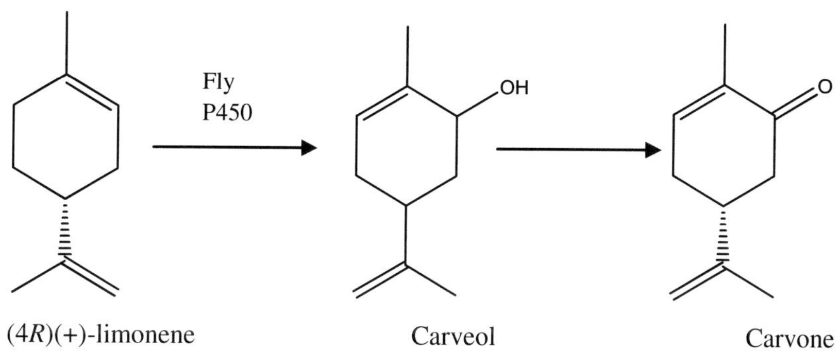

Figure 1. Conversion of (4*R*)(+)-limonene to carveol and carvone mediated by fly cytochrome P450.

Table 1. Relative amount of terpenes recovery from dead flies after treatment with *Citrus sinensis* EO or (4*R*)(+)-limonene with or without piperonyl butoxide (PBO)

SPME analysis of	Relative amount (%)[a,b]				
	(4*R*)(+)-limonene	α-pinene	β-pinene	carveol	carvone
C. sinensis EO	97.0 ± 1.5	0.7 ± 0.2	2.2 ± 0.1	nd	nd
flies dead by action of *C. sinensis* EO	50 ± 1	6.2 ± 0.1	12.5 ± 0.3	6.3 ± 0.1	25 ± 0.5
flies dead by action of *C. sinensis* EO + PBO	62.5 ± 1	6.3 ± 0.1	12.5 ± 0.3	nd	18.7 ± 0.5
(4*R*)(+)-limonene	99 ± 0.5				
flies dead by action of (4*R*)(+)- limonene	46.2 ± 1.4			15.3 ± 0.1	38.5 ± 0.2
flies dead by action of (4*R*)(+)- limonene + PBO	66.6 ± 2.1			6.7 ± 0.1	26.7 ± 0.2

[a] Percentages were calculated by a standard internal method. [b] nd: undetected with a limit of quantification of 0.3 μg/ vial.

It was also demonstrated that *M. domestica* transformed (4*R*)(+)-limonene to carveol and carvone by the P450 oxidative detoxification pathway. Such compounds as α-pinene and β-pinene were detected in the flies in a larger proportion than in EO, suggesting a selective absorption of these terpenes (Table 1) and indicating as well, that they were not metabolized.

Toxicity of Metabolites

The LC_{50} of (4*R*)(+)-limonene was equivalent to 6.2 mg/dm^3[4], while the LC_{50} of carveol and carvone was 1122 and 19 mg/dm^3, respectively [24]. This means that carveol and carvone are 181 and 3 times, respectively, less toxic against *M. domestica* adults than (4*R*)(+)-limonene (Table 2) [24]. Compounds α- and β-pinene were also toxic against *M. domestica* with LC_{50} of 11.5 and 6.4, respectively (Table 2) [4]. In agreement with the LC_{50} values of the terpenes absorbed and produced by the fly metabolism and with the proportion of each of them in the insect, (4*R*)(+)-limonene would be the principal toxicant, followed by α- and β-pinene. Carveol and carvone, rather contribute to decrease the toxicity of (4*R*)(+)-limonene.

Table 2. LC_{50} of *Citrus sinensis*, (4*R*)(+)-limonene, (±)-α-pinene, (1*S*)(-)β-pinene, carveol[a], carvone[a] and deltamethrin[b] with or without PBO against *Musca domestica* in fumigant bioassay

Essential oil or terpene	Mean LC_{50} in mg/dm^3 (95% confidence interval)	Slope	X^2
C. sinensis	3.9 (1.2-13)	2.5	6.532
C. sinensis + PBO	2.4 (0.9-6.6)	3.1	1.746
(4*R*)(+)-Limonene	6.2 (1.7–23)	6.4	0.404
(4*R*)(+)-Limonene+PBO	3.6 (1.4-9.8)	2.2	1.432
(±)-α-Pinene	11.5 (3.6 - 37.3)	6.5	1.741
(1*S*)(-)β-Pinene	6.4 (2.4 - 17.4)	8.4	0.740
Carveol *[a]*	1122 (972-1290)		
Carvone *[a]*	19.0 (15.5-23.2)		
Deltamethrin *[b]*	9.2 (2.8-29.5)	1.1	0.920
Deltamethrin+PBO *[b]*	1.5 (0.2-11.4)	0.7	0.168

[a] Taken from Rice and Coats [24]. *[b]* Applied topically and LC_{50} expressed in µg/fly. X^2: chi-square.

The stronger toxicity of *C. sinensis* EO compared with that of (4*R*)(+)-limonene is possibly explained by the presence of α-pinene and β-pinene which contribute to (4*R*)(+)-limonene toxicity. The carveol and carvone formation resulted from the reaction of (4*R*)(+)-limonene with P450 oxidative system. In insects, cytochromes P450 are involved in a wide range of metabolic processes, from hormone syntheses to activation or degradation of xenobiotics [27]. Few studies have been made about the metabolism of (4*R*)(+)-limonene in insects. When this terpene was mixed with an artificial diet of *Spodoptera litura* larvae at a concentration of 1 mg/g, (4*R*)(+)-limonene was transformed mainly into uroterpenol (52%) and perillic acid (43%) [28]. The oxidation of (4*R*)(+)-limonene by cytochrome P450 has been previously described for some organisms, including microbials [29], plants [30] and rats

[31]. Microalga *Oocystis pusilla* transforms (4*R*)(+)-limonene into carveol, carvona and limonene oxide [32]. In rats, (+)- and (−)-limonene were found to be oxidized to their respective carveol and perillyl alcohol derivatives [31].

Determination of PBO Synergistic Effect

In order to demonstrate the participation of *M. domestica* P450 oxidizing system in the metabolism of *C. sinensis* and of (4*R*)(+)-limonene, the LC_{50} of both the EO and of the terpene were determined in flies previously treated with PBO, a recognized P450 inhibitor [33]. In the presence of this inhibitor, the toxicity of *C. sinensis* EO increased twice (LC_{50} with PBO = 2.4 mg/dm^3) (Table 2), whereas the LC_{50} of (4*R*)(+)-limonene diminished from 6.2 to 3.6 mg/dm^3, raising its toxicity level nearly twice. This result shows the same tendency demonstrated for the toxicity (topical) of deltamethrin against flies treated with PBO, where deltamethrin was 6 times more toxic to PBO treated flies than to untreated ones [20].

The SPME analysis of the flies that died by the action of *C. sinensis* EO plus PBO showed the presence of (4*R*)(+)-limonene, α-pinene, β-pinene and carvone at 62.5%, 6.3%, 12.5% and 18.7%, respectively, while the metabolite carveol was not detected (Table 1). The decrease in the formation of carveol and carvone in *M. domestica*, as well as the decrease of LC_{50} (from 3.9 to 2.4 mg/dm^3) are in agreement with the participation of P450 in the metabolism of *C. sinensis* EO. Such participation leads to a smaller formation of less toxic terpenes (carveol and carvone), thus avoiding the detoxification of (4*R*)(+)-limonene and provoking the death of flies at smaller doses of EO or (4*R*)(+)-limonene. In the fumigation experiments of (4*R*)(+)-limonene against PBO treated flies, the relative amounts of carveol and carvone were reduced, ranging from 15.3% to 6.7% and from 38.5% to 26.7%, respectively (Table 1). These results confirm that the changes in LC_{50} registered for these compounds were due to a lower yield of (4*R*)(+)-limonene metabolites.

The other EO components absorbed by the flies, α- and β-pinene, were not metabolized by the P450 system, being detected in *M. domestica* treated with and without PBO in the same proportion (Table 1). However, it has been reported that α-pinene is converted by the P450 of some insects into pheromones or polar metabolites [34]. This result may suggest that in *M. domestica*, (4*R*)(+)-limonene reacts faster with P450, decreasing or avoiding the reaction of α- and β-pinene with this oxidation system.

The results of this and other studies [20] suggest that once a terpene goes inside the fly, the P450 system detoxifies it. Terpenes like (4*R*)(+)-pulegone and menthone are oxidated by P450, transforming them into more toxic terpenes [20]. In contrast, (4*R*)(+)-limonene is turned into less toxic metabolites. However, when (4*R*)(+)-pulegone is mixed with (4*R*)(+)-limonene, for example, in the essential oil of *Minthostachys verticillata*, the former is oxidized but the latter is not [20]. Terpenes such as α-pinene [34] and β-pinene [35] are known to be transformed by some insects, but they are not metabolized by *M. domestica* P450 when they go into the fly together with (4*R*)(+)-limonene. These findings suggest that P450 may actually react only with the most abundant terpene, while the other terpenes present in the EO could positively contribute to the toxicity of the mix. As a result of these findings, it was suggested that when *C. sinensis* EO (or (4*R*)(+)-limonene) is used as a commercial insecticide against flies, it should be formulated with a P450 substrate or inhibitor, with the aim of increasing *C. sinensis* EO toxicity.

Influence of Temperature on *C. sinensis* EO and (4*R*)(+)-Limonene Action

As temperature is the most important environmental factor influencing the action of fumigants on insects, the role of this parameter during fumigation was examined.

The effectiveness of EOs depends on various factors such as the rate of vapor release, level of sorption, uptake of vapors by insects, efficacy of detoxification systems, spontaneous release, all of them depending on temperature [36]; so *C. sinensis* EO fumigant action during 30 min was studied against *M. domestica* at 18°C, 26°C, 30°C and 35°C [37] (Table 3). LC_{50} of *C. sinensis* EO decreased with the increase in temperature from 18°C to 26°C. From this last point, increasing LC_{50} values (lower toxicity) were observed when temperature increased. A similar tendency was observed in treatments with (4*R*)(+)-limonene (Table 3), although the minimum LC_{50} value was observed at 30°C. Comparing the curve of response (Figure 2) of both the EO and the terpene, it can be noted that they showed a similar mode of action, with bigger LC_{50} at lower and higher temperatures and a smaller LC_{50} at 26°C and 30°C, respectively. The temperature coefficient of *C. sinensis* EO (Table 3) [38] was positive between 18°C and 26ºC, but negative values were observed between 26-35ºC, reflecting the second-order temperature dependence of the LC_{50}. (4*R*)(+)-Limonene presented positive temperature coefficients between 18°C and 30°C, and a negative one between 30°C and 35ºC.

The effect of temperature on the toxicity of synthetic insecticides has also been studied in many pests such as *Trichoplusia ni* and *Spodoptera frugiperda* [39, 40], *Heliothis virescens* [41], *Anthonomus grandis grandis* [42], *M. domestica* [43], *Blattella germanica* [44], etc. The toxicity have been shown to be positively correlated with temperature for most organophosphorus and carbamate insecticides, thus showing a positive temperature coefficient [42, 45].

On the other hand, DDT and pyrethroids have been reported to possess a negative temperature coefficient since insects were more sensitive to these insecticides at lower temperatures, although no second order dependence was observed [43, 46].

Table 3. LC_{50} (in mg/dm^3) of *Citrus sinensis* and (4*R*)(+)-limonene at different temperatures for 30 minutes exposure

Temperat. (°C)	*C. Sinensis* EO LC_{50} (95% confidence interval)	Temperature coefficient[a]			(4*R*)(+)-limonene LC_{50} (95% confidence interval)	Temperature coefficient[a]		
		8ºC	4ºC	5ºC		8ºC	4ºC	5ºC
18	6.0 (2.9-12.3)				10.7 (5.5-20.7)			
26	3.9 (1.2-13)	+1.6			6.2 (1.7–23)	+1.7		
30	7.0 (3.9-12.7)		-0.5		5.7 (1-31.8)		+1.1	
35	9.8 (5.5-17.3)			-0.7	6.3 (3.2-12.3)			-0.9

[a] Temperature coefficients for differences of 4, 8 and 5°C of temperature; (+) positive, (-) negative.

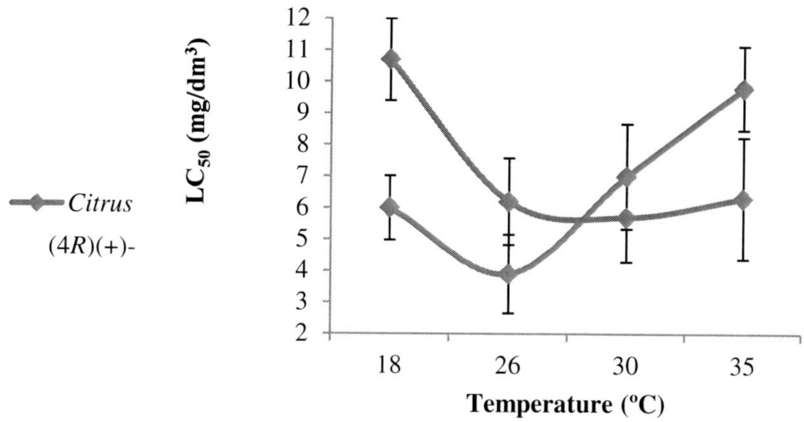

Figure 2. LC_{50} (mg/dm^3) vs. temperature (°C) of *Citrus sinensis* and (4*R*)(+)-limonene.

Previously reported data of Papachristos and Stamopoulos [36] on fumigant toxicity of essential oils from *Lavandula hybrida*, *Rosmarinus officinalis* and *Eucalyptus globulus* against the larvae and pupae of *Acanthoscelides obtectus,* revealed that intermediate temperatures (10ºC, 18 ºC and 26ºC) enhanced the efficacy of the fumigants with respect to higher (32 ºC and 36ºC) or lower ones (4ºC). These findings are in accord with our observations for *C. sinensis* EO against *M. domestica*.

Lee et al. [22] reported that the fumigant LC_{50} of pulegone, l-fenchone, and perillaldehyde against *T. castaneum* tended to decrease at higher temperatures (from 24°C to 40ºC). Another study consistent with these results tested the fumigant activity of eighteen essential oils derived from species of the *Myrtaceae* family against adult females and eggs of *Tetranychus urticae* at 5ºC, 15ºC and 25ºC, where some EOs showed higher toxicity at 25ºC than at 5°C [47].

The *C. sinensis* EO toxicity may be interpreted as the consequence of the influence of different factors such as the insect uptake of vapors, the spontaneous release from the insect and the level of P450 activity [36]. The uptake of vapors is expected to have a positive linear dependence with the temperature because more vapors are available as the temperature increases, the spontaneous release, in turn, is likely to increase with temperature rise while metabolism occurs more rapidly at higher temperatures. The variation of LC_{50} between 26ºC and 35°C could be explained by an enhanced metabolism or spontaneous release with respect to the uptake, whereas between 18°C and 26°C, even when the last variable would be more influencing than release and metabolism, are not enough to explain the inverse dependence with temperature. As demonstrated above, P450 activity changes the level of toxicant when *M. domestica* is fumigated with *C. sinensis* EO, so we wonder about the variation of P450 activity with temperature in *M. domestica*. Unfortunately, not many studies in this matter have been published. Brattsen et al. reported a higher activity of P450 in *Spodoptera eridania* at low temperatures (15ºC) [48] compared with activity at 30°C. Consequently, larvae grown at 15°C were less susceptible to insecticides than those reared at 30°C due to an enhanced detoxification rate of the insecticide. If flies had the same enzymatic response to temperature, the lower enzyme activities at 26ºC compared with 18°C could be the cause of higher toxicity at 26ºC because the metabolization of (4*R*)(+)-limonene would be relatively diminished at this temperature. Therefore less detoxification products would be formed and a lower LC_{50} would be observed. However, this does not explain the variation between 26°C and 35°C. Taking into account all these analyses, we can conclude that the observed variation of toxicity of *C. sinensis* EO against flies could be due to the convergence of many variables which are in turn a function of temperature and one of them likely has a second order dependence with it.

NEUROTOXIC ACTION OF *C. SINENSIS* ESSENTIAL OIL

Anti-Acetylcholinesterase Activity

During fly exposure to *C. sinensis* EO and (4*R*)(+)-limonene in bioassays, progressive neurotoxic symptoms were observed in each individual. Insects showed excitation (increasing their locomotor activity moving from excitation to hyperexcitation), incoordination (the insect was altered in its locomotor activity), convulsions and tremors followed by paralysis (knockdown), similar to those symptoms produced by synthetic insecticides such as organophosphates and carbamates [14, 49]. Some authors have proposed that the mode of action of essential oils is due to a reversible competitive inhibition of the acetylcholinesterase enzyme [18, 23, 50-52]. These results were obtained after performing tests with AChE isolated from electric eels and from heads of houseflies, cockroaches and head lices [18, 23, 50-52]. However, in these studies the effect against acetylcholinesterase activity *in vivo* was not correlated with its activity *in vitro* [18, 23, 50-52].

We have observed that (4*R*)(+)-limonene presented a low activity at inhibiting AChE (from electric eel) when it was assayed according to Ellman's method [53]. A low level of AChE inhibition corresponding to 22.6% was observed even at the high dose of 0.61 M (equivalent to 84 mg/mL or 100 μL/mL). Compounds with important AChE inhibition such as physostigmine show an IC_{50} of 0.0028 mg/mL [54]. Even when the AChE used in these experiments has minimum sequence differences as that from insect source [56], the low level of effectiveness observed would also result in a low activity in the insect AChE. This statement could be sustained by the findings of Oliveira Marques et al. [56], who observed the same sensitivity towards methamidophos pesticide by AChE from *Drosophila melanogaster* and the commercial electric eel AChE.

Miyazawa et al. found that (+)-limonene and (-)-limonene inhibited 30 to 40% the activity of AChE obtained from bovine erythrocytes at 1.2 mM [52]. The AChE inhibitory effect of (+)-limonene was also studied by Kostyukovsky [18]. This terpene did not inhibit enzyme activity of electric-eel AChE at a concentration of 1 mM. AChE extracted from *Rhyzopertha dominica* was also tested with (+)-limonene, diminishing only 2% of the enzyme activity at 1 mM [18]. Therefore, the toxic action of limonene could be mediated through other pathways such as γ-aminobutyric acid (GABA) or octopaminergic receptors [18, 57-59]. The relation between chemical structure and AChE inhibition seems to show that monoterpenoid ketones provoke a stronger inhibition due to the presence of conjugated double bonds [52]. Abdelgaleil et al. demonstrated that monoterpenes as cuminaldehyde, 1,8-cineole, (-)-limonene and (L)-fenchone have potent AChE inhibitory activity against *Sitophilus oryzae* at 0.01 and 0.05 M but, except 1,8-cineole, they performed as weak insecticides [60]. Keane and Ryan mentioned that *in vitro* inhibition of AChE should be additionally validated by demonstrating an appropriate effect *in vivo* study. These authors also pointed out that it was important to not exclude the additional modes of action of monoterpenoids [61].

Biogenic Amine Levels

Another possible target for EOs activity is the octopaminergic and dopaminergic system of insects [62, 63]. Biogenic amines, octopamine, dopamine, serotonin, tyramine and histamine act as neurotransmitters, neurohormones and neuromodulators in invertebrate systems. The amino acid tyrosine is the starting point for the synthesis of both dopamine and octopamine. Tyramine is the product of direct decarboxylation of tyrosine through tyrosine decarboxylase (TDC). Subsequent reactions of tyramine with the tyramine-β-hydroxylase (TβH) yield octopamine. Tyrosine can also be turned into 3,4-dihydroxyphenylalanine (DOPA) via the tyrosine hydroxylase (TH) pathway and subsequently to dopamine via the 3,4-dihydroxyphenylalanine-decarboxylase pathway [64, 65] (Figure 3).

The levels of tyrosine, dopamine, tyramine and octopamine in *M. domestica* head after fumigation with *C. sinensis* EO were analyzed by HPLC and compared with the corresponding levels of untreated flies. Fumigation with *C. sinensis* EO or (4*R*)(+)-limonene increased the levels of dopamine 8 times but did not affect the concentration of octopamine, compared with control group (Table 4). The level of tyrosine was enhanced 3.3 and 3.6 times, when flies were fumigated with *C. sinensis* EO and (4*R*)(+)-limonene, respectively (Table 4).

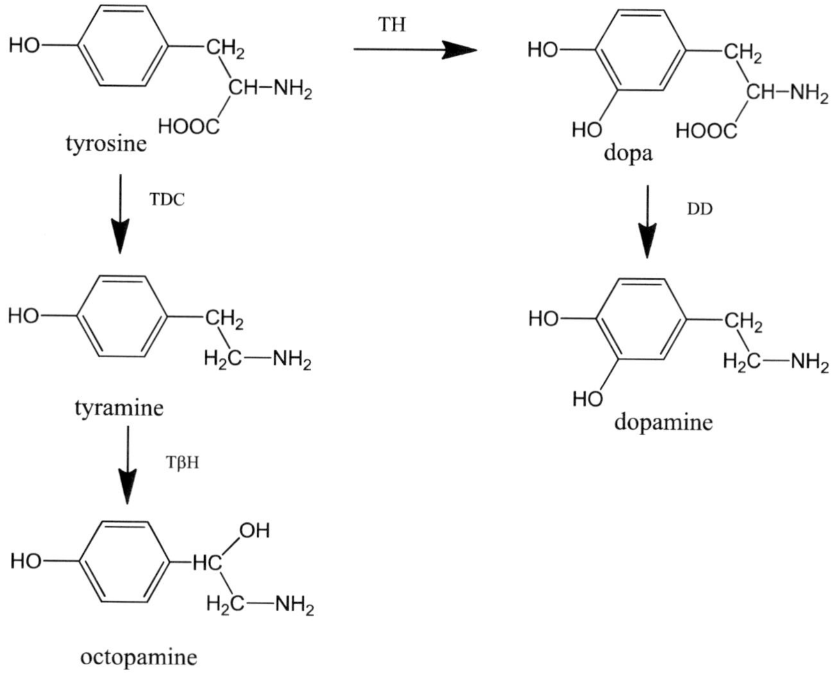

Figure 3. Synthesis of dopamine and octopamine in insects [61, 62]. TH: tyrosine hydroxylase; TDC: tyrosine decarboxylase; DD: dopa decarboxylase; TβH: tyramine β-hydroxylase.

Table 4. Biogenic amines levels measured on 100 heads of *Musca domestica*

	Tyrosine ng/g head	Dopamine ng/g head	Tyramine ng/g head	Octopamine ng/g head
Control Flies	12000 a	12000 a	0*	4000 a
Flies fumigated with *C. sinensis* EO	39400 b	93400 b	0*	6000 a
Flies fumigated with (4*R*)(+)-limonene	42600 b	80000 b	0*	2000 a

*: Limit of detection: 300 ng/g head. Limit of quantification: 700 ng/g. Values in columns, with different letters are significantly different ($p \leq 0.05$).

The acute and sub-lethal behavioral effects of EOs on insects, as well as their low toxicity in vertebrates suggest action on octopaminergics receptors, neurological system restricted to invertebrates [64]. In agreement with the obtained results, the action of EO on the dopaminergic system would indicate the interaction of (4*R*)(+)-limonene with dopamine receptors, causing an increased level of this neurotransmitter in fly heads. Kostyukovsky analyzed the effects of (+)-limonene on *R. dominica* abdominal segments, recording intracellular cyclic adenosine monophosphate (cAMP) levels as indicator of octopaminergic effect, but (+)-limonene had no significant effect at 10^{-7} M [18].

Conclusion

C. sinensis EO can be included as part of a new generation of highly active natural compounds for insect control. However, its insecticidal action may be considerably influenced by many factors, both endogenous and exogenous to the target insect. The components of *C. sinensis* EO, (4*R*)(+)-limonene, α-pinene and β-pinene are absorbed by flies exposed to it; acting as a potent fumigant mixture against *M. domestica*. Flies metabolize (4*R*)(+)-limonene into carveol and carvone, which show less toxicity than their precursor. This fact suggests that flies use oxidation reactions for the detoxification of (4*R*)(+)-limonene. The toxicity of EO and (4*R*)(+)-limonene increases when a P450 inhibitor is used in combination with any of them, suggesting that P450 monooxygenase mediated this detoxification. The toxicity of *C. sinensis* EO was higher at 26ºC, which could be possible due to that the P450 activity is minimum at this temperature, thus diminishing the formation of metabolites. Neurotoxic symptoms observed in flies fumigated with *C. sinensis* EO or (4*R*)(+)-limonene, were associated with a high level of dopamine, suggesting that the disturbance in this pathway is the responsible for the effect rather than a neurotoxicity by inhibition of AChE, which activity was no influence by the application of both tested compounds.

All these findings suggest that *C. sinensis* EO acts as an excellent fumigant against *M. domestica* and probably can also be an invaluable insecticide against some other species due to its mechanism of action. Its toxicity was enhanced by P450 inhibitors; therefore, these substances have to be seriously considered at the time of formulating *C. sinensis* EO as a commercial insecticide.

REFERENCES

[1] Choi, H.-S., (2006). Lipolytic Effects of Citrus Peel Oils and Their Components. *J. Agr. Food Chem.,* 54, 3254-3258.

[2] Kumar, P., Mishra, S., Malik, A., Satya, S., (2012). Insecticidal Evaluation of essential oils of *Citrus sinensis* L. (Myrtales: Myrtaceae) against housefly, *Musca domestica* L. (Diptera: Muscidae). *Parasitol. Res.,* 110, 1929-1936.

[3] Shalaby, A. A., Allam, K. A., Mostafa, A. A., Fahmy, S. M., (1998). Insecticidal properties of citrus oils against *Culex pipiens* and *Musca domestica. J. Egypt. Soc. Parasitol.,* 28, 595-606.

[4] Palacios, S., Bertoni, A., Rossi, Y., Santander, R., Urzúa, A., (2009). Efficacy of essential oils from edible plants as insecticides against the house fly, *Musca domestica* L. *Molecules,* 14, 1938-1947.

[5] Anaso, H. U., Ilouno, L. E., Onuorah, D., Umerie, S. C., (1990). Potency of orange peel as a mosquito fumigant. *Biol. Waste,* 34, 83-88.

[6] Warikoo, R., Ray, A., Sandhu, J. K., Samal, R., Wahab, N., Kumar, S., (2012). Larvicidal and irritant activities of hexane leaf extracts of *Citrus sinensis* against dengue vector *Aedes aegypti* L. *Asia-Pac. J. Mol.Biol.,* 2, 152-155.

[7] Michaelakis, A., Papachristos, D., Kimbaris, A., Koliopoulos, G., Giatropoulos, A., Polissiou, M., (2009). Citrus essential oils and four enantiomeric pinenes against *Culex pipiens* (Diptera: Culicidae). *Parasitol. Res.*, 105, 769-773.

[8] Shaaya, E., Ravid, U., Paster, N., Juven, B., Zisman, U., Pissarev, V., (1991). Fumigant toxicity of essential oils against four major stored-product insects. *J. Chem. Ecol.,* 17, 499-504.

[9] Rajendran, S., Sriranjini, V., (2008). Plant products as fumigants for stored-product insect control. *Journal of Stored Products Research,* 44, 126-135.

[10] Ezeonu, F. C., Chidume, G. I., Udedi, S. C., (2001). Insecticidal properties of volatile extracts of orange peels. *Bioresource Technol.,* 76, 273-274.

[11] Förster, M., Klimpel, S., Mehlhorn, H., Sievert, K., Messler, S., Pfeffer, K., (2007). Pilot study on synanthropic flies (e.g. *Musca, Sarcophaga, Calliphora, Fannia, Lucilia, Stomoxys*) as vectors of pathogenic microorganisms. *Parasitol. Res.,* 101, 243-246.

[12] Kumar, P., Mishra, S., Malik, A., Satya, S., (2012). Compositional analysis and insecticidal activity of *Eucalyptus globulus* (family: Myrtaceae) essential oil against housefly (*Musca domestica*). *Acta Trop.,* 122, 212-218.

[13] Acevedo, G., Zapater, M., Toloza, A., (2009). Insecticide resistance of house fly, *Musca domestica* (L.) from Argentina. *Parasitol. Res.,* 105, 489-493.

[14] Isman, M. B., (2000). Plant essential oils for pest and disease management. *Crop. Prot.,* 19, 603-608.

[15] Isman, M. B., (2006). Botanical insecticides, deterrents, and repellents in modern agriculture and an increasingly regulated world. *An. Rev. Entomol.,* 51, 45-66.
[16] Brattsten Lena, B., (1983). Cytochrome P-450 involvement in the interactions between plant terpenes and insect herbivores. In: *Plant Resistance to Insects.* American Chemical Society. pp. 173-195.
[17] Coats, J., Karr, L., Drewes, C., (1991) Toxicity and neurotoxic effects of monoterpenoids in insects and earthworms. In: Hedin, P. A., (editor). *Naturally Occurring Pest Bioregulators.* Washington: ACS; 1991. p. 306–316.
[18] Kostyukovsky, M., Rafaeli, A., Gileadi, C., Demchenko, N., Shaaya, E., (2002). Activation of octopaminergic receptors by essential oil constituents isolated from aromatic plants: possible mode of action against insect pests. *Pest Manag. Sci.,* 58, 1101-1106.
[19] Rice, P. J., Coats, R., (1994). Insecticidal Properties of Several Monoterpenoids to the House Fly (Diptera: Muscidae), Red Flour Beetle (Coleoptera: Tenebrionidae), and Southern Com Rootworm (Coleoptera: Chrysomelidae). *J. Econ. Entomol.,* 87, 1172-1179.
[20] Rossi, Y. E., Canavoso, L., Palacios, S. M., (2012). Molecular response of *Musca domestica* L. to *Mintostachys verticillata* essential oil, (4*R*)(+)-pulegone and menthone. *Fitoterapia,* 83, 336-342.
[21] Lee, S., Tsao, R., Peterson, C., Coats, J. R., (1997). Insecticidal Activity of Monoterpenoids to Western Corn Rootworm (Coleoptera: Chrysomelidae), Twospotted Spider Mite (Acari: Tetranychidae), and House Fly (Diptera: Muscidae). *J. Econ. Entomol.,* 90, 883-892.
[22] Lee, S., Peterson, C. J., Coats, J. R., (2003). Fumigation toxicity of monoterpenoids to several stored product insects. *J. Stored Prod. Res.,* 39, 77-85.
[23] Picollo, M. I., Toloza, A. C., Mougabure Cueto, G., Zygadlo, J., Zerba, E., (2008). Anticholinesterase and pediculicidal activities of monoterpenoids. *Fitoterapia,* 79, 271-278.
[24] Rice, P. J., Coats, R. Structural Requirements for Monoterpenoid Activity against Insects. In: *Bioregulators for Crop Protection and Pest Control.* American Chemical Society, Washington. 1994. pp. 92-108.
[25] García, M., Donadel, O. J., Ardanaz, C. E., Tonn, C. E., Sosa, M. E., (2005). Toxic and repellent effects of *Baccharis salicifolia* essential oil on *Tribolium castaneum. Pest Manag. Sci.,* 61, 612-618.
[26] Rossi, Y. E., Palacios, S. M., (2013). Fumigant toxicity of *Citrus sinensis* essential oil on *Musca domestica* L. adults in the absence and presence of a P450 inhibitor. *Acta Trop.,* 127, 33-37.
[27] Feyereisen, R., (1999). Insect P450 enzimes. *An. Rev. Entomol.,* 44, 507-533.
[28] Miyazawa, M., Wada, T., Kameoka, H., (1998). Biotransformation of (+)- and (−)-limonene by the larvae of common cutworm (*Spodoptera litura*). *J. Agri. Food Chem.,* 46, 300-303.
[29] Lerin, L., Toniazzo, G., Oliveira, D.d., Rottava, I., Dariva, C., Cansian, R. L., et al., (2010). Microorganisms screening for limonene oxidation. *Ciencia Tecnol. Alime.,* 30, 399-405.
[30] Wüst, M., Little, D. B., Schalk, M., Croteau, R., (2001). Hydroxylation of limonene enantiomers and analogs by recombinant (−)-limonene 3- and 6-hydroxylases from

mint (*Mentha*) species: evidence for catalysis within sterically constrained active sites. *Archives of Biochemistry and Biophysics,* 387, 125-136.

[31] Miyazawa, M., Shindo, M., Shimada, T., (2001). Sex Differences in the Metabolism of (+)- and (−)-Limonene Enantiomers to Carveol and Perillyl Alcohol Derivatives by Cytochrome P450 Enzymes in Rat Liver Microsomes. *Chemical Research in Toxicology,* 15, 15-20.

[32] Ghasemi, Y., Mohagheghzadeh, A., Moshavash, M., Ostovan, Z., Rasoul-Amini, S., Morowvat, M., et al., (2009). Biotransformation of monoterpenes by *Oocystis pusilla. World J. Microbiol. Biotechnol.,* 25, 1301-1304.

[33] Kasai, S., Scott, J. G., (2000). Overexpression of cytochrome P450 CYP6D1 is associated with monooxygenase-mediated pyrethroid resistance in house flies from Georgia. *Pestic. Biochem. Phys.,* 68, 34-41.

[34] Tillman, J. A., Seybold, S. J., Jurenka, R. A., Blomquist, G. J., (1999). Insect pheromones—an overview of biosynthesis and endocrine regulation. *Insect. Biochem. Mol. Biol.,* 29, 481-514.

[35] Renwick, J. A. A., Hughes, P. R., Ty, T. D., (1973). Oxidation products of pinene in the bark beetle, *Dendroctonus frontalis. J. Insect Physiol.,* 19, 1735-1740.

[36] Papachristos, D. P., Stamopoulos, D. C., (2002). Toxicity of vapours of three essential oils to the immature stages of *Acanthoscelides obtectus* (Say) (Coleoptera: Bruchidae). *J. Stored Prod. Res.,* 38, 365-373.

[37] Rossi, Y., Palacios, S. M., editors. Influence of temperature in action of fumigant natural insecticides. IOCD 2009 International Symposium: Biology, Chemistry, Pharmacology and Industrial Applications of Plants of the Americas; 2009; Viña del Mar, Chile.

[38] Fan, H., Cheng, H., Richards, A., (1948). The temperature coefficients of DDT action in insects. *Physiol. Zool.,* 21, 48-59.

[39] Toth Jr., S. J., Sparks, T. C., (1988). Influence of Treatment Technique on the Temperature-Toxicity Relationships of cis- and trans-Permethrin in the Cabbage Looper (Lepidoptera: Noctuidae). *J. Econ. Entomol.,* 81, 115-118.

[40] Sparks, T. C., Shour, M. H., Wellemeyer, E. G., (1982). Temperature-Toxicity Relationships of Pyrethroids on Three Lepidopterans. *J. Econ. Entomol.,* 75, 643-646.

[41] Sparks, T. C., Pavloff, A. M., Rose, R. L., Clower, D. F., (1983). Temperature-Toxicity Relationships of Pyrethroids on *Heliothis virescens* (F) (Lepidoptera: Noctuidae) and *Anthonomus grandis grandis* Boheman (Coleoptera: Curculionidae). *J. Econ. Entomol.,* 76, 243-246.

[42] Norment, B. R., Chambeas, H. W., (1970). Temperature relationships in organophosphorus poisoning in Boll Weevils 1,2. *J. Econ. Entomol.,* 63, 502-504.

[43] Scott, J. G., Georghiou, G. P., (1984). Influence of temperature on knockdown, toxicity, and resistance to pyrethroids in the house fly, Musca domestica. *Pestic. Biochem. Phys.,* 21, 53-62.

[44] Wadleigh, R. W., Koehler, P. G., Preisler, H. K., Patterson, R. S., Robertson, J. L., (1991). Effect of Temperature on the Toxicities of Ten Pyrethroids to German Cockroach (Dictyoptera: Blattellidae). *J. Econ. Entomol.,* 84, 1433-1436.

[45] Chalfant, R. B., (1973). Cabbage Looper: Effect of Temperature on Toxicity of Insecticides in the Laboratory. *J. Econ. Entomol.,* 66, 339-341.

[46] Gammon, D. W., (1978). Effects of DDT on the cockroach nervous system at three temperatures. *Pestic. Sci.,* 9, 95-104.
[47] Lim, E., Lee, B. H., Park, C. G., (2012). Fumigant activity of essential oils and their components from *Eucalyptus codonocarpa* and *E. dives* against *Tetranychus urticae* (Acari: Tetranychidae) at three temperatures. *J. Appl. Entomol.,* 136, 698-703.
[48] Brattsten, L. B., Gunderson, C. A., Fleming, J. T., Nikbahkt, K. N., (1986). Temperature and diet modulate cytochrome P-450 activities in southern armyworm, *Spodoptera eridania* (Cramer), caterpillars. *Pestic. Biochem. Phys.,* 25, 346-357.
[49] Houghton, P. J., Ren, Y., Howes, M.-J., (2006). Acetylcholinesterase inhibitors from plants and fungi. *Nat. Prod. Rep.,* 23, 181-199.
[50] Grundy, D. L., Still, C. C., (1985). Inhibition of acetylcholinesterases by pulegone-1,2-epoxide. *Pestic. Biochem. Physiol.,* 23, 383-388.
[51] Ryan, M. F., Byrne, O., (1988). Plant-insect coevolution and inhibition of acetylcholinesterase. *J. Chem. Ecol.,* 14, 1965-1975.
[52] Miyazawa, M., Watanabe, H., Kameoka, H., (1997). Inhibition of Acetylcholinesterase Activity by Monoterpenoids with a p-Menthane Skeleton. *J. Agric. Food Chem.,* 45, 677-679.
[53] Ellman, G. L., Courtney, K. D., Andres jr., V., Featherstone, R. M., (1961). A new and rapid colorimetric determination of acetylcholinesterase activity. *Biochem. Pharmacol.,* 7, 88-95.
[54] Carpinella, M. C., Andrione, D. G., Ruiz, G., Palacios, S. M., (2010). Screening for acetylcholinesterase inhibitory activity in plant extracts from Argentina. *Phytother. Res.,* 24, 259-263.
[55] Pang, Y.-P., (2006). Novel acetylcholinesterase target site for malaria mosquito control. *PLoS ONE,* 1, e58.
[56] de Oliveira Marques, P. R. B., Nunes, G. S., dos Santos, T. C. R., Andreescu, S., Marty, J.-L., (2004). Comparative investigation between acetylcholinesterase obtained from commercial sources and genetically modified *Drosophila melanogaster*: Application in amperometric biosensors for methamidophos pesticide detection. *Biosens. Bioelectron.,* 20, 825-832.
[57] Enan, E., (2001). Insecticidal activity of essential oils: octopaminergic sites of action. *Comp. Biochem. Physiol. C: Pharmacol. Toxicol. Endocrinol.,* 130, 325-337.
[58] Priestley, C. M., Williamson, E. M., Wafford, K. A., Sattelle, D. B., (2003). Thymol, a constituent of thyme essential oil, is a positive allosteric modulator of human $GABA_A$ receptors and a homo-oligomeric GABA receptor from *Drosophila melanogaster. British J. Pharmacol.,* 140, 1363-1372.
[59] López, M. D., Pascual-Villalobos, M. J., (2010). Mode of inhibition of acetylcholinesterase by monoterpenoids and implications for pest control. *Ind. Crop. Prod.,* 31, 284-288.
[60] Abdelgaleil, S. M., Mohamed, M. E., Badawy, M. I., El-arami, S. A., (2009). Fumigant and contact toxicities of monoterpenes to *Sitophilus oryzae* (L.) and *Tribolium castaneum* (Herbst) and their Inhibitory effects on acetylcholinesterase activity. *J. Chem. Ecol.,* 35, 518-525.
[61] Keane, S., Ryan, M. F., (1999). Purification, characterisation, and inhibition by monoterpenes of acetylcholinesterase from the waxmoth, *Galleria mellonella* (L.). *Insect Biochem. Molec.Biol.,* 29, 1097-1104.

[62] Blenau, W., Baumann, A., (2001). Molecular and pharmacological properties of insect biogenic amine receptors: Lessons from *Drosophila melanogaster* and *Apis mellifera*. *Arch. Insect Biochem. Physiol.*, 48, 13-38.

[63] Marg, S., Walz, B., Blenau, W., (2004). The effects of dopamine receptor agonists and antagonists on the secretory rate of cockroach (Periplaneta americana) salivary glands. *J. Insect Physiol.*, 50, 821-830.

[64] Roeder, T., (2005). Tyramine and Octopamine: Ruling Behavior and Metabolism. *An. Rev. Entomol.*, 50, 447-477.

[65] Hardie, S. L., Hirsh, J., (2006). An improved method for the separation and detection of biogenic amines in adult *Drosophila* brain extracts by high performance liquid chromatography. *J. Neurosci. Methods*, 153, 243-249.

In: Citrus
Editor: Khizar Hayat
ISBN: 978-1-63117-985-3

Chapter 10

THE POTENTIAL OF D(+)-LIMONENE TO IMPROVE PLA-PHB BLENDS PROPERTIES

***M. P. Arrieta*[1,4,*]*, J. López*[1]*, A. Hernández*[2] *and E. Rayón*[3]**

[1]Instituto de Tecnología de Materiales, Universitat Politècnica de València, Plaza Ferrandiz y Carbonell 1, Alicante, Spain

[2]Servicio de Microscopía Óptica y Confocal, Centro de Investigación Príncipe Felipe, Eduardo Primo Yúfera, Valencia, Spain

[3]Instituto de Tecnología de Materiales, Universitat Politècnica de València, Valencia, Spain

[4]Analytical Chemistry, Nutrition and Food Sciences Department, University of Alicante (UA), Alicante, Spain

ABSTRACT

In the recent years multifunctional biocompatible materials based on poly-lactic acid (PLA) have gain great interest in biomedical applications for its biocompatibility in the human body. However, some PLA properties have to be enhanced such as its low crystallinity and its mechanical properties. The introduction of other materials to reinforce PLA matrix as well as the addition of active additives to reduce the microorganism growth on the final material has been also suggested to obtain a final material with active properties. The addition of 25 wt% of poly-3-hydroxybutyrate (PHB) into PLA matrix has shown a positive reinforcement effect by maintaining the biocompatibility of the final formulation. The use of natural terpene D-(+)-limonene (D-(+)-Lim) to improve the compatibility between two polymer matrixes has been also proposed. The introduction of citrus essential oil as a component in biocompatible polymeric matrices opens new perspectives for biomedical applications.

Keywords: Poly-lactic acid (PLA), Poly-hydroxybutyrate (PHB), D-(+)-limonene; Biobased materials, Polymer blends

* Corresponding author address: Instituto de Tecnología de Materiales, Universitat Politècnica de València, Plaza Ferrandiz y Carbonell 1, 03801 Alcoy, Alicante, Spain. Tel.: +34-966528433; fax: +34-966528433. E-mail address: marrieta@itm.upv.es.

Introduction

The strategy to obtain multifunctional biobased materials for biomedical applications with specific properties by blending biocompatible materials, has gained a lot of interest during the last two decades. Moreover, biopolyesters such as poly-lactic acid (PLA) and poly-hydroxybutyrate (PHB) have attracted wide attention for their potential applications in implanted medical devices due to their biocompatibility in the human body.

The selection of constituents to be used for the development of biomedical materials intended to be in contact with the human body is a key point for their successful use with desirable properties. In this sense, PLA is one of the most attractive biocompatible polymers due to its acceptable mechanical properties, it is typically melt processed and its degradation produces lactic acid, which naturally occurs during metabolism [1]. PLA is a thermoplastic polyester produced from lactic acid, which is derived from the fermentation of corn starch and other polysaccharide sources [2]. It has been demonstrated that PLA is biocompatible and degrade into non-toxic components with a controllable degradation rate *in-vivo* [3]. As a consequence, it has been approved by the Food and Drug Administration (FDA) for clinical uses [1] such as in degradable surgical sutures [3], in some kind of medical implants and in drug-delivery systems [1]. However, PLA presents slow crystallization rate [4], brittleness and also shows low processing properties [5].

PHB is one of the best known poly-hydroxyalkanoates (PHA) made by controlled bacterial fermentation [6]. The PHB enzymatic polymerization leads to the formation of macromolecules with highly ordered stereochemical structure, as a result PHB is a highly crystalline bio-based polymer [7], which is also a fully biodegradable and biocompatible thermoplastic [8]. However, the main drawbacks of PHB are its brittleness and its low degradation temperature being very close to its melting temperature [5, 6]. PHB brittleness is attributed to its large spherulitic size and secondary crystallization [5], and therefore its processing is restricted.

It has been reported that changing PHB compositions is possible to obtain favorable mechanical, biocompatible and degradation times under specific physiological conditions [9]. Likewise, PLA properties could be improved by blending it with others biopolymers. In this sense, blending 75 wt.% of PLA with 25 wt.% of PHB allows producing a synergic effect, since PHB produces a reinforcement effect on PLA matrix [6], whereas PLA improves mechanical properties of PHB [10]. It should be noticed that PLA and PHB could be blended due to the fact they have similar melting point, which allows obtaining a blend in the melt state [11] avoiding any thermal degradation of the biopolymers during processing.

However, it is known that the application of this kind of implanted biomedical devices are limited since they often cause bacterial infections [12]. A possible strategy to reduce the bacterial growth in polymeric biomedical devices is the incorporation of an antimicrobial agent into the polymer matrix. The use of essential oils as natural additives to produce multifunctional materials with antimicrobial properties is a common practice in the development of active polymer materials [13]. D-(+)-limonene is the most abundant naturally occurring monoterpene, representing more than 90% of citrus fruits peel oil [14]. D-(+)-limonene has been proposed as a novel monomer to obtain polylimonene [16] and also it has been blended with PLA [15]. Furthermore, it was found that D-(+)-limonene present antimicrobial activity against gram positives and gram negatives bacteria [17]. The strategy to blend D-(+)-limonene with a biocompatible polymer matrix may represent an innovative approach to obtain materials with antimicrobial properties suitable for biomedical applications.

In this chapter the potential of natural D-(+)-limonene to improve the compatibility between PLA and PHB in PLA-PHB blends is highlighted and PLA-PHB-D(+)-Lim blends are proposed as novel materials for biomedical applications since they may offer some advantages such as their biocompatible nature, enhanced mechanical properties and with potential antimicrobial activity.

D-(+)-LIMONENE

Limonene is the most abundant monocyclic monoterpene in nature and represents more than 90% of orange peel oil [14]. The molecule has a chiral centre and thus it exists as two optical isomers, D-(+)-Limonene and L-(-)-Limonene (Figure 1). The main chemical compound found in nature and of greater interest in industrial applications is D-(+)-Limonene which is commercialized with a purity of about 90–98% [18]. It is known that D-(+)-Limonene essential oil possesses antifungal, bacteriostatic and bactericidal properties [19]. Thus, it has been widely used as food preservative because it is generally recognized as safe (GRAS) by the Food and Drug Administration (FDA) [20]. Moreover, the cytotoxic activity of D-(+)-limonene has been proven in some bacterium such as *Staphylococcus epidermidis, Escherichia coli, Pseudomonas aeruginosa* and *Klebsiella pneumonia* [21] as well as in a yeast *Cryptococcus neoformans* [22] which are microorganisms that can affect the human health. In the field of polymer science, D-(+)-Limonene is widely used for the synthesis of polymers [23]. The use of limonene as a novel monomer to obtain polyterpenes has also been proposed [16]. In previous works the effectiveness of D-(+)-Limonene as a plasticizer for biopolymers such as PLA [15] and PHB [24] has been recently demonstrated. The use of D-(+)-Limonene for materials intended to be applied in biomedical devices seems to be safe because of D-(+)-Limonene is readily metabolized in the human body [18].

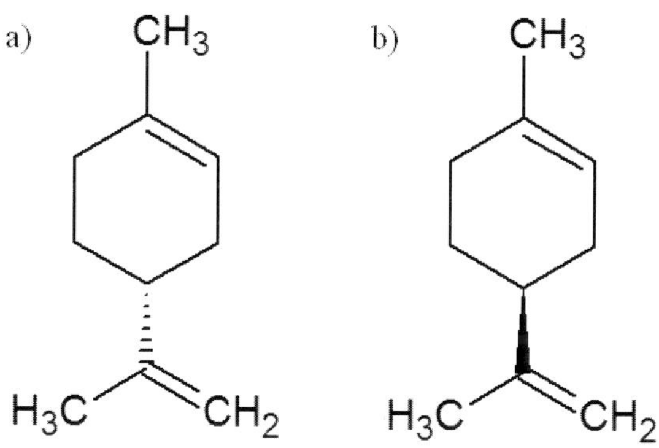

Figure 1. Chemical structure of (a) *D*-(+)-Limonene and (b) *L*-(-)-Limonene.

Elaboration of PLA-PHB Blends

The temperature used during PLA-PHB blend preparation has significant influence on the miscibility between both biopolymers. It is known that PLA and PHB are fully miscible in the melt state [25] and as a consequence, the most common processing condition currently used for the preparation of PLA-PHB blends is by melt blending. Moreover, melt blending process is a common and relatively simple approach to tuning the physical and mechanical properties of biopolymers [26]. Thus, PLA-PHB blends are commonly prepared by melt blending using 75 wt.% of PLA and 25 wt.% of PHB [24, 27, 28], since, in these proportions materials have shown improved final properties [6]. The temperature needed to overcome rigidity and to reach enough processability is between 170-180°C [6, 24, 26-28]. To avoid humidity PLA pellets have to be dried overnight at 80 °C [29, 30] while PHB pellets [24] and D-(+)-limonene [15, 24] must be dried at 40°C for at least 4 h before processing.

Miscibility between Different Blend Components

The miscibility between different polymer matrix is mainly dependent on the chemical structure and it could be predicted comparing their solubility parameters (δ) [29, 30]. Solubility parameter is dependent on the group molar cohesive energy. The solubility parameter for PLA, PHB and limonene are 19.5 $MPa^{0.5}$, 18.5 $MPa^{0.5}$ and 14.3 $MPa^{0.5}$, respectively. PLA and PHB present similar solubility parameters, therefore, they should be miscible. The δ of D-(+)-limonene is lower than those of the PLA and PHB, however, it is still in the same order of magnitude. Moreover, the miscibility also depends on the proportion used for each component.

Several investigations have studied the compatibility between both polymers in PLA-PHB blends and their full characterization could be found elsewhere [6, 26, 31]. Zhang and Thomas studied different proportion of PLA-PHB blends (100:0, 75:25, 50:50, 25:75 and 0:100) and demonstrated that the best synergic effect was obtaining by blending 75 wt.% of PLA with 25 wt.% of PHB due to the ability of PHB to act as a reinforcement agent for PLA [6] and thus this proportion had shown improved final properties of particular interest in its application.

Morphological Aspects

It is widely known that the Scanning Electron Microscopy (SEM) observations of neat PLA show that PLA has smooth and uniform fracture surface [15, 27, 29] while neat PHB has an irregular fracture surface due to its crystalline structure nature [24, 27]. Zhang and Thomas studied the microstructure of PLA-PHB in different proportions (100:0, 75:25, 50:50, 25:75 and 0:100) by SEM and showed that all PLA-PHB blends consisted of two phases, which indicated that PLA-PHB blends were not miscible. But in PLA-PHB (75:25), the micrograph showed that PHB particles were dispersed as fillers in PLA matrix, which could improve the mechanical properties of the final formulation [6]. Abdelwahab et al. demonstrated that the introduction of a Lapol 108 in PLA-PHB (75:25) produced a plastic deformation due to the plasticizer effect of Lapol 108 and they concluded that the different fracture directions obtained in plasticized materials required more energy with respect with unplasticized PLA-PHB (75:25) blends and thus the materials with plasticizer would have better toughness [27]. Similarly, the effectiveness of D-(+)-Limonene as a PLA plasticizer has been reported [15]. In a previous work we introduced D-(+)-Limonene into PLA-PHB (75:25) blend and a better interaction between PLA and PHB was achieved due to the D-(+)-Limonene presence, and in addition, a plastic behavior was observed showing the effectiveness of D-limonene to plasticize the PLA-PHB blend [24]. Figure 2 and 3 show optical and confocal microscopy images, respectively, of PLA, PLA-D(+)Lim, PLA-PHB and PLA-PHB-D(+)Lim. PLA and PLA-D(+)Lim surfaces appear smooth and uniform (Figure 2 a and b), meanwhile some signs of roughness were detected with the presence of PHB in PLA-PHB and PLA-PHB-D(+)Lim samples (Figure 2 c and d). This result was in agreement with the profiles measurements and images acquired by the extended depth of field (EDF) technique (Figure 2 A, B, C and D). Samples containing PHB presented more irregular surface profiles than their PLA counterparts.

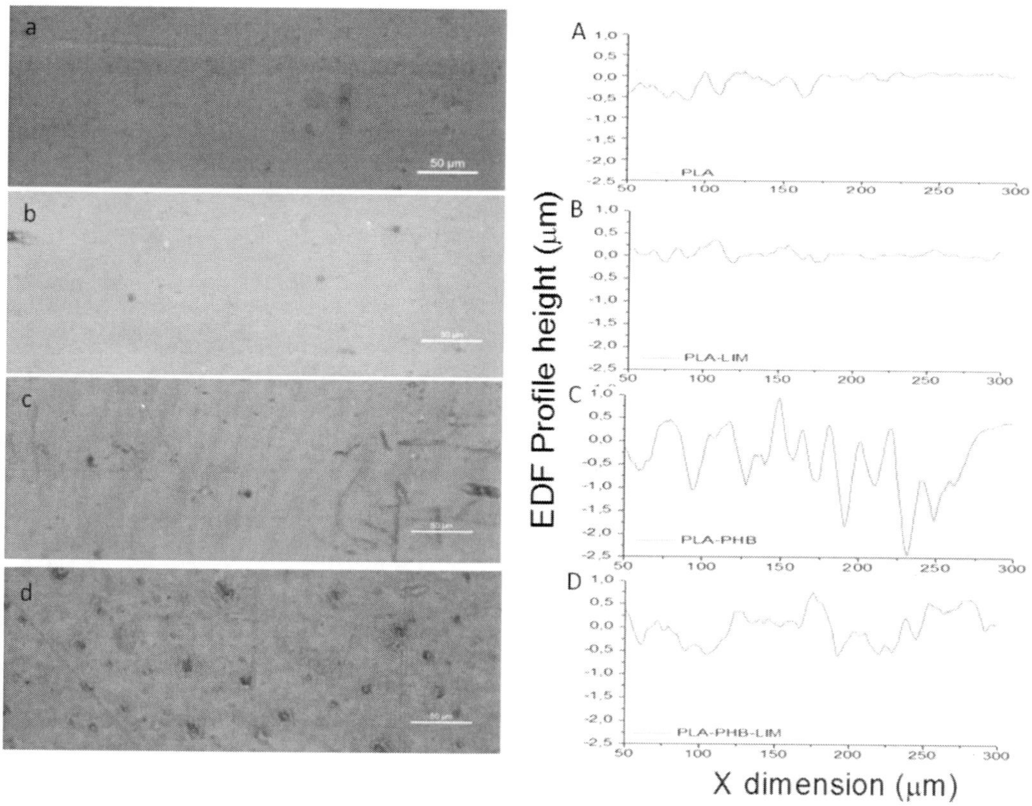

Figure 2. Surfaces optical micrographs of samples (20 x) [(a) PLA, (b) PLA D(+)Lim, (c) PLA-PHB and (d) PLA-PHB- D(+)Lim] and EDF-z profile [(A) PLA, (B) PLA-D(+)Lim, (C) PLA-PHB and (D) PLA-PHB- D(+)Lim].

This behavior could be ascribed to the ability of PHB to increase the degree of crystallinity of PLA [6]. Moreover, the morphology studied by confocal observations (Figure 3) confirms that surfaces of samples with PHB were rougher than samples without it.

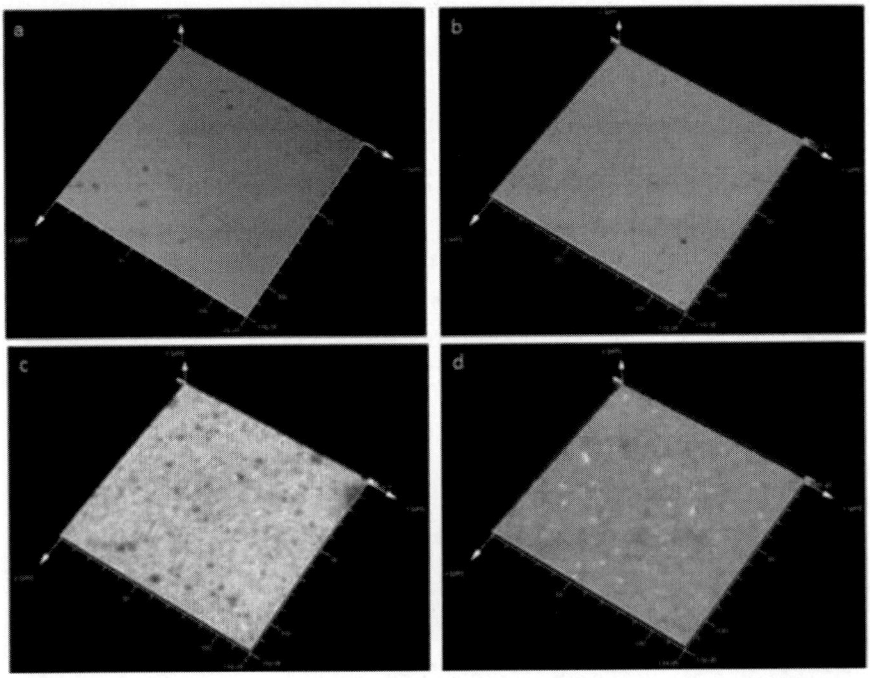

Figure 3. Confocal images of (a) PLA, (b) PLA-D(+)Lim, (c) PLA-PHB and (d) PLA-PHB- D(+)Lim.

THERMAL PROPERTIES

The thermal stability of materials is of a great importance in view of the fact that materials should be thermally stable at the processing conditions as well as during their intended uses. PLA thermal degradation can be attributed to hydrolysis, depolymerization, random-chain scission, inter and intramolecular transesterification, resulting in the formation of lactide monomer and oligomers [1]. On the other hand, the main drawback of the addition of essential oils into polymer matrices is their poor thermal stability. In this sense, somewhat loss of D-(+)-Limonene is expected during processing because the boiling point of D-Limonene is around 176ºC [18]. The thermal degradation of polymers is commonly studied by thermogravimetric analysis (TGA). The thermal degradation of PLA has been widely studied and it occurs in a single degradation process in the temperature range between 270ºC and 400ºC [2, 15]. Meanwhile, the thermal degradation of PHB occurs in two steps, between 250ºC and 300ºC [24]. The thermal degradation of PLA, PLA-PHB blends with and without D-(+)-limonene investigated by thermo gravimetric analysis (TGA) is shown in Figure 4. While, PLA degrades in only one step, the rest of samples exhibited a multi step thermal degradation showing their multi component nature, binary systems in the case of PLA-D(+)Lim and PLA-PHB and ternary systems for PLA-PHB-D(+)Lim. PLA presents the maximum degradation rate at 364ºC [12, 15, 29] and the initial decomposition temperature was resolved at 332ºC. PLA-D(+)Lim showed two degradation steps, the first one has been related with the degradation of D-(+)-limonene [15]. Therefore, PLA-D(+)Lim showed the initial degradation temperature at 106ºC. The second step centered at 378ºC corresponds to the degradation of the PLA itself. It is interesting to notice that the maximum degradation rate was slightly shifted to higher temperature showing a good interaction between D-(+)-Limonene and PLA. For samples containing PHB, it is clear that PHB started the decomposition before the PLA (Figure 4 c and d), as expected, showing the maximum degradation at 293ºC for PLA-D(+)Lim and at 282ºC for PLA-PHB-D(+)Lim.

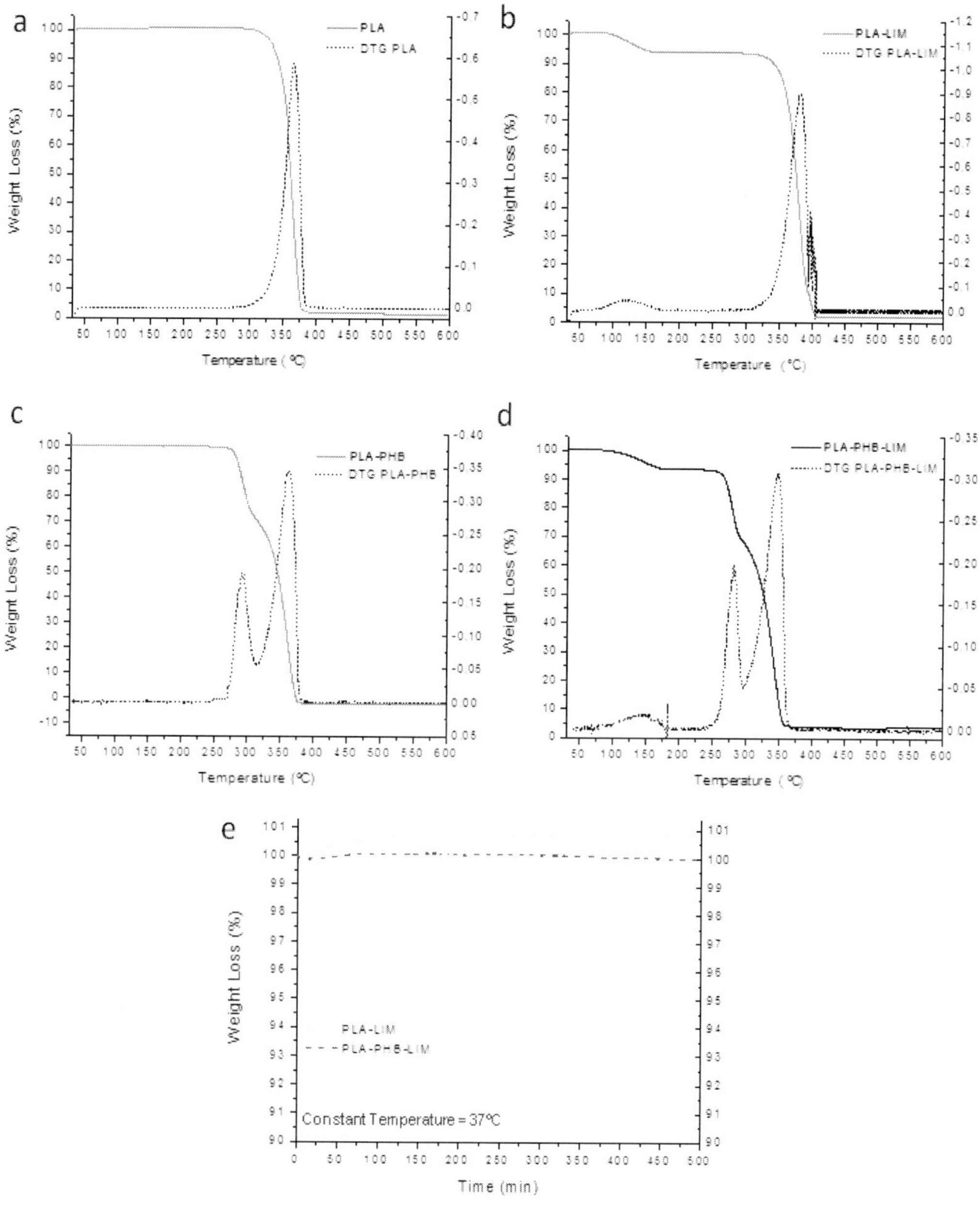

Figure 4. Dynamic thermal degradation of (a) PLA, (b) PLA-D(+)Lim, (c) PLA-PHB and (d) PLA-PHB-D(+)Lim. (e) Isothermal degradation of PLA-D(+)Lim and PLA-PHB-D(+)Lim.

Nevertheless, the initial degradation temperatures were 272ºC and 111ºC, respectively suggesting that PLA blended with PHB is somewhat more efficient to retain D-(+)-Limonene. The loss of D(+)-Limonene during processing should be taken into account because of it has been shown that PLA-D(+)-Lim (85:15) lost approximately 40% of D(+)-limonene [15] while PLA-PHB (75:25) blend added with 15 wt.% of D(+)-Limonene lost approximately 30% of D(+)-limonene during processing [24]. Isothermal experiments carried out at 37 ºC corroborate the stability of the PLA-D(+)-Lim and PLA-PHB-D(+)-Lim at the physiological temperature (Figure 4 e). As a conclusion, ternary PLA-PHB-D(+)Lim shows adequate stability at the recommended processing temperature for PLA-PHB blends (170-180ºC) as well as during the intended use in biological applications.

The thermal properties of PLA-PHB blends could be significantly affected by the crystallization characteristics of each component on the blend. Differential Scanning Calorimetry (DSC) has been extensively used to demonstrate the ability of PHB to recrystallize PLA. Particularly, PLA-PHB blend in 75:25 proportion has shown a strong recrystallization behavior due to the small finely dispersed PHB crystals acting as nucleating agents in PLA matrix [6]. This behavior is because of the crystal structure of PHB in the PLA-PHB (75:25) blend from interactions between PLA and PHB, where the crystal growth rate of PHB are higher and faster than those of PLA [27]. Meanwhile, D-(+)-Limonene has shown an increase in polymer chain mobility due to its plasticization effect in PLA [15] as well as in PLA-PHB blends [24]. Figure 5 shows the DSC curves of PLA and PLA-PHB (75:25) blends with 15 wt.% of D-(+)-Limonene. PLA showed the T_g at 60ºC, the cool crystallization at 99.8ºC and two melting peaks at 167ºC and 173ºC.

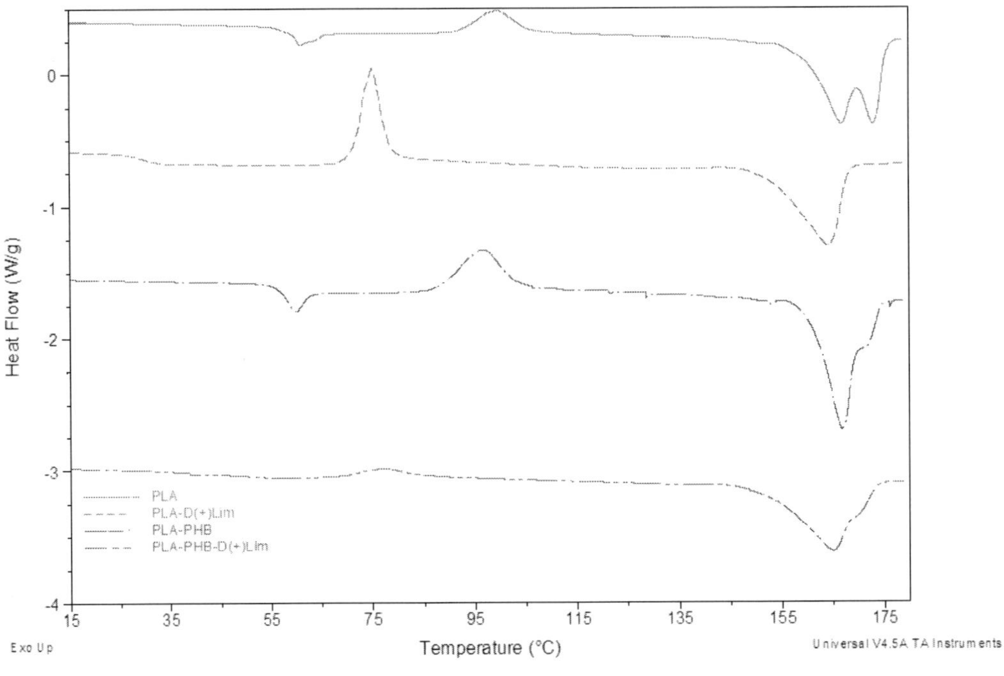

Figure 5. DSC thermograms of PLA, PLA-D(+)Lim, PLA-PHB and PLA-PHB- D(+)Lim.

An endothermic peak observed just before the T_g indicates that the material is suffering a physical ageing due to the relaxation of materials stored at temperatures below of T_g [29, 32]. The physical ageing is also observed in PLA-PHB blend with a T_g at 59°C. However, this relaxation did not appeared in PLA-PHB-D(+)Lim, with a T_g at 40°C, showing a good interaction between the three components. The introduction of D-(+)-Limonene to PLA matrix provoked a reduction in the T_g value (30.3°C). It also reduced the crystallization temperature and melting point to 75°C and 164°C, respectively. The two melting points of PLA have been attributed to PLA-D-isomer which has poor ability to crystallize and therefore presents residual crystallinity [29]. PLA-PHB and PLA-PHB-D(+)Lim samples presented the cold crystallization at 96.8°C and 78°C while the melting points were centered at 167°C and 165°C, respectively. The higher melting peak observed in PLA-PHB-D(+)Lim confirms the ability of PHB to favor the nucleation and crystal growth of PLA.

Mechanical and Nanomechanical Properties

The improvement in mechanical properties of PLA is one of the major issues concerning the use of PLA in biomedical applications. As it was commented previously, melt-blending PLA with PHB is a relatively simple approach to improve the mechanical properties of PLA.

The mechanical properties of biopolymers are commonly investigated by tensile test. The tensile test showed that PLA-PHB (75:25) blend presents better mechanical properties than neat PLA and neat PHB [6]. This findings has been attributed to the finely dispersed PHB crystals acting as a filler in PLA matrix enhancing the mechanical performance of the final formulation [6]. The addition of a third component is mainly focused on the improvement of the interaction between both biopolymers. For instance, the addition of plasticizers has shown to improve the interaction between PLA-PHB blends while increasing the elongation at break of PLA-PHB blends [24, 27].

The mechanical performance of materials could be also studied at the nanometer scale by means a nanoindenter equipment. The nanoindentation is a powerful technique to determine the Hardness (*H*) and Elastic Modulus (*E*) of polymers [33]. Hardness is calculated by using the following equation:

$$H = \frac{P_{max}}{A(h_c)} \qquad \text{Eq. (1)}$$

being P_{max} the applied load for each penetration depth reached and $A(h_c)$ is the area of the polymer assayed. The area of the indenter in contact with polymer sample is calculated knowing that a Berkovich diamond indenter shows a semi-angle of $\theta = 65.27^{o}$. The effective elastic modulus (*E*) is calculated by means of the following formula:

$$E = \frac{1}{\beta} S \frac{\sqrt{\pi}}{2} \frac{1}{\sqrt{A}} \qquad \text{Eq. (2)}$$

in which β is a geometrical constant factor that for Berkovich (β =1,034), *S* is the contact stiffness and *A* is the contact area. The stiffness acquired by Continuous Stiffness Measurement (CSM) method avoids the Oliver & Pharr method limitation for materials with creep behavior [34], such as polymers. The CSM technique resolved the stiffness for all depths reached during the experiment, which implies that the entire profile in-depth of *H* and *E* is obtained. This solution was adopted in order to avoid the roughness and tip roundness effects at low penetration depths, while the possible creep effect was avoided at higher loads. Figure 6 shows the *E* and *H* average values calculated between 100 and 200 nm applying 70 Hz of harmonic oscillation frequency with 2 nm harmonic amplitude. Similar values were observed in nanohardness and modulus being the lowest values for the ternary nanocomposite PLA-PHB-D(+)Lim with an *E* of 4.2 GPa and an *H* of 260 MPa. Meanwhile, PLA and PLA-PHB showed the highest values of *E* at approximately 4.5 GPa and also showed the highest values of *H* between 260 and 290 MPa. In a previous work, it has been shown that the addition of common PLA plasticizers, such as poly-ethylene glycol (PEG) and acetyl-tri-n-butyl citrate (ATBC), reduces both, the *E* and *H* values, the nanomechanical parameters of PLA and PLA-PHB blends, due to the ability of plasticizers to reduced the inherent brittleness of both biopolymers [28]. Similarly, the plasticizer role of D(+)-Limonene has been also observed by nanoindentation technique in PLA and in PLA-PHB blends [24]. Therefore, the nanomechanical parameters showed in Figure 6 suggest that the presence of D-(+)-limonene into PLA and PLA-PHB matrices induce an increment of the free volume between polymer chains and thus the resultant materials become somewhat weak.

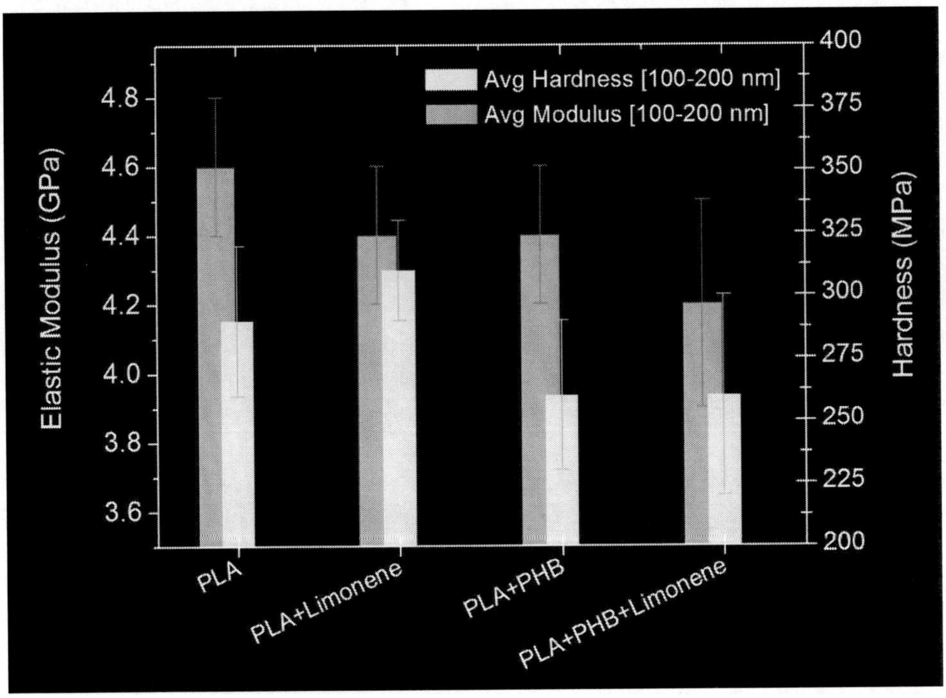

Figure 6. Nanohardness (*H*) and reduced modulus (*E*) of PLA, PLA-D(+)Lim, PLA-PHB and PLA-PHB- D(+)Lim.

CONCLUSION

The new generation of biomedical materials is expected to be made by materials coming from renewable sources, biocompatible and containing active components. Bio-materials based in PLA, PHB and D-(+)-Lim are proposed as biopolymers with active properties for biomedical applications. PHB presence increases the roughness of material surfaces at the same time as it favors the nucleation and crystal growth in PLA matrix, while, D-(+)-Lim decreases the T_g of the systems and improves the compatibility between both biopolymers. In correlation, a increase of ductility in blends is obtained when D(+)limonene is present. Thus, the combination of the addition of 25 wt.% of PHB into PLA matrix to enhance the crystallinity and mechanical properties with the presence of 15 wt.% of D-(+)-limonene as natural active agent could lead to interesting bio-active materials for biomedical applications. Furthermore, studies should be conducted on the functional properties such as antibacterial or antifungal activity as well as the biodegradable properties in characteristics physiological mediums of these bio-based formulations.

ACKNOWLEDGMENTS

Authors thank Spanish Ministry of Science and Innovation for the financial support. (MAT2011-28468-C02-01 and MAT2011-28468-C02-02). M.P. Arrieta is granted by Santiago Grisolía program (GRISOLIA/2011/007).

REFERENCES

[1] Armentano, I., Bitinis, N., Fortunati, E., Mattioli, S., Rescignano, N., Verdejo, R., Lopez-Manchado, M. A., Kenny, J. M., (2013). Multifunctional nanostructured PLA materials for packaging and tissue engineering. *Prog. Polym. Sci.* 38 (10–11), 1720-1747.

[2] Fortunati, E., Armentano, I., Iannoni, A., Kenny, J. M., (2010). Development and thermal behaviour of ternary PLA matrix composites. *Polym. Degrad. Stabil.* 95 (11), 2200-2206.

[3] Armentano, I., Dottori, M., Fortunati, E., Mattioli, S., Kenny, J. M., (2010). Biodegradable polymer matrix nanocomposites for tissue engineering: A review. *Polym. Degrad. Stabil.* 95 (11), 2126-2146.

[4] Tri, P. N., Domenek, S., Guinault, A., Sollogoub, C., (2013). Crystallization behavior of poly(lactide)/poly(β-hydroxybutyrate)/talc composites. *J. Appl. Polym. Sci.* 129 (6), 3355-3365.

[5] Chang, L., Woo, E. M., (2012). Crystallization of poly(3-hydroxybutyrate) with stereocomplexed polylactide as biodegradable nucleation agent. *Polym. Eng. Sci.* 52 (7), 1413-1419.

[6] Zhang, M., Thomas, N. L., (2011). Blending polylactic acid with polyhydroxybutyrate: The effect on thermal, mechanical, and biodegradation properties. *Adv. Polym. Tech.* 30 (2), 67-79.

[7] Imre, B., Pukánszky, B., (2013). Compatibilization in bio-based and biodegradable polymer blends. *Euro. Polym. J.* 49 (6), 1215-1233.

[8] Erceg, M., Kovacic, T., Klaric I., (2005). Thermal degradation of poly(3-hydroxybutyrate) plasticized with acetyl tributyl citrate. *Polym. Degrad. Stabil.* 90 (2), 313-318.

[9] Chen, G. Q., (2011). Biofunctionalization of polymers and their applications. *Adv. Biochem. Eng. Biotechnol.* 125, 29-45.

[10] Vogel, C., Wessel, E., Siesler, H. W., (2008). FT-IR imaging spectroscopy of phase separation in blends of poly(3-hydroxybutyrate) with poly(L-lactic acid) and poly(epsilon-caprolactone). *Biomacromolecules.* 9 (2), 523-527.

[11] Arrieta, M. P., Fortunati, E., Dominici, F., Rayón, E., López, J., Kenny, J. M., (2014) Multifunctional PLA-PHB/cellulose nanocrystal films: Processing, structural and thermal properties. *Carbohyd. Polym.* http://dx.doi.org/10.1016/j.carbpol.2014.02.044

[12] Fortunati, E., Latterini, L., Rinaldi, S., Kenny, J. M., Armentano, I., (2011). PLGA/Ag nanocomposites: In vitro degradation study and silver ion release. *J, Mater, Sci-Mater M.* 22 (12), 2735-2744.

[13] Sánchez-González, L., Vargas, M., González-Martínez, C., Chiralt, A., Cháfer, M. (2011). Use of Essential Oils in Bioactive Edible Coatings: A Review. *Food Eng. Rev.* 3 (1), 1-16.

[14] Bicas, J. L., Pastore, G. M., (2007). Isolation and screening of D-limonene-resistant microorganisms. *Braz. J. Microbiol.* 38 (3), 563-567.

[15] Arrieta, M. P., López, J., Ferrándiz, S., Peltzer, M. A., (2013). Characterization of PLA-limonene blends for food packaging applications. *Poly. Test.* 32 (4), 760-768.

[16] Singh, A., Kamal, M., (2012). Synthesis and characterization of polylimonene: Polymer of an optically active terpene. *J. Appl. Polym. Sci.* 125 (2), 1456-1459.

[17] Palá-Paúl, J., Velasco-Negueruela, A., José Pérez-Alonso, M., Sanz, J., (2002). Antimicrobial activity profiles of the two enantiomers of limonene and carvone isolated from the oils of Mentha spicata and Anethum sowa. *Flavour Frag. J.* 17 (1), 59-63.

[18] World Health Organization., (1998). Concise international chemical assessment document nº 5, Limonene. 1-32.

[19] Espina, L., Gelaw, T.K., de Lamo-Castellví, S., Pagán, R., García-Gonzalo, D., (2013). Mechanism of bacterial inactivation by (+)-Limonene and its potential use in food preservation combined processes. *PLoS ONE.* 8 (2).

[20] Fisher, K., Phillips, C., (2008). Potential antimicrobial uses of essential oils in food: is citrus the answer? *Trends Food Sci. Technol.* 19 (3), 156-164.

[21] Bakkali, F., Averbeck, S., Averbeck, D., Idaomar, M., (2008). Biological effects of essential oils – A review. *Food Chem. Toxicol.* 46 (2), 446-475.

[22] Van Vuuren, S. F., Viljoen, A. M., (2007). Antimicrobial activity of limonene enantiomers and 1,8-cineole alone and in combination. *Flavour Frag. J.* 22 (6), 540-544.

[23] Yao, K., Tang, C. (2013). Controlled polymerization of next-generation renewable monomers and beyond. *Macromolecules.* 46 (5), 1689-1712.

[24] Arrieta, M. P., López, J., Hernández, A., Rayón, E. (2014). Ternary PLA-PHB-Limonene blends intended for biodegradable food packaging applications. *Eur. Polym. J.* 50 (1), 255-270.

[25] Blümm, E., Owen, A. J., (1995). Miscibility, crystallization and melting of poly(3-hydroxybutyrate)/ poly(l-lactide) blends. *Polymer*. 36 (21), 4077-4081.

[26] Bartczak, Z., Galeski, A., Kowalczuk, M., Sobota, M., Malinowski, R., (2013). Tough blends of poly(lactide) and amorphous poly([R,S]-3-hydroxy butyrate) - Morphology and properties. *Eur. Polym. J.* 49 (11), 3630-3641.

[27] Abdelwahab, M. A., Flynn, A., Chiou, B. S., Imam, S., Orts, W., Chiellini, E., (2012). Thermal, mechanical and morphological characterization of plasticized PLA-PHB blends. *Polym. Degrad. Stabil.* 97 (9), 1822-1828.

[28] Arrieta, M. P., López, J., Rayón, E., Jiménez, A., (2014). Disintegrability under composting conditions of plasticized PLA-PHB blends. *Polym. Degrad. Stabil.* http://dx.doi.org/10.1016/j. polymdegradstab.2014.01.034

[29] Burgos, N., Martino, V. P., Jiménez, A., (2013). Characterization and ageing study of poly(lactic acid) films plasticized with oligomeric lactic acid. *Polym. Degrad. Stabil.* 98 (2), 651-658.

[30] Martino, V. P., Ruseckaite, R. A., Jiménez, A. (2006). Thermal and mechanical characterization of plasticized poly (L-lactide-co-D,L-lactide) films for food packaging. *J. Therm. Anal. Calorim.* 86 (3), 707-712.

[31] Furukawa, T., Sato, H., Murakami, R., Zhang, J., Duan, Y. X., Noda, I., Ochiai, S., Ozaki, Y., (2005). Structure, dispersibility, and crystallinity of poly(hydroxybutyrate)/ poly(L-lactic acid) blends studied by FT-IR microspectroscopy and differential scanning calorimetry. *Macromolecules*. 38 (15), 6445-6454.

[32] Soto-Valdez, H., Auras, R., Peralta, E., (2011). Fabrication of poly(lactic acid) films with resveratrol and the diffusion of resveratrol into ethanol. *J. Appl. Polym. Sci.* 121 (2), 970-978.

[33] Roa, J. J., Rayon, E., Morales, M., Segarra, M. (2012). Contact mechanics at nanometric scale using nanoindentation technique for brittle and ductile materials. *Recent Pat. Eng*. 6 (2), 116-126.

[34] Oliver, W. C., Pharr, G. M., (2004). Measurement of hardness and elastic modulus by instrumented indentation: Advances in understanding and refinements to methodology. *J. Mater. Res*. 19 (1), 3-20.

INDEX

B

C

D

E

F

G

H

I

J

K

L

M

N

O

P

Q

R

S

T

U

V

W

X

Y

Z